Mechanisms
of Disease

spital

Mechanisms of Disease

An Introduction to Clinical Science

Second Edition

Stephen Tomlinson

Cardiff Univeristy, UK

Anthony M. Heagerty

Univeristy of Manchester, UK

Anthony P. Weetman

University of Sheffield, UK

Rayaz A. Malik

University of Manchester, UK

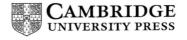
CAMBRIDGE
UNIVERSITY PRESS

CAMBRIDGE UNIVERSITY PRESS
Cambridge, New York, Melbourne, Madrid, Cape Town, Singapore, São Paulo, Delhi

Cambridge University Press
The Edinburgh Building, Cambridge CB2 BRU, UK

Published in the United States of America by Cambridge University Press, New York

www.cambridge.org

Information on this title: www.cambridge.org/9780521818582

First published 2008

Printed in the United Kingdom at the University Press, Cambridge

A catalogue record for this publication is available from the British Library.

Library of Congress Cataloguing-in-Publication Data

Mechanisms of disease : an introduction to clinical science / Stephen Tomlinson ... [et al.] – 2nd ed.
    p. ; cm.
  Includes bibliographical references and index.
  ISBN 978-0-521-81858-2 (hardback) – ISBN 978-0-521-52318-9 (pbk.)
  1. Physiology, Pathological. 2. Pathology, Molecular. 3. Pathology, Cellular. I. Tomlinson, S. (Stephen), 1994–
  [DNLM: 1. Disease. 2. Clinical Medicine–methods. 3. Pathology–methods. QZ 140 M486 2008]
RB113 M38 2008
613.07 – dc22   2007050395

ISBN 13: 978-0-521-81858-2 hardback
ISBN 13: 978-0-521-52318-9 paperback

Contents

Colour plate section follows page 114.

Contributors

Andrew J. M. Boulton, MD FRCP
Faculty of Medical and Human Sciences
School of Medicine
Manchester Royal Infirmary
Manchester, UK

Mamta H. Buch
MRI Central Manchester and
Manchester Children's University Hospitals
Manchester Royal Infirmary
Manchester, UK

Timothy M. Cox, MA MSc MD FRCP FMedSci
University of Cambridge and
Department of Medicine,
University of Cambridge NHS Hospitals
    Foundation Trust
Cambridge, UK

Julian R. E. Davis, MD PhD FRCP
Endocrine Sciences Research Group
School of Clinical & Laboratory Sciences
University of Manchester
Manchester, UK

Adam Greenstein, BSc (Hons) ChB MRCP
Faculty of Medical and Human Sciences
School of Medicine
Manchester Royal Infirmary
Manchester, UK

George E. Griffin, BSc PhD FRCP (Lon,E) FMedSci
St George's, University of London
London, UK

Else Guthrie, MSc MD MBChB FRCPsych
Manchester Royal Infirmary
Manchester, UK

Anthony M. Heagerty
Cardiovascular Research Group
Division of Cardiovascular and Endocrine
    Sciences
University of Manchester
Manchester, UK

Sudhesh Kumar, MD FRCP
Clinical Sciences Research Institute
Warwick Medical School
University of Warwick
Coventry, UK

Stephen D. Lawn, BMedSci MB BS MRCP MD DTM&H Dip HIV Med
The Desmond Tutu HIV Centre
Institute of Infectious Disease and Molecular
    Medicine
Faculty of Health Sciences
University of Cape Town
South Africa
and
Clinical Research Unit
Department of Infectious and Tropical Diseases
London School of Hygiene and Tropical
    Medicine
London, UK

Michael E. J. Lean, MA MD FRCP
University of Glasgow and
Glasgow Royal Infirmary
Glasgow, UK
and
University of Otago
Dunedin, New Zealand

P. G. McTernan
Division of Clinical Sciences
Warwick Medical School
University of Warwick
Coventry, UK

Rayaz A. Malik, MD ChB FRCP PhD
Division of Cardiovascular Medicine and
    Endocrine Sciences
University of Manchester
Manchester, UK

Wasat Mansoor, MBChB MRCP PhD
Christie Hospital
Manchester, UK

Moaz Mojaddidi, MB ChB
Faculty of Medical and Human Sciences
School of Medicine
Manchester Royal Infirmary
Manchester, UK

Malcolm E. Molyneux, MD
Malawi–Liverpool-Wellcome Trust Clinical Research
    Programme
College of Medicine
University of Malawi
Blantyre, Malawi

Ludwig Neyses, MD
University of Manchester
Manchester, UK

James Neuberger, DM FRCP
Queen Elizabeth Hospital and
University of Birmingham
Birmingham, UK

Nick Payne
Wythenshawe Hospital
Manchester, UK

Richard S. H. Pumphrey, MD
Honorary Consultant Immunologist
Manchester Royal Infirmary
Manchester, UK

Jerard Ross
The Department of Clinical Neurosciences
Western General Hospital
Edinburgh, UK

Nancy J. Rothwell, FRS FMedSci
Faculty of Life Sciences
University of Manchester
Manchester, UK

J. Shakher
Diabetes & Endocrine Centre
Birmingham Heartlands Hospital
and
University of Birmingham
Birmingham, UK

Craig J. Smith
Division of Medicine and Neuroscience–Hope
University of Manchester
Hope Hospital
Salford, UK

Pippa J. Tyrrell
Division of Medicine and Neuroscience – Hope
University of Manchester
Hope Hospital
Salford, UK

Anthony P. Weetman, MD DSc FMedSci
School of Medicine & Biomedical
    Sciences
University of Sheffield
Sheffield, UK

David W. Yates, MD MCh FRCP FRCS FCEM
University of Manchester
Manchester, UK

Preface to the first edition

This book reflects innovative approaches to the learning of core subjects and provides opportunities for in-depth study in undergraduate medicine, emphasising the understanding of principles rather than simply memorising facts. Our approach follows the direction of curricular development throughout the UK and the expressed educational aim of the General Medical Council. In addition, higher medical training at the postgraduate level will be increasingly based on the principles of clinical science; given the accelerating pace of advances in biomedical knowledge, requirements of continuing education are likely to have a strong scientific component.

The introductory section of the book sets out the essentials of molecular and cellular biology as they relate to mechanisms of disease. There is also a brief description of some established and more recently developed methodologies used in molecular and cell biology.

The book then outlines leading-edge scientific knowledge and demonstrates how this is fundamental to the practice of up-to-date clinical medicine. Each chapter focuses on one or more clinically important exemplar topics where science has helped to develop clinical practice or improved understanding of the basis of disease.

Each chapter falls broadly into two parts: the first is devoted to basic mechanisms and the second to the application of knowledge of these basic mechanisms to the understanding of the pathogenesis and diagnosis of an exemplar condition. Although the emphasis is on mechanisms of disease, aspects of treatment are also included where they have explanatory value in understanding disease processes. Authors have usually focused on one specific exemplar condition, but where appropriate, there is comment on other diseases relevant to the section 'mechanism'.

The overriding aim of the book is to meet the need for new approaches to learning medicine; it also provides information for students undertaking special study modules, encouraging self-directed learning by the study in depth of specific subjects chosen by the students themselves.

We are especially grateful to Professor David R. London, Registrar of the Royal College of Physicians of London, for the chapter on the historical development of concepts of disease, which we believe sets the scene for succeeding chapters.

S. Tomlinson, A. M. Heagerty and P. Weetman

Preface to the second edition

This second edition of *Mechanisms of Disease* builds on our original aims of providing a mechanistic, as opposed to traditional, list-based approach to medicine. This is in keeping with the huge transformation in both undergraduate and postgraduate teaching and learning and is in accord with the aims of the General Medical Council (GMC) described in *Tomorrow's Doctors* (1993, 2003).

This book provides the essential knowledge required for the core curriculum and is delivered by leading clinicians and scientists. In keeping with one of the major remits of the GMC on delivering the core curriculum, *factual information* has been 'kept to the essential minimum that students need at this stage of medical education'. The use of principles of disease combined with an appropriate exemplar approach provides learning opportunities that help the student to explore knowledge and evaluate and integrate evidence critically, motivating them to develop the necessary skills for self-directed learning. The use of exemplars provides students with clinical information relevant to their special study modules and *student-selected components*, allowing them to study particular areas in depth. Again in keeping with the change from simply 'learning lists' to establishing principles of disease, each chapter provides knowledge of the sciences and scientific methods on which medicine is based.

Finally, to integrate theory with clinical practice, each chapter includes a series of clinical scenarios, followed by questions.

Molecular and cell biology

Julian R. E. Davis

Key points

- The human genome functions through transcription of coding regions (exons) of DNA to messenger RNA (mRNA) and translation of mRNA into protein.
- Normal cell function and growth are controlled by intracellular signalling systems that couple external stimuli to cellular responses.
- Gene expression can be studied *in vitro* by cloning of DNA, sequence analysis, analysis of DNA–protein interactions *in vivo* and by gene transfer, including the use of transgenic animals.
- Such studies have led to the identification of genetic defects in diseases such as cystic fibrosis and the genetic events underlying cancer formation; they have also directed the first applications of gene therapy.
- Molecular and cell biology, as techniques used to elucidate normal cellular mechanisms, are themes that run through each chapter of this book as mechanisms of disease are explored.

Molecular biology

The human genome and gene structure

The genome comprises all the inherited material passed on from one generation to the next. In humans, it consists of the 23 pairs of chromosomes in the nucleus together with a small amount of mitochondrial DNA. Chromosomal DNA is a tightly packaged array of genes (the units of inheritance) together with long tracts of intergenic DNA whose function is still largely unknown. The overall organisation and structure of the human genome is under intense study at present, and this chapter focuses only on small parts of this overall structure in order to describe some of the essential elements of molecular biology involved in mechanisms of disease. In Chapter 3, changes in chromosomes and genes relating to hereditary diseases are described. Later sections of this chapter outline intracellular signalling systems, especially as they relate to the control of gene expression and regulation of growth. Finally, some of the methods of analysis currently used in molecular and cell biology are reviewed.

The basic chemical composition of chromosomes – DNA and protein – was generally understood long before it was clear which functioned as genes. Work by Griffith and Avery showed that DNA was the most likely candidate, and experiments by Hershey and Chase in 1952 showed that only DNA from bacteriophages entered the host cell and initiated the production of viral particles. The double helix structure of DNA, defined by Watson and Crick, comprising two antiparallel strands with the sugar phosphate backbones on the outside and the purine–pyrimidine base pairs (bps) on the inside, forms the basis of our concepts of the replication and utilisation of genes. A consequence of this hydrogen-bonded pairing of the two DNA strands is that the strands can be separated by conditions that break hydrogen bonds (heat or extremes of pH) and then allowed to rejoin or anneal under less stringent conditions. Because of the obligatory complementary binding, strands that are complementary in sequence will bond to form a double helix. This is the basis of many of the experimental studies that allow related genes to be identified and probes of known sequence to be 'annealed' or bound to sections of DNA (see below).

The linear sequence of nucleotides forms a genetic code in which triplets of nucleotides code for each amino acid. The possible permutations of nucleotides allow some degeneracy (more than one code for an amino acid) and for start and stop codons.

Chromosomes are generally organised in pairs – one inherited from each parent – and in each pair, genetic material undergoes rearrangement by the crossing over of paired segments during meiosis in paternal or maternal gametes. Thus, each chromosome contains newly arranged genetic material, but with conserved overall structure in homologous pairs of chromosomes. Most genes will be represented by a maternal and a paternal 'allele', (alternative forms of the same gene), which in turn can undergo pairing in meiosis to form the next generation of gametes.

Genes contain structural information that ultimately dictates the sequence of a protein; for example, a peptide hormone, an enzyme, or a structural protein. The linear sequence of deoxynucleotides determines the properties of the gene and its protein product. However, this protein-coding information is not an unbroken stretch of DNA but instead consists (in most mammalian genes) of separate coding regions, exons interspersed with non-coding introns. Each gene also contains characteristic flanking sequences both upstream and downstream of the coding region (Fig 1.1).

The function of much of the intergenic DNA is unknown: it occupies a large percentage of the genome, proportionately more in humans than in simpler organisms. Some of this material has obvious structural functions; for example, several megabases of DNA in the centromere of most chromosomes are involved in the formation of the mitotic spindle in cell division. Other parts of chromosomes contain long stretches of repetitive non-coding sequences, such as tandem repeats, whose function is still unknown.

Repetitive sequences have, in some cases, been found to have major significance, as illustrated by the discovery of genetic alterations in repetitive DNA in a number of disorders, exemplified by Huntington's disease. The Huntington's disease gene on chromosome 4 contains an expanded unstable region of DNA comprising a series of CAG repeats whose overall length changes during gamete formation: this repetitive DNA stretch is longer in patients with Huntington's disease than in non-affected people, and the more CAG repeats that occur, the earlier the disease develops. Such alterations in the length of this DNA region may favour the assembly of *nucleosomes*. These are complexes of chromosomal DNA with histone proteins that hinder the access of regulatory proteins to control elements of genes; hence

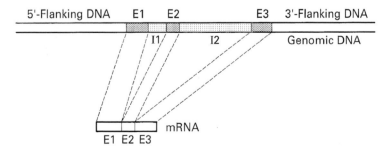

Figure 1.1 Gene structure. Exons (E1, E2 and E3) contain the sequences that code for proteins. Exons are separated by regions of non-coding DNA, introns (I1 and II2).

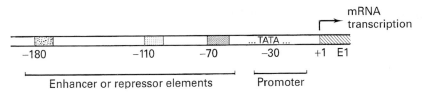

Figure 1.2 Structure of the 5′-flanking DNA. Boxes represent DNA elements to which diffusible protein factors can bind. These occur at different points upstream of the transcriptional start site (right-angled arrow), which is known as nucleotide +1. Transcription of the exon occurs from +1. The non-coding region is numbered back from the start site with nucleotides numbered –1 upwards.

they will mediate general repression of gene transcription.

The non-coding DNA that is closely associated with genes themselves, upstream and downstream flanking regions, are now known to be the major regulatory elements that modulate both gene transcription and the stability of mRNA; this is considered in more detail in the following section.

Gene transcription

The upstream flanking DNA in most genes contains sequences involved in regulation of transcription. This stretch of DNA contains a number of specific sequences, known as *cis* elements because they can affect only adjacent genes that bind diffusible nuclear proteins (*trans* elements) involved in transcription. The minimal upstream element necessary for transcription to occur is in many cases a clearly defined region of less than 30 base pairs of DNA and is termed the gene's *promoter*. Additional upstream elements may stimulate or inhibit the process of transcription and are termed *enhancers* or *repressors* (Fig. 1.2). The transcription of mRNA from the genomic DNA occurs via the enzyme RNA polymerase II, which starts the process at a point on the gene determined by specific sequences in the promoter region, such as a TATA motif (the TATA box). A complex of protein transcription factors (designated TFIIA, TFIIB, etc.) is established at this transcriptional start site, initiated by the binding of the factor TFIID, which binds to the TATA element itself. The cluster of TF proteins thus built up then allows RNA

polymerase II to bind tightly as part of this transcriptional initiation complex (Fig. 1.3)

Upstream of the minimal promoter, enhancer elements may be extensive. These are often several thousand base pairs distant and contain a large number of characteristic sequences that serve as recognition motifs for other transcription factors. Enhancers have the ability to influence the rate of gene transcription at a variable distance and in either orientation relative to the promoter. Their transcription factors modulate the rate of transcription of the gene: some are specific to the cell type whereas others are ubiquitous but tightly regulated by intracellular signalling systems. The nature of their interaction with the transcription initiation complex is not fully understood, but it probably involves looping of DNA in order to bring distant enhancer elements into proximity with the promoter to modulate the function of the transcriptional machinery (Fig. 1.3).

Transcription factors

A series of families of transcription factors have been described with distinct regions of the protein (domains) involved in DNA binding or in transcriptional activation. Several different classes of DNA-binding domains are now recognised, including 'zinc fingers', 'leucine zippers' and helix-turn-helix motifs; more are being identified.

Zinc fingers

These are found in many transcription factors, including steroid receptors, and consist of peptide

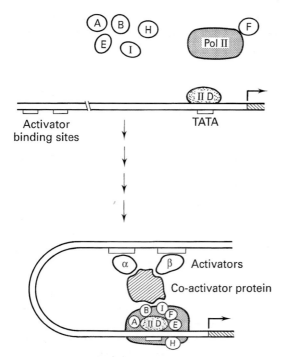

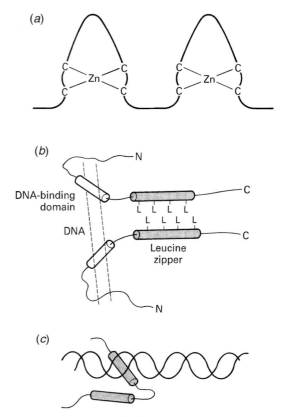

Figure 1.3 Simplified model of the transcriptional initiation complex. Transcription factors TFIID, TFIIA, TFIIB, etc. sequentially bind at the TATA box and stabilize RNA polymerase II (Pol II) attachment. Upstream DNA–bound transcription factors (α, β) may interact directly or indirectly (via a co-activator) with the transcriptional complex. This probably involves some form of DNA looping.

Figure 1.4 Transcription factor structures. (*a*) Zinc fingers. (*b*) Leucine zipper, allowing dimerisation of two factors. (*c*) Helix-turn-helix motif orientated against a DNA helix.

loops in which an atom of zinc is tetrahedrally co-ordinated by cysteine and histidine residues at the base of the finger (Fig. 1.4*a*). Usually, there are several zinc fingers in transcription factor proteins, and the tips of the fingers (containing basic amino acids) are thought to contact the acidic DNA by poking into the major groove of the double helix.

Leucine zippers
These domains have been identified in several transcription factors (e.g. Jun, Fos and Myc) and are regions in which every seventh amino acid is leucine. In an α-helical structure, the leucines occur every second turn, and their long side chains can interdig-

itate with those of an analogous helix in a second protein, like a zipper, allowing dimerisation of the two proteins (Fig. 1.4*b*). Leucine zippers are important not only for transcription factor dimerisation but also for DNA binding; they allow the formation of either homo- or heterodimers among related proteins, for example, Jun–Jun and Jun–Fos.

Helix-turn-helix motifs
These comprise two α helices separated by a β turn. One of the helices, the 'recognition helix', lies in the major groove of the DNA and provides the DNA sequence specificity of binding, the second lies across the major groove and probably stabilises the

DNA contact (Fig. 1.4c). An example of this type of transcription factor is the pituitary-specific factor Pit-1/GHF-1.

Activation domains

These are less clearly defined in transcription factors than the DNA-binding structures but may contain characteristic acidic domains or proline- or glutamine-rich domains. Their function has been confirmed by 'domain-swap' experiments in which chimaeric factors are constructed with the DNA-binding region of one factor linked to the activation domain of another. The mechanism of transcriptional activation is still not well understood but may involve direct contact between the activation domains and the components of the transcription initiation complex (e.g. TFIID, TFIIB, or RNA polymerase II itself) or, in some cases, indirect contact via intermediate adaptor proteins.

Repression

Although most transcription factors seem to be activators, in some cases they can *repress* gene transcription, and several mechanisms are possible. For example, a negatively acting factor can simply interfere with the effect of an activator by occupying the activator protein's binding site (or a closely adjacent site) on the target DNA. In other cases, two factors may interact such that a positively acting factor is sequestered by dimerisation. For example, the glucocorticoid receptor can be prevented from *trans*-activating target genes by becoming complexed with the factor AP-1.

Regulation of gene transcription by intracellular signalling systems is an important aspect of transcriptional control and this is one of the best characterised systems. Most of the steps between an external stimulus and a cellular response have been defined. This is discussed in more detail later in this chapter.

Control of transcription: tissue specificity

Differentiation of tissues with a variety of distinct phenotypes requires the expression of particular genes in a cell type–specific manner; a number of tissue-specific transcription factors have recently been identified in addition to those that are ubiquitous. For example, the factor MyoD is a transcription factor expressed only in differentiating myoblast cells, and artificial expression of MyoD alone in undifferentiated fibroblast cell lines can induce this differentiation process. MyoD can either form transcriptionally active homodimers or it can heterodimerise by helix-loop-helix interaction with other proteins with varying effects. One such protein, Id, is a negative regulator that lacks a DNA-binding domain and so prevents MyoD from binding to DNA. Levels of Id decline during differentiation; therefore the overall effect of the tissue-specific factor MyoD will depend on its interaction with changing levels of other factors, such as Id, that determine its transcriptional activity.

Another tissue-specific transcription factor is Pit-1/GHF-1, which is expressed in the differentiating fetal pituitary gland. This factor is necessary not only for pituitary-specific expression of the peptide hormones prolactin and growth hormone but also for the development of the respective lactotroph and somatotroph cell types. Recently, a number of cases have been described of loss-of-function mutations of Pit-1/GHF-1 in which patients are hypopituitary, with pituitary hypoplasia as well as prolactin and growth hormone deficiency.

mRNA and protein synthesis

The process of gene transcription occurs by complementary base pairing from the genomic DNA template to form a primary transcript of heterogeneous nuclear RNA (hnRNA), which contains both exonic and intronic sequences. This RNA forms the precursor to mRNA, whose message is carried in the genetic code of nucleotide triplets (codons), each specifying one of the usual 20 amino acids. The hnRNA is then processed to form mature messenger RNA (mRNA) by a series of steps (Fig. 1.5).

1. A methylated guanosine residue (m^7Gppp) is added at the 5′ end (the 5′ cap) at the start of the first exon's untranslated leader sequence; the

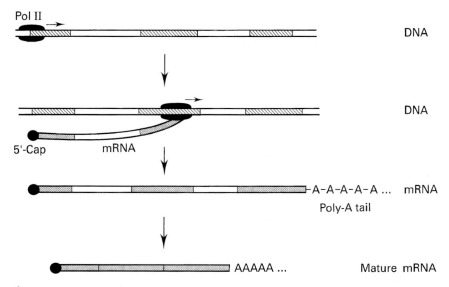

Figure 1.5 Formation of mature mRNA. Double-stranded DNA is transcribed by RNA polymerase II (Pol II) and the mRNA is modified at its 5′-end by the addition of a G residue with a triphosphate bond (Gppp) that is methylated (5′-cap). Splicing removes intronic sequences and a 'poly-A tail' is added.

end of this untranslated region is marked by an AUG initiation codon encoding the first methionine residue of the protein.

2. Intronic regions are removed and the exons spliced together by a 'spliceosome' complex of small ribonucleoproteins, the splice sites being marked by characteristic GU and AG splice donor and acceptor sites at the beginning and end of intron transcripts.

3. A long tract of 100 or more A residues (the 'poly-A tail') is added at the 3′ end, signalled by characteristic polyadenylation sequences (such as AAUAAA) downstream of the stop codon (UGA, UAA, or UAG) that terminates protein translation.

These features of mature mRNA are important for stability and translocation. In particular, the structure of the 5′ and 3′ untranslated regions appears to be significant, with secondary structures such as hairpin and cruciate loops affecting the rate of peptide translation in the ribosome. The process of splicing also appears to have a significant function, allowing the cell to select which exons will be represented. Therefore alternative splicing of the primary transcript can generate alternative gene products, as in the case of calcitonin and the calcitonin gene–related peptide (CGRP), which are encoded by one gene. The gene encoding the transcriptional repressor CREM (cyclic AMP-response element modulator; see pages 11–12) similarly can be alternatively spliced to produce two forms of the factor with different DNA-binding domains.

Protein synthesis: mRNA translation

mRNA is translated into protein in the cytoplasm by a complex process of matching nucleotide sequences to amino acids. These are polymerised to form the polypeptide chain at the ribosomes.

Ribosomes

These are large multimolecular complexes of many different proteins associated with several structural

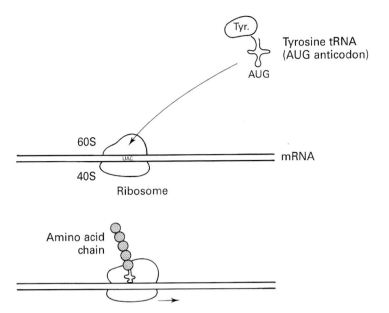

Figure 1.6 Translation of mRNA. tRNAs enter the ribosome and bind to the mRNA by matching of their anticodons. Peptide bonds are formed between the amino acids to give a growing amino acid chain with its sequence defined by the nucleotide sequence of the mRNA.

RNA (ribosomal RNA, rRNA) molecules. These complexes act to position transfer RNA (tRNA) molecules sequentially to match the triplet code of mRNA. Each ribosome comprises two subunits, one large and one small. The small 40S subunit contains a single (18S) rRNA molecule with over 30 proteins, and the large 60S subunit contains three different rRNAs and over 40 proteins. The overall assembly has a molecular weight of 4.5 million daltons (Da) and forms a particle visible by electron microscopy. The three-dimensional structure allows this molecular machine to engage both a strand of mRNA and a growing peptide chain (Fig. 1.6).

tRNA

Molecules of tRNA are essentially adaptors that recognise both a mRNA nucleotide sequence *and* an amino acid sequence. They are single polynucleotide chains, 70 to 90 bases in length, that undergo inter-nal base pairing to form a complex with exposed nucleotide loops. One such loop contains the 'anti-codon' that can base-pair with the corresponding codon in mRNA, while the exposed 3′ end of the tRNA molecule is attached covalently to a specific amino acid (Fig. 1.6).

Translation

The process of translation is rapid, a single ribosome taking only 1 min to polymerise over 1000 amino acids. The ribosome binds to a specific site on the mRNA, allowing the first 'initiator tRNA' to bind to the AUG initiation codon and start the peptide chain with the initial methionine residue. Subsequently, the ribosome moves along the mRNA translating codon by codon with a series of tRNAs adding amino acids to the growing peptide chain. When the end of the message is reached at the stop codon, the ribosome subunits are released along with the newly made peptide.

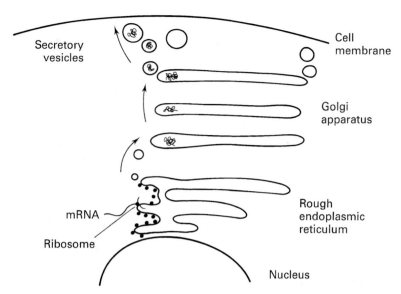

Figure 1.7 Cellular organelles involved in protein synthesis. Ribosomes attached to rough endoplasmic reticulum synthesise peptide chains that contain signals allowing entry to the endoplasmic reticulum. These leader sequences are later cleaved off and the protein is routed through the Golgi apparatus to secretory vesicles or other cellular destinations.

Protein secretion

The fate of the protein product of mRNA translation depends upon the nature of the protein and the cell type. For proteins such as peptide hormones that are exported by the cell into the extracellular fluid, specialised secretory processes are involved. Cells can secrete hormones 'constitutively', in a continuous manner unaffected by external stimuli and dependent only on the rate of transcription and translation, or via a 'regulated' pathway, using secretory granules to package and store hormone until an external or internal stimulus causes exocytosis.

Secreted proteins are synthesised on ribosomes attached to rough endoplasmic reticulum. They then enter the lumen of the endoplasmic reticulum by the binding of a hydrophobic leader sequence of the peptide with a 'signal recognition particle' to a docking protein on the endoplasmic reticulum surface. The proteins are then transported to the Golgi complex, where they undergo post-translational modifi-cation, such as glycosylation, before being concentrated into granules which are pinched off from the Golgi membrane (Fig. 1.7). Finally, under the influence of secretory stimuli, the granules 'marginate' and fuse with the cell membrane, allowing their contents to be released into the extracellular fluid, a process known as exocytosis.

Post-translational processing

Post-translational processing of proteins is an important regulating process that modifies the biological activity of many proteins. It occurs largely in the endoplasmic reticulum, the Golgi apparatus, and the cytoplasm, but it can also occur within the secretory granule.

An important initial modification is the *three-dimensional folding* of the new polypeptide chain, which is largely determined by the array of hydrophobic or hydrophilic amino acid side chains.

Particular patterns of protein folding have been confirmed by X-ray crystallography to occur in many different proteins, namely the α *helix*, a rigid cylinder formed by a spiral of amino acid residues, and the β *sheet*, formed by alignment of antiparallel or parallel straight chains of amino acids.

The folded protein conformation may be stabilised by the formation of covalent bonds between or within chains by *disulphide bridges* between nearby cysteine-SH groups.

Further covalent post-translational modifications include *phosphorylation*, catalysed by protein kinases that transfer a high-energy phosphate group from ATP to specific amino acid sequences in proteins, and *glycosylation*, the addition of complex carbohydrates to particular residues, often asparagine (N-linked oligosaccharides) or the hydroxy groups of serine or threonine (O-linked oligosaccharides). Other modifications include the aggregation of protein subunits to form multimers, the attachment of co-enzymes such as biotin to some enzymes, and acetylation and hydroxylation of certain amino acids.

Cellular signalling and growth regulation

Cells respond to a series of extracellular stimuli such as hormones, growth factors, and neurotransmitters. Some agents, such as steroid and thyroid hormones, are able to enter the cell and bind to intracellular receptors that in turn bind to DNA as transcription factors, directly altering the transcription of target genes. However, many other factors (such as peptide hormones) are unable to enter the cell and instead must stimulate a receptor on the cell membrane to trigger an intracellular 'second messenger'. This then generates a cellular response. This process is termed signal transduction, and a variety of intracellular signalling processes have been discovered.

The systems are complex and can be viewed as molecular cascades comprising receptors, transducing proteins (G proteins), effector proteins, second-messenger molecules, protein kinases and kinase substrates. The complexity of these systems allows for great amplification within the cell of an initial extracellular signal, and also for interaction and co-regulation of parallel signalling pathways. The corollary is that the genes for some of the many proteins involved are subject to mutations that result in human disease, including tumour formation. Indeed these genes are in many cases known as 'proto-oncogenes', the normal cellular homologues of viral 'oncogenes' that cause cancers (see pages 18–21).

Membrane receptors

Peptide hormones, catecholamines, growth factors and neurotransmitters bind to specific cell surface receptors, which are coupled to intracellular signalling pathways in a variety of ways.

G protein–linked receptors

A very large number of membrane receptors are coupled to second messenger–generating systems via intermediate *transducers*, 'G proteins' (see below), which in turn are linked to *effector* molecules that generate the intracellular second messenger. Molecular cloning has shown that these G protein–linked receptors belong to a superfamily of proteins that have similar structures. They are characterised by seven hydrophobic α helices traversing the membrane, with an extracellular amino-terminal and an intracellular carboxy-terminal, three intracellular loops thought to couple to the G proteins, and three extracellular loops involved in ligand binding (Fig. 1.8). The G protein–linked receptors in general operate to initiate the generation of diffusible small molecules such as cyclic adenosine monophosphate (cAMP), which in turn activate protein kinases.

G protein–independent receptors

Not all receptors are linked to G proteins, and a number of transmembrane receptors possess intrinsic intracellular effector domains without intermediate transducing proteins. Some such receptors, such as the epidermal growth factor (EGF) receptor,

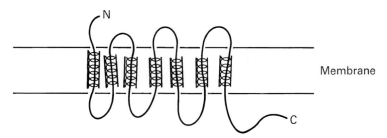

Figure 1.8 A membrane receptor with seven α-helical transmembrane domains.

have a single polypeptide chain, while others, such as the insulin receptor, have linked α and β subunits. Some of these receptors possess intrinsic tyrosine kinase activity, allowing them to phosphorylate (and hence activate) target intracellular proteins, while others are closely associated with separate tyrosine kinase proteins – for example, the 'Janus kinases' such as Jak-2, linked to the erythropoietin and growth hormone receptors. Thus, these receptors are able directly or indirectly to initiate a cascade of protein phosphorylation as their mechanism of action without necessarily generating intermediate second messengers. A typical phosphorylation cascade of this sort is illustrated in Fig. 1.9.

Nuclear receptors

Steroid and thyroid hormones, vitamin D and retinoic acid are small lipophilic molecules that are membrane-soluble and interact directly with intracellular receptor proteins. These receptors exist in the cytoplasm complexed with 'chaperone' molecules (for example, heat-shock protein 90, or hsp-90), from which they dissociate on activation by the hormonal ligand. After dissociation, they change conformation and translocate to the nucleus.

Again, molecular cloning has shown that there is a large superfamily of nuclear receptors that function as ligand-activated transcription factors. Some of these receptors have no identifiable ligand and have been termed 'orphan receptors'. Nonetheless, despite having widely differing ligands, the nuclear receptors have remarkable structural similarity, with six identifiable domains (A to F), including con-

served DNA-binding domains with two zinc-finger motifs (see above) and a hormone-binding domain (Fig. 1.10).

The receptors for oestrogen and glucocorticoid activate gene transcription as homodimers bound to short, palindromic DNA response elements (for example, a typical oestrogen response element would be 5'-GGTCAnnnTGACC-3', the palindrome being apparent on the complementary strand in the reverse direction). The other members of the family form heterodimers with a different protein, the retinoid X receptor (RXR), whose ligand is 9-*cis*-retinoic acid; the nature of the complexes that form on DNA is determined by the arrangement of the response elements in the enhancer regions of gene promoters, usually as short direct-repeat or inverted-repeat sequences with variable spacing of one to five nucleotides.

G proteins

G proteins are a large family of membrane-associated transducing proteins that are linked to transmembrane receptors, as described above. G proteins are so named because they bind guanosine triphosphate (GTP) and are themselves members of a larger superfamily of GTP-binding proteins (which includes the *ras* proto-oncogene product p21) whose general function in cells is proposed to be one of molecular switching. The receptor-associated G proteins fulfil exactly this role, conveying an 'on' signal from a newly occupied receptor to switch an intracellular effector protein into its activated state.

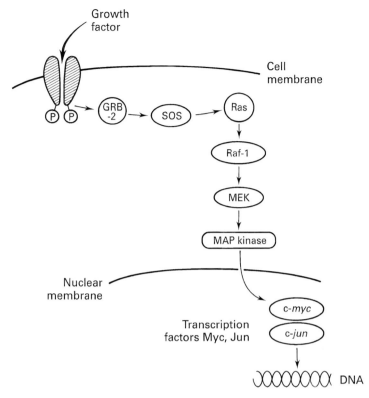

Figure 1.9 A typical cascade of protein activation induced by growth factor binding to a transmembrane receptor.

G proteins are heterotrimers, consisting of α, β, γ subunits. The β and γ subunits are tightly associated and function as a single β-γ complex; the α subunit binds GTP and possesses intrinsic GTPase activity (Fig. 1.11). Hormone activation of a G protein–linked receptor allows the α subunit to exchange a GDP molecule for GTP; this results in its dissociation from the β-γ complex and enables the α subunit to change to its active configuration to switch on or off the effector protein to which it is coupled. In some cases the β-γ complex appears to have a signalling function in its own right.

Different types of G protein are coupled to different intracellular signalling systems: for example, Gs is the stimulatory G protein that activates adenylate cyclase to form cAMP (3′, 5′-cyclic adenosine monophosphate); G_i inhibits adenylate cyclase; G_q stimulates phospholipase C to hydrolyse phosphatidylinositol bisphosphate; while other proteins are linked to ion channels. In some cases, a particular type of receptor can be linked to different intracellular effectors via different G proteins; for example, the dopamine D_2 receptor can be linked either to adenylate cyclase via G_i or to phospholipase C via G_q.

Second messengers: the cAMP/protein kinase A system

Cyclic AMP

Cyclic AMP is one of several small diffusible molecules produced as a result of receptor–G protein

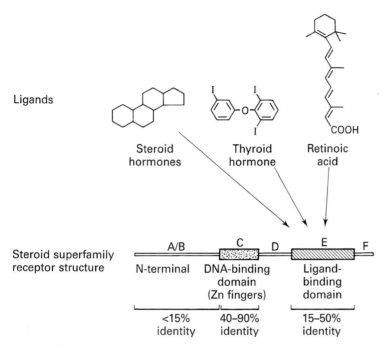

Figure 1.10 Nuclear receptors. Widely differing hormonal ligands bind to conserved members of the steroid receptor superfamily; the conservation of structure resides in the DNA-binding domains.

activation of effector proteins. The production of these small molecules allows for amplification and diffusion of the initial signal.

The formation of cAMP from ATP (adenosine triphosphate) is catalysed by the enzyme adenylate cyclase, whose activity is modulated by extracellular signals via receptor-associated G proteins. Levels of cAMP are tightly controlled, rising within seconds of activation of the cyclase enzyme; the cAMP signal is also rapidly terminated by cellular phosphodiesterases, which hydrolyse cyclic AMP to inactive 5′ adenosine monophosphate (5′ AMP).

Protein kinase A

A number of protein kinases are activated by cAMP, the best-understood of which is protein kinase A. This is an inactive holoenzyme complex compris-

ing two regulatory (R) subunits and two catalytic (C) subunits: the C subunit is highly conserved, but the R subunit varies among different cell types. Binding of cyclic AMP to the R subunit allows dissociation and activation of free C subunits, which rapidly translocate to the cell nucleus, where they phosphorylate substrate proteins such as the cAMP response element–binding protein (CREB) transcription factor (see below) (Fig. 1.12).

Second messengers: the phospholipid/calcium signalling system

Inositol lipid signalling

Phosphoinositide (PI) molecules are components of membrane phospholipids comprising a lipid moiety, diacylglycerol, from the inner leaflet of the membrane lipid bilayer, linked by a phosphodiester bond

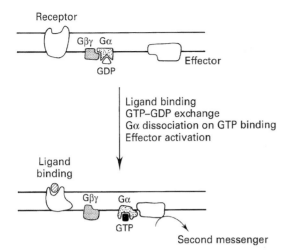

Figure 1.11 Model for activation of an effector molecule by an activated receptor via a G-protein. The heterotrimer ($G\alpha$/$G\beta$/$G\gamma$) dissociates such that $G\alpha$, binding GTP, will activate (or inhibit) the production of an intracellular signal by the effector protein (e.g. the production of cyclic AMP by adenylate cyclase).

to an inositol sugar head group. A variety of enzymes are able to phosphorylate or dephosphorylate the inositol head group. The PI3 kinase enzymes comprise a series of family members, which can phosphorylate inositol lipids on the inositol head group. Dephosphorylation steps are catalysed by a network of phosphoinositide phosphatases. The phosphatidylinositol molecule can therefore have a variety of configurations: $PI(4,5)P_2$ is a substrate for cleavage by phospholipase C, which is coupled to a series of membrane receptors via the G protein G_q, and this hydrolysis step yields free diacylglycerol (DAG) in the plasma membrane and a soluble sugar-phosphate, inositol -1,4,5-triphosphate (IP_3), both of which have identifiable signalling pathways; see below). $PI(3,4)P_2$ and $PI(3,4,5)P_3$ are present in very small amounts in resting cells but increase rapidly and transiently after hormonal stimulation, and a variety of downstream targets for PI3 kinases have now been identified. Phosphatidylinositol 4,5-bisphosphate (PIP2) is a minor component of membrane phospholipids, which nonetheless has a

crucial role in intracellular signalling. It is formed by the phosphorylation of phosphatidylinositol (PI) and is rapidly turned over in the membrane after stimulation by certain hormones and growth factors. A large number of membrane receptors are coupled via the G protein G_q to *phospholipase C*, which hydrolyses PIP2 to form two important second messengers: namely, the membrane lipid *diacylglycerol* (DAG) and a hydrophilic sugar phosphate molecule *inositol 1,4,5-triphosphate (IP$_3$)*. DAG remains in the membrane and activates protein kinase C, while IP_3 is released into the cytoplasm and mobilises calcium from intracellular stores (see Fig. 1.13).

Protein kinase C and DAG

DAG formed in the cell membrane directly activates the phospholipid-dependent calcium-activated kinase protein kinase C. There is, in fact, a family of protein kinase C molecules, derived from alternative splicing of several different genes. DAG increases the affinity of protein kinase C for calcium, rendering the kinase highly active. The effect of DAG may be mimicked pharmacologically by tumour-promoting phorbol esters such as 12-O-tetradecanoylphorbol-13-acetate (TPA); this allows detailed studies of the role of protein kinase C. It has a wide range of effects in different cell types, including regulation of hormone secretion, modulation of ion channels and gene transcription – although only in the last have the mechanisms been dissected in detail, as described below.

DAG may be metabolised to generate further second-messenger lipid molecules, including arachidonic acid, which in turn may be metabolised to yield active substances, such as prostaglandins, leukotrienes and thromboxanes.

IP$_3$, intracellular calcium and calmodulin

Inositol -1,4,5-triphosphate (IP_3) binds to a specific tetrameric protein receptor located on the endoplasmic reticulum, which is the major store of intracellular calcium. The IP_3 receptor is homologous to the ryanodine receptor found in muscle cells, and

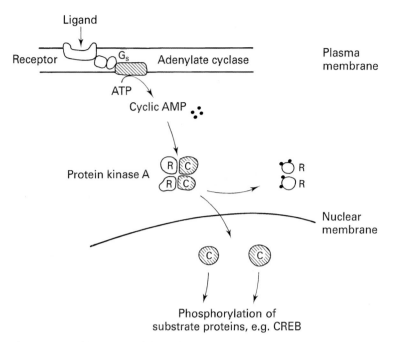

Figure 1.12 Activation of protein kinase. A by cyclic AMP. The kinase holoenzyme complex dissociates so that free catalytic subunits can diffuse into the nucleus to phosphorylate proteins such as the CREB transcription factor.

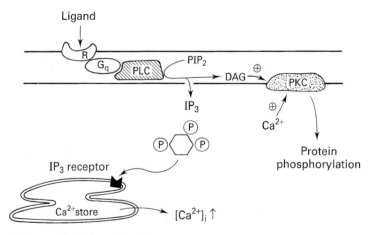

Figure 1.13 The phosphatidylinositol signalling system. Activation of phospholipase C (PLC) results in the hydrolysis of the membrane lipid PIP_2 to from DAG and IP_3. DAG is a lipid and remains in the membrane to activate protein kinase C (PKC); IP_3 is water soluble and diffuses into the cytoplasm to mobilise calcium from intracellular stores.

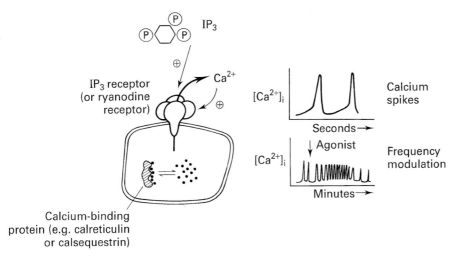

Figure 1.14 Mobilisation of intaracellular free calcium by IP_3. Activation of the tetrameric IP_3 receptor allows efflux of free calcium from intracellular organelles, where it exists in equilibrium with protein-bound calcium.

both are calcium-sensitive, so that an initial release of calcium induced by IP_3 may promote further calcium release, thus amplifying the initial signal. Ryanodine receptors are thought to be activated by cyclic adenosine diphosphate-ribose (cADPR), which may prove to be an important second messenger parallel to cAMP in certain cell types.

Measurements of single-cell intracellular calcium concentrations using fluorescent dyes and high-resolution microscopy have shown that calcium levels fluctuate rapidly in response to stimulation by extracellular signals. Calcium concentrations rise rapidly in one part of the cell, and this calcium 'spike' propagates across the cell as a wave. The frequency of the calcium spikes is proportional in many cases to the concentration of the agonist, suggesting that the calcium signal is frequency-modulated, not amplitude-modulated (Fig. 1.14).

The initiation of a full calcium spike depends on *calcium entry*, as well as mobilisation from intracellular stores. Calcium entry occurs through a series of membrane calcium channels, which may be voltage-operated channels (VOCs, opened by cell depolarisation), receptor-operated channels (ROCs, opened by agonist binding to membrane receptors) or second messenger–operated channels (SMOCs, affected by other intracellular signals such as cAMP).

Calcium within the endoplasmic reticulum is released from calcium-sequestering proteins, such as calreticulin and calsequestrin, in a quantal manner, which can be visualised using fluorescent dyes in muscle cells as localised 'calcium sparks'. The frequency of this localised sparking is increased by entry of extracellular calcium until a critical point is reached and a full calcium wave is irreversibly triggered.

Calcium exerts its intracellular effects through binding to one or more calcium-binding proteins, the best known of which is calmodulin. Calmodulin is a highly conserved protein found in all mammalian cells: it is a single-chain peptide with four calcium-binding sites and activates a number of calcium/calmodulin-dependent protein kinases, such as calmodulin dependent kinase-II (CaMK-II), myosin light-chain kinase and adenylate cyclase itself.

IP_3 is removed from the cytoplasm by progressive dephosphorylation to form free inositol, which is recycled to form phosphatidylinositol. In some cases, IP$_3$ is further phosphorylated to form inositol 1, 3, 4, 5-tetrakisphosphate, which has been implicated in calcium influx into the cell and the replenishment of calcium stores.

Effects of signalling pathways on gene transcription

The end points of the signalling cascades described above have been defined most completely in terms of the regulation of gene expression. The techniques of molecular biology have been used first to locate signal-responsive elements within regulatory regions of DNA that control gene transcription and then to use these DNA sequences to isolate and characterise the protein transcription factors that are activated by signalling pathways. Two of the signal transduction pathways described above, namely the cAMP–protein kinase A pathway and the DAG–protein kinase C pathway, have been analysed in such a way, leading to the identification of the CREB and AP-1 transcriptional regulators.

Cyclic AMP and CREB

Analysis of the promoters of cAMP-regulated genes has revealed that their cAMP responsiveness could be attributed to short DNA sequences, termed 'cAMP response elements' (CREs). The classical CRE contains a conserved 8-bp palindromic sequence (5'-TGACGTCA-3'), the identification of which led to the discovery of a 43-kDa CRE-binding protein termed CREB. CREB is a transcription factor and contains a typical leucine zipper, allowing it to form homo- and heterodimers. It is phosphorylated by protein kinase A, which promotes its dimerisation and increases its transcriptional activity (Fig. 1.15). In fact, CREB has proved to be one member of a large family of related factors, including a series of activating transcription factors (ATFs 1 to 8), and CRE-modulator proteins (CREMs) that repress transcription.

In summary, the complete cAMP signalling pathway can now be described, in which an external hormonal stimulus can trigger a molecular cascade (receptor–Gs protein–adenylate cyclase–protein kinase–CREB), with the final end point of posttranslational modification of a transcription factor altering the transcriptional rate of a target gene.

Protein kinase C and activator protein-1

Activation of protein kinase C increases the transcription of a number of genes; the mechanism of

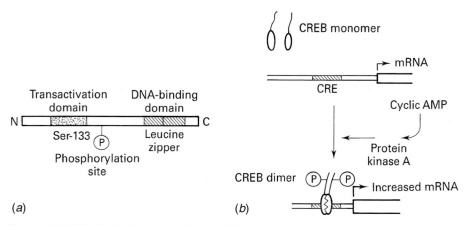

Figure 1.15 CREB: the binding protein that modulates genes responsive to cyclic AMP levels by binding to cyclic AMP response elements (CREs). (*a*) structure of CREB showing the phosphorylation site at Ser-133. (*b*) Activation of transcription by CREB phosphorylation and dimerisation at the CRE.

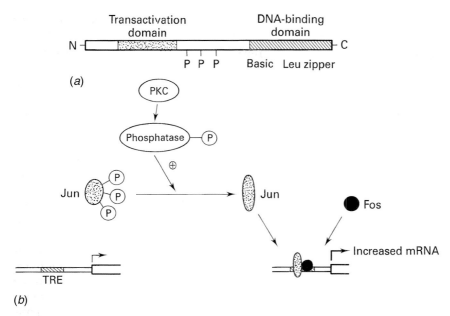

Figure 1.16 Activator protein 1 and c-*jun*. (*a*) The structure of Jun. (*b*) Jun is activated by dephosphorylation. This is catalysed by a phosphatase which is itself activated by protein kinase C (PKC). The activated Jun can form a heterodimer with FOS at a phorbol ester response element (TRE) that activates gene transcription.

this activation has been analysed using phorbol esters such as TPA as specific pharmacological activators of protein kinase C. Promoter analysis revealed that the TPA responsiveness of these genes could be attributed to a specific 7-bp 'TPA-response element' (TRE) very similar to the CRE (5'-TGAGTCA-3'). This TRE binds a transcription factor complex of 44 to 47 kDa termed activator protein-1, or AP-1, which contains the protein *Jun*.

Jun is the protein product of the cellular *proto-oncogene* c-*jun*, which is the normal cellular homologue of the *oncogene* v-*jun* found in avian sarcoma virus (ASV-17). Like CREB, Jun is a 'bZip' transcription factor, containing both a conserved basic domain and a leucine zipper that allows dimerisation. Therefore Jun can heterodimerise with Fos, the product of the c-*fos* proto-oncogene (again a normal cellular homologue of an oncogene, v-*fos*, found in the FBJ murine sarcoma virus). Jun and Fos heterodimers bind to TREs with high affinity, but their activity depends on intracellular signalling pathways (Fig. 1.16).

Jun is activated both by amino-terminal phosphorylation (induced via other proto-oncogenes such as *ras*) and by carboxy-terminal dephosphorylation, probably by phosphatases activated by protein kinase C. Levels of c-*jun* mRNA are normally low in unstimulated cells but rise rapidly after exposure to growth factors and in response to several 'transforming' proto-oncogenes, such as *src*, *ras* and *mos*.

In summary, it is now clear that signalling pathways can interact at the level of transcription factors themselves. A variety of signals converge on the Jun transcription factor in addition to its activation by the classical protein kinase C pathway. Furthermore, the composition and activity of heterodimers is variable; Jun interacts not only with Fos (which is cAMP-regulated) but also with CREB.

Alterations of signalling pathways in human disease

The complex cascades of signalling molecules are susceptible to alteration, and many components have been identified as responsible for a series of human diseases. A whole cascade may be activated or blocked by abnormal stimulation of a receptor (for example, by immunoglobulins that bind to a hormone receptor), or any one of the proteins involved in the cascade may be mutated, with damaging consequences. Indeed, many of the proteins have been identified as 'proto-oncogenes', which may be susceptible to oncogenic mutation that can either impair or enhance their function and lead to tumour formation.

Membrane receptors

G protein–coupled membrane receptors are the largest family of membrane receptors; some examples illustrate the potential for activating of these proteins by mutations. The receptor for thyroid-stimulating hormone (TSH) controls thyroid cell function and growth, and activating mutations affecting the structure of its third intracellular loop produce functioning *thyroid neoplasms* and hyperthyroidism. Activating mutations in the gene for the receptor for the pituitary gonadotrophin luteinising hormone (LH) are responsible for abnormal sensitivity of the testis to LH, resulting in *precocious puberty*. In the hereditary disease *retinitis pigmentosa*, which leads to blindness, germ cell mutations have been found that constitutively activate rhodopsin, a light-responsive retinol-binding receptor in the human retina.

G protein–independent receptors such as growth factor receptors may also be constitutively activated by mutation, and several viral oncogenes represent tumour-inducing counterparts of normal cellular proteins; for example the c-*erbB* product is the EGF receptor, while v-*erbB* is responsible for avian erythroleukaemia.

Loss-of-function mutations may affect the insulin receptor, giving severe *insulin resistance*, and the growth hormone receptor is disrupted in *Laron-type dwarfism*, which explains the failure of these patients to respond to therapy with growth hormone.

G proteins

The G_s-α subunit of the heterotrimeric G_s-protein complex coupled to the cyclic AMP system has been found to be mutated in several human tumours, notably endocrine tumours. These '*gsp*' oncogenic mutations occur in somatic cells after embryogenesis and result in constitutive activation of adenylate cyclase. The high levels of intracellular cAMP stimulate not only differentiated cell function but also cell proliferation: for example, in some cases of acromegaly, growth hormone hypersecretion occurs from a pituitary tumour.

A major example of a related GTP-binding protein involved in human disease is that produced by the *ras* proto-oncogene. This protein is part of the signal transduction pathway linked to several growth factor receptors such as the EGF receptor. Oncogenic mutations result in permanent activation of Ras and are commonly found in human cancers.

Kinases

The role of spontaneous kinase mutations in human disease is less clear, although mutations of protein kinase C have been detected in certain endocrine tumours. However the c-*src* proto-oncogene is the cellular homologue of the v-*src* oncogene, found in the Rous sarcoma virus and responsible for sarcoma formation in chickens.

The c-*abl* proto-oncogene produces a cytosolic tyrosine kinase (see below for its involvement in apoptosis), and this has been found to be involved in a chromosomal translocation that results in *chronic myeloid leukaemia*. The translocation on the 'Philadelphia chromosome' results in part of the coding region of c-*abl* (chromosome 9) being spliced onto part of the *bcr* gene on chromosome 22. The Bcr–Abl fusion protein is oncogenic, possibly because Bcr is able to autophosphorylate and activate the Abl portion of the hybrid oncogene.

Nuclear receptors and transcription factors

Mutations in genes for intracellular receptors have been found in a series of hormone-resistance syndromes. For example, single-base substitutions can result in impaired ligand binding to the androgen receptor, and the resulting resistance to androgen action in a genetic male can result in a spectrum of effects, from the profound changes of a female phenotype (as in the androgen insensitivity syndrome, formerly termed *testicular feminisation* syndrome) to mild infertility.

Similar mutations have been identified in the genes for the vitamin D receptor (leading to vitamin D–resistant rickets), the thyroid hormone receptor (giving thyroid hormone resistance), and the glucocorticoid receptor (giving cortisol resistance), all with major phenotypic consequences. In many cases, these mutations are in the area coding for the hormone-binding domain, but in others they may affect the zinc fingers in the DNA-binding domain or produce truncated mRNAs. Pit-1 is an example of a tissue-specific transcription factor that may have loss-of-function changes in the DNA-binding domain; these are responsible for loss of development of certain pituitary cell types, resulting in hypopituitarism and growth failure.

Summary: signalling, proto-oncogenes, and oncogenes

A series of proteins are involved in intracellular signalling, and they are mutated in many different types of human disease (see box). In some cases, loss-of-function mutations generate hormone-resistant states, while in others, gain-of-function mutations give rise to tumours. In the latter case, many of the proteins involved have come to be termed 'cellular proto-oncogenes' because of their homology with tumour-generating viral oncogenes. These include receptors, G proteins, kinases, intracellular receptors, and transcription factors (see Fig. 1.17). Oncogenes may be derived from proto-oncogenes by gain-of-function mutations that increase activity or level of expression. Oncogenic viruses either carry onco-genes or, in some cases, activate normal cellular proto-oncogenes.

Cell cycle and growth regulation

Normal mammalian cells undergo a 'cell cycle' of replication, with protein synthesis, DNA synthesis, and mitosis occurring in defined phases. *Mitosis* (M phase) of a somatic cell generates two daughter cells, each with a full genetic complement of chromosomes. After mitosis, cells enter G_1 *phase*, representing a 'gap' during which RNAs and proteins are synthesised and then enter *S phase*, when DNA synthesis (i.e. replication of the genome) starts. Finally, there is a further 'gap', termed G_2 *phase*, before the cell enters mitosis. Cells may withdraw from the cycle during the G_1 phase into a non-cycling state termed G_0 (Fig. 1.18).

The cell cycle is subject to control by a series of cell cycle genes (best characterised in yeasts) whose activity is affected by phosphorylation and dephosphorylation. Homologues for some of these genes have been found in humans, and a series of *cyclin* proteins have been cloned that appear to have important evolutionarily conserved functions, with sequential activation through different stages of the cell cycle.

Tumour suppressor genes

Tumour suppressors are identified by the fact that loss-of-function mutations give rise to increased cell proliferation.

p53

The best known example of a tumour suppressor is p53, which was originally thought to be an oncogene because mutations were associated with cancers. In fact, these mutations are largely mis-sense (i.e. loss-of-function) mutations, inhibiting the action of normal p53 produced by the unaffected allele. As a nuclear phosphoprotein, p53 has a variety of discrete activities. It is a transcription factor, binding to target sequences in normal DNA, but its functions also include induction of growth arrest and of apoptosis. It binds to proteins involved in the cell cycle,

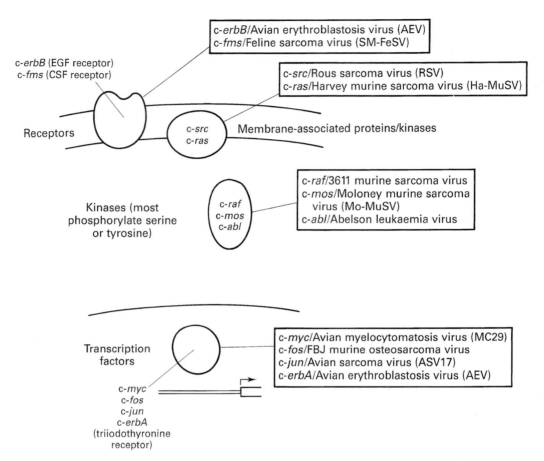

Figure 1.17 Examples of cellular proto-oncogenes whose products are involved in different steps in signal transduction. The viral oncogenic homologues are shown in the boxes and the protein products in parentheses.

notably mdm2 and SV40 T antigen, and also binds to damaged DNA through its C terminal. Mutant p53 molecules are unable to bind the SV40 virus large T tumour antigen: normal p53 binds to T antigen and prevents it from replicating the SV40 genome. Therefore it has been proposed that normal cells contain a homologue of the large T antigen and that this function is lost in cells with mutant p53, allowing uncontrolled cell growth.

The retinoblastoma gene (Rb). This is another tumour suppressor gene. It was first identified in the childhood retinal tumour retinoblastoma, where both copies of the gene are inactivated or deleted;

however, Rb gene deletions have now been demonstrated in a series of human tumours apart from retinoblastoma – for example, small cell lung cancer. The tumour itself contains no Rb protein, usually because of a loss of gene expression rather than point mutations affecting protein function. The Rb protein, a nuclear phosphoprotein, is unphosphorylated in resting (G_0-phase) cells but undergoes phosphorylation at the end of the G_1 phase, probably by a cyclin E–dependent protein kinase. The Rb protein is once again dephosphorylated at the end of mitosis. The unphosphorylated protein is able to bind several cell-cycle proteins, such as the E2F transcription

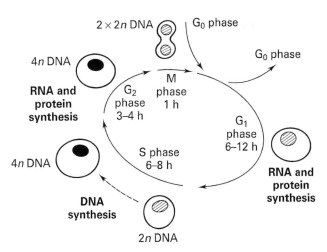

Figure 1.18 Stages of the cell cycle. The normal diploid complement of genetic material is given as $2n$ DNA; $4n$ is the tetraploid content just before mitosis.

factor and cyclin D; this places a block on the cell entering the cell cycle by preventing these proteins from being released.

Apoptosis

Cell population number is affected not only by proliferation but also by cell death. Apoptosis is an active, regulated form of cell death, unlike necrosis, and is central to embryogenesis and development as well as homeostasis of adult tissues. Abnormally regulated apoptosis has recently been implicated in several human diseases including cancer and neurodegeneration.

Apoptosis was first identified microscopically as a distinctive reduction in cell volume and condensation of nuclear chromatin. The nucleus then breaks into smaller fragments, but other organelles remain intact. Eventually the endoplasmic reticulum fuses with the plasma membrane, and round apoptotic bodies are released and rapidly phagocytosed. Intracellular events accompanying apoptosis include characteristic internucleosomal fragmentation of DNA resulting from regulated endonuclease activity. A number of genes have been identified

that control the initiation of these processes, notably *ced-3* and *myc*, which promote apoptosis, and *bcl-2* and c-*abl* (see above), which can suppress it *in vitro*.

Molecular biology: methods of investigation

Studies of the molecular basis of disease depended initially on identifying an abnormal product, such as a protein. The development of techniques to manipulate DNA made it possible to utilise information from characterised proteins to clone and identify genes, from which further information about the disorder could be found. A further development is the isolation and cloning of genes likely to be involved in a disease and using these to produce and identify abnormal proteins (see box).

Enzymes

The development of modern molecular biology was made possible with the discovery of a series of enzymes that allowed specific (usually sequence-specific) manipulations of DNA and RNA. This made it possible to produce DNA fragments reproducibly

(*a*)

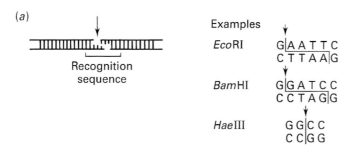

(*b*)

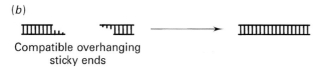

Compatible overhanging
sticky ends

Figure 1.19 Examples of DNA-modifying enzymes. (*a*) Endonucleases.
(*b*) Ligases.

from a variety of tissues and, in particular, allowed the generation of new DNA molecules by recombining fragments from different sources.

Endonucleases (restriction endonucleases)

These are bacterial enzymes that cleave double-stranded DNA at specific symmetrical (palindromic) sequences, leaving fragments with characteristic patterns, either blunt-ended or with overhanging ends of specific bases ('sticky ends') (Fig. 1.19*a*). A huge number of enzymes is now available. Each one recognises and cleaves at a specific DNA sequence usually 4 to 6 bp in length. Using different endonucleases, specific DNA fragments can be produced and then cloned by inserting them into plasmid or bacteriophage vectors for propagation in bacteria, as described below.

Ligases

These enzymes catalyse the formation of a DNA molecule from two fragments with compatible termini (as shown in Fig. 1.19*b*).

Polymerases

Polymerases catalyse the generation of a new DNA or RNA molecule by assembling nucleotides linearly along a pre-existing DNA or RNA template. This property can be used to incorporate radiolabelled nucleotides into a molecule – for example, in the production of labelled DNA or RNA probes and for sequence analysis.

Reverse transcriptase

This enzyme can be used to transcribe mRNA to produce a complementary DNA (cDNA) molecule that can be used for direct cloning or for polymerase chain reaction (PCR) amplification as described below.

cDNA synthesis

One of the most powerful uses of endonucleases and other enzymes is the synthesis of DNA molecules that are complementary to a DNA or RNA template. cDNA can be produced from a template of unknown or only partly known mRNA, propagated in bacteria, and then sequenced and its function analysed in detail. This process is summarised in Fig. 1.20. Essentially, polyA-rich RNA (i.e. mRNA) is extracted from a suitable tissue or cell line and a synthetic DNA sequence is added that contains a series of T residues. This 'oligo-dT primer' anneals to the poly-A tail of the mRNA, after which the enzyme reverse transcriptase

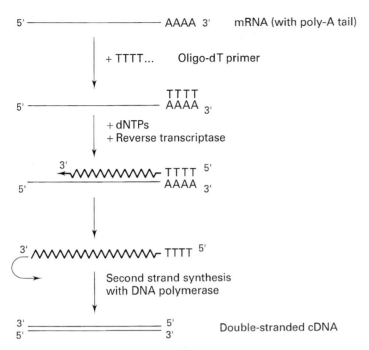

Figure 1.20 Synthesis of cDNA from RNA.

can be used to synthesise a new DNA molecule by the base pairing of nucleotides with the mRNA template. A second strand of DNA can be made from the first strand using DNA polymerase. The final product is a new double-stranded DNA molecule that can be inserted into a vector for cloning, as outlined below.

Cloning

Vectors

The discovery of specific enzymes for DNA and RNA manipulation has allowed the cloning of recombinant DNA fragments such as cDNA in *vectors*, which can carry such foreign sequences in host bacteria. Bacterial plasmids have been widely used as vectors: they are circular double-stranded DNA molecules that are normally found in bacteria, and although not an integral part of the host genome, they can replicate within the bacterium. The plasmids can be iso-

lated and artificially introduced into special strains of bacteria developed for experimental use that are unable to grow outside of laboratory conditions; in this way, the bacteria can be used to propagate large amounts of DNA. Plasmids were originally discovered because they conferred resistance to antibiotics, and this property can be used to select only those bacteria that have successfully taken up the plasmid DNA. The principles of cloning are summarised in Fig. 1.21.

The technology of using vectors for cloning has advanced rapidly, and a great variety of tools is now available, including plasmids with synthetic sequences incorporating multiple restriction endonuclease recognition sites ('polylinkers', or multiple cloning sites). Plasmid vectors have been developed to incorporate promoter sequences to allow *in vitro* transcription of the cloned DNA or *in vivo* expression of the protein product in living cells. Other types of vector also include bacteriophage

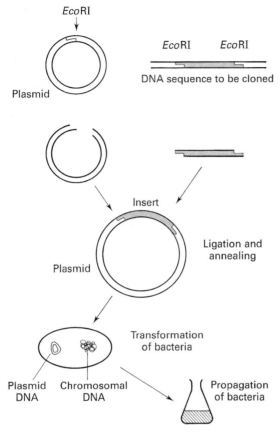

Figure 1.21 Principles of cloning DNA in bacteria.

lambda (λ), a bacterial virus that multiplies rapidly within its host and can carry large amounts of DNA.

Libraries

Using cloning techniques, it is possible to prepare DNA from a human tissue, digest it into fragments using one or more endonucleases, insert the fragments into a vector, and propagate them as a 'library' in bacteria. Total genomic DNA can be prepared in this way, in which case the transformed bacteria will carry a 'genomic library'; alternatively, cDNA pre-

pared from the mRNA expressed by a given cell type can be used to generate a 'cDNA library'.

Nucleic acid libraries contain many millions of sequences, and in order to identify bacteria bearing specific DNA fragments of interest, a series of screening procedures are used.

In the case of genomic libraries, fragments of DNA can be screened, for example, to identify upstream regulatory elements of specific genes for studies of transcriptional regulation. cDNA libraries can be screened to identify sequences encoding newly discovered proteins.

Library screening

Recombinant bacterial clones in a cDNA library can be screened with antibodies or with DNA probes. Antibody screening requires that the library be constructed in an *expression vector* that contains promoter sequences to direct transcription and translation of the cloned DNA in the bacteria. The bacteria are lysed to expose the intracellular protein and transferred to a membrane that is then incubated with the antibody. Positive colonies can be selected from the bacterial cultures for selective propagation and further rounds of screening. Screening of cDNA libraries with small known sequences of DNA – probes – is simpler because it does not require synthesis of an immunoreactive peptide, but it does require some prior knowledge of the DNA sequence being sought.

Subtractive hybridisation

A number of approaches have been developed to enrich cDNA libraries for sequences that are specifically found in certain tissues or that are associated with differentiation. Two cDNA libraries are prepared, a [+]cDNA from a tissue that expresses the factor of interest, and a [–]cDNA from a tissue that does not. The [+]cDNA is prepared with specific restriction endonuclease recognition sites at each terminus so that it can be cloned, and it is then allowed to hybridise with the [–]cDNA. Those [+]cDNAs that fail to hybridise with [–]cDNA represent species that are only present in the [+] tissue; they can be selectively cloned, resulting in a library that has been enriched by the 'subtraction' of irrelevant [−] clones.

Nucleic acid analysis

Gel electrophoresis

DNA and RNA molecules can be separated by electrophoresis through gels of agarose or polyacrylamide, migrating towards the anode because of the negatively charged phosphates along the DNA backbone. As the charge/mass ratio of DNA of different lengths is the same, the rate of migration through a gel is determined by the size of the molecule – up to about 50 kilobases (kb) (Fig. 1.22). However the conformation of DNA alters its electrophoretic mobility, so that molecules such as supercoiled closed circular plasmids migrate faster than linear DNA of the same base length because of their different hydrodynamic radii. The concentration of gels can be adjusted to give optimal separation of fragments varying in length from 20 to 20 000 bp.

(a) Electrophoresis

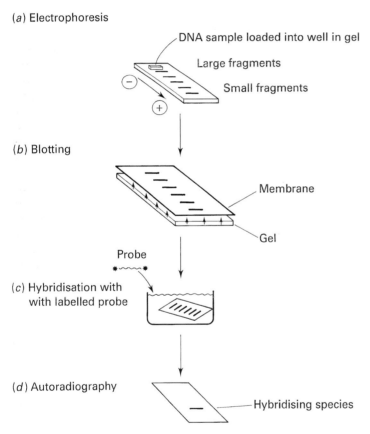

(b) Blotting

(c) Hybridisation with with labelled probe

(d) Autoradiography

Figure 1.22 Principles of nucleic acid analysis. (a) Electrophoresis separates DNA by fragment size and shape. (b) Blotting techniques allow the separated fragments to be transferred to a membrane for analysis. (c) The fragments are labelled by hybridisation with probes. (d) Autoradiography indicates the position of positive fragments where probe has bound to target DNA.

Larger molecules (25 000 to over 150 000 bp) can be separated by more complex techniques such as *pulsed field gel electrophoresis* (PFGE). In this technique, an electrophoretic gel is subjected to alternating-angle electric fields. This discriminates between the differing abilities of very large DNA molecules to alter their conformation rapidly on changing the electric field (which varies with molecular size); this determines their speed of migration.

Blotting techniques

DNA or RNA, once separated in a gel, may be transferred to a membrane for easier analysis by a number of 'blotting' techniques. The first technique to be widely used was developed by E. M. Southern and involving the transfer of DNA from gels onto nitrocellulose membranes by capillary blotting; this has become known as Southern blotting (Fig. 1.22). Various processes of macromolecule transfer from gels to membranes have since been applied to RNA (non-eponymously called Northern blotting) and to protein (usually for analysis with antibodies, Western blotting). Once transferred, nucleic acids can be fixed covalently onto membranes by baking or ultraviolet cross-linking and subjected to analysis.

Labelling nucleic acids

DNA and RNA, once separated by electrophoresis, can be visualised directly by incorporation of the dye ethidium bromide. This intercalates between the stacked bases of the nucleic acid and fluoresces orange under ultraviolet light. Analysis of specific DNA or RNA sequences relies on labelling of a known sequence – a 'probe' – and allowing it to hybridise with separated nucleic acids that have been transferred onto a membrane. Probe labelling is commonly achieved with radioactive phosphorus (^{32}P), although non-radioactive methods are becoming popular.

Short sequences of DNA, such as oligonucleotides of 20 to 40 bp, can be end-labelled by transfer of a ^{32}P-labelled γ-phosphate group from ATP to the 5'-hydroxyl terminus of a DNA molecule using the enzyme T4 polynucleotide kinase. Longer DNA molecules require 'body labelling', and a widely used method uses random-sequence hexamer primers to prime synthesis of a new DNA strand from a single-stranded DNA or RNA template: the primers anneal at multiple sites on a long DNA template and can prime second-strand DNA synthesis, incorporating radiolabelled nucleotides, in the presence of DNA polymerase.

Identification

The fragments of DNA and RNA that have hybridised with the probes are identified by autoradiography.

Sequencing

DNA sequencing relies on the separation of a series of radiolabelled oligonucleotides that differ by a single base using high-resolution denaturing polyacrylamide gels (sequencing gels). A set of single-stranded oligonucleotides is generated that all have one fixed end but terminate in each successive base of the template DNA sequence. Four separate reactions are used to generate oligonucleotides that terminate in A, T, G, or C. The reaction products are resolved on the gel such that four 'ladders' are seen, and the sequence can be read directly from the autoradiograph (see Fig. 1.23).

Two techniques are used in most sequencing reactions – namely, the dideoxy or enzymatic method, originally developed by Sanger, and the chemical method developed by Maxam and Gilbert. These techniques form the basis of the rapid sequencing equipment that has dramatically reduced the time involved in sequencing DNA fragments. The complementary development of computer programs to store, examine and compare sequences has allowed the ambitious genome projects, to define genomes from major species groups, to be carried out.

In the dideoxy method, 2′, 3′-dideoxynucleotide triphosphates are used to terminate the elongation of a newly synthesised DNA molecule made from a synthetic primer annealed to the template DNA under study. Thus, ddATP can be utilised by DNA polymerase to extend a DNA chain, but further deoxynucleotides cannot be added; therefore

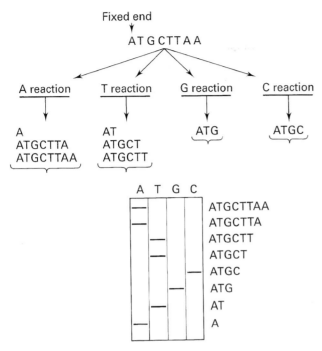

Figure 1.23 DNA sequencing. A set of radiolabelled oligonucleotides is generated in four different reactions, resulting in a terminal A, T, G or C, respectively. The DNA fragments are separated on a gel and the sequence of the substrate DNA is read directly from the autoradiograph.

random stops in the extension occur, depending on the ddNTP used. Four different ddNTPs are used to generate the four reactions whose products are visualised on the gel.

In the chemical method, a labelled single-stranded DNA molecule is subjected to a set of base-specific cleavage reactions: again the reaction results in a set of oligonucleotides, all labelled at one end, but with different termini (A, T, G or C) according to the chemical cleavage, and the products are visualised in the same way as a set of ladders on a gel.

Polymerase chain reaction

Since its first description in 1986, the polymerase chain reaction (PCR) has revolutionised the practice of molecular biology by allowing rapid enzymatic amplification of specific DNA fragments in large amounts from very small amounts of starting material, even single cells. RNA can be amplified by converting it first to DNA using reverse transcriptase. A huge variety of applications has been found for PCR, including direct cloning of genomic DNA or cDNA, engineering of new recombinant fragments, forensic analysis of small tissue samples, prenatal diagnosis and detection of pathogenic DNA from microorganisms (e.g. viruses and mycobacteria) in diseased human tissues.

The technique requires a double-stranded DNA template and a pair of single-stranded oligonucleotide primers that are complementary to sequences flanking the region of interest, so defining the ends of the region. The template DNA strands are denatured by heating, and the primers, added in large excess, anneal, on cooling, to the respective opposite strands of DNA. New DNA synthesis is then catalysed by DNA polymerase in the presence of deoxynucleotide triphosphates (dNTPs). The resulting new double-stranded molecules are in turn denatured and form new templates for the next round of DNA synthesis, again using the oligonucleotide primers (Fig. 1.24).

(*a*) Denature (heat for 60 s)

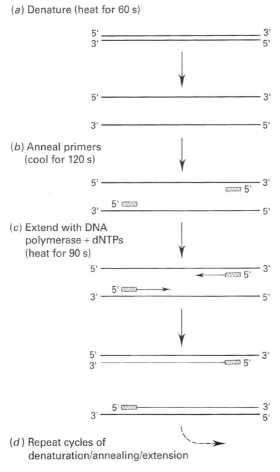

(*b*) Anneal primers
(cool for 120 s)

(*c*) Extend with DNA
polymerase + dNTPs
(heat for 90 s)

(*d*) Repeat cycles of
denaturation/annealing/extension

Figure 1.24 The principle of PCR. A single cycle consists of three steps (a)–(c) at the end of which there is twice the amount of target DNA. Repeating the cycle once gives four times the DNA and so on.

The technique relies on successive cycles of denaturation, annealing and DNA synthesis, and exponential amplification of DNA is possible, such that, in principle, 30 cycles would result in almost 270 000 000-fold (2^{28}-fold) amplification. With the discovery of thermostable DNA polymerases (such as that from the thermophilic bacterium *Thermus aquaticus*, Taq polymerase) and technological advances in the development of thermal cycler machines, it is possible to perform multiple simultaneous PCR reactions in just a few hours.

The specificity of PCR can be increased by using 'nested' primers, which are complementary, to sequence between the two original primer sites. This technique is used to prevent closely related DNA sequences from being amplified along with the desired sequence.

Application of molecular techniques

Analysis of gene transcription

The techniques of nucleic acid analysis described above have been extensively applied to studies of gene expression, and this has led to a detailed understanding of transcriptional control as outlined in the first section of this chapter. Here, some of the approaches currently used are briefly illustrated.

mRNA analysis

RNA can be isolated for analysis by a variety of methods. In general, strict precautions must be taken to avoid degradation of the mRNA by ribonucleases, and it must be separated from contaminating DNA and proteins. Either total RNA (which comprises more than 90% ribosomal RNA) or poly-A-enriched RNA (i.e. mRNA) is purified and subjected to hybridisation analysis with labelled probes. Membrane blotting of electrophoresed RNA (Northern blotting) is commonly used before hybridisation, but alternative techniques involve solution hybridisation followed by electrophoresis of RNA–probe hybrid molecules (e.g. ribonuclease protection assays). In some cases, the mRNA species under study are rare transcripts and may be reverse-transcribed (using reverse transcriptase) to make cDNA, which is then amplified by PCR to provide amounts of material sufficient for more detailed analysis (reverse transcription PCR, or rt-PCR).

This type of mRNA analysis has led to detailed definition of the patterns of gene expression in different tissues, and it has become clear that this expression involves tissue-specific mechanisms as well as regulation by external stimuli such as hormones.

Mechanisms of regulation: gene promoter analysis

Analysis of the mechanisms of mRNA regulation has required detailed investigation of the function of genomic DNA associated with a series of coding genes. A typical approach is outlined here as an example of the molecular dissection of genetic control.

In principle, alteration in the level of mRNA in a cell may depend either on changes in the rate of gene transcription or on altered stability of the mRNA. Both mechanisms have been found to operate, but most progress has recently been made in our understanding of transcriptional control, which in most cases is a function of upstream (5′) elements in the gene's promoter and enhancer regions.

Genomic DNA libraries are commonly used as the starting material from which a stretch of putative upstream regulatory DNA can be isolated. This DNA is first sequenced and the sequence searched for typical consensus motifs to which known transcription factors may bind, such as the TATA and CAAT boxes, and for recognition sequences for other factors such as AP-1 and steroid hormone receptors. In addition, sequencing is useful for defining potential endonuclease sites that may be valuable for engineering new DNA constructs for functional studies. In this way, a physical map of the promoter is built up, but the significance of particular sequences now requires direct experimental confirmation.

In order to determine whether a given stretch of DNA really functions as transcriptional regulator, it may be isolated from its genomic context and linked to a 'reporter gene' in a new synthetically engineered plasmid; the new plasmid construct is then introduced into a living cell. Systems include the *Xenopus* oocyte, bacterium or yeast cell, or mammalian cell lines. A reporter gene is one that encodes a protein product that is easily measured in living cells, usually a protein not normally produced by those cells. For example, the firefly luciferase gene encodes a protein not found in mammalian cells that catalyses the production of light from the substrate luciferin. If a plasmid containing the luciferase gene is introduced into a cell by a process of 'transfection', then the amount of luciferase produced is determined by the activity of the promoter element to which it is linked. Then, when cell extracts are made and incubated with luciferin and adenosine triphosphate (ATP), the amount of light produced is a measure of promoter activity.

A series of techniques is now available for the introduction of DNA into mammalian cells, including calcium phosphate transfection and diethylaminoethyl (DEAE)–dextran transfection (which each promote DNA attachment to the cell surface, allowing endocytotic uptake), liposome-mediated transfection and electroporation. In each case, the cell type for study must be carefully chosen and the actual transfection procedure carefully optimised (see Fig. 1.25).

Using these techniques, a functional map can now be produced of the important control elements that modulate transcription of a given gene. DNA elements responsible for conferring cell type–specific transcription or intracellular signal-mediated transcription can be closely defined, and those sequences can then, in turn, be used as tools with which to identify the protein transcription factors to which they bind. For example, double-stranded synthetic oligonucleotide probes containing multimers of a critical DNA sequence can be used to screen a cDNA expression library for DNA-binding proteins and hence characterise new factors (see Latchman, 2005).

Transgenic animals

Gene function can be studied by genetic manipulation of whole animals using a series of 'transgenic'

(*a*) Isolate putative regulatory DNA

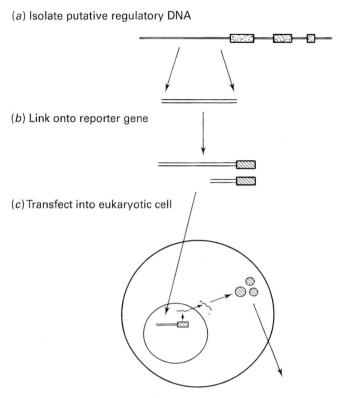

(*b*) Link onto reporter gene

(*c*) Transfect into eukaryotic cell

(*d*) Analyse cell for expression of reporter gene product

Figure 1.25 Gene promoter analysis. The segment of putative regulatory DNA is isolated (*a*) and linked to a reporter gene (*b*). Deletions may by introduced into the regulatory DNA to define critical regions involved in transcriptional control. After transfection (*c*), the cell is analysed to assess the level of expression of the reporter gene. This is a function of the activity of the promoter under examination.

approaches. Essentially, transgenic animals are produced by incorporation of an exogenous 'transgene' into the genome of an early-stage embryo. This routinely involves microinjection of the exogenous gene construct of interest into a pronuclear-stage embryo where it integrates into the host DNA of the fertilised oocyte. The foreign DNA is integrated at random in the recipient genome, which may result in loss of expression of host genes, changed expression patterns of the foreign DNA because of its modification by host gene-controlling elements or its control by a strong constitutive host promoter, or no expression of the foreign DNA because it integrated into a transcriptionally quiet region. If possible, the inclusion of as much as is possible of the human gene's controlling elements will avoid these problems.

The alternative approach to the production of transgenic animals involves transfection of embryonic stem (ES) cells. These cell lines are derived from the inner cell mass of an early blastocyst embryo, which are transfected with the exogenous gene construct of interest: those cells positive for the

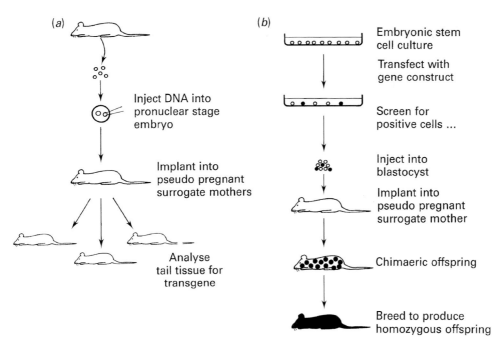

(a)

Inject DNA into
pronuclear stage
embryo

Implant into
pseudo pregnant
surrogate mothers

Analyse
tail tissue for
transgene

(b)

Embryonic stem
cell culture

Transfect with
gene construct

Screen for
positive cells ...

Inject into
blastocyst

Implant into
pseudo pregnant
surrogate mother

Chimaeric offspring

Breed to produce
homozygous offspring

Figure 1.26 Strategies for producing transgenic mice. (*a*) Pronuclear injection. (*b*) Embryonic stem cell transfection.

transgene can be identified, and the mutant clones are then microinjected into a normal blastocyst to produce chimaeric animals.

The resulting modified embryonic cells produced by either approach are capable of differentiation into any tissue, including germ cells in the gonads; hence animals that are chimaeric in their germ line can be bred to produce offspring that are heterozygous for the transgene throughout their somatic cells. These animals can, in turn, be interbred to produce homozygous offspring if desired (see Fig. 1.26).

The pronuclear injection approach has been widely used to study the tissue-specific activation of promoter regions by examining the expression of reporter genes and also to study the targeted expression of specific proteins using well-characterised promoters. For example, the activation of homeodomain gene promoters in embryonic development has been studied using the β-galactosidase reporter gene, the expression of which is easily

detected in whole embryos. If a tissue-specific promoter is used, expression can be targeted to a certain cell type. For example, pituitary-specific promoters have been used to target high-level expression of mutant CREB to the pituitary in order to demonstrate the role of CREB in the development and function of pituitary cells. Other applications of the latter technique include achieving the targeted expression of the herpesvirus-1 thymidine kinase (HSV-TK) gene in specific tissues, which then become uniquely sensitive to drugs whose metabolites kill dividing cells (a 'TK oblation system').

Gene targeting by homologous recombination

Transgenic mice have recently been used to produce animals with mutations in any desired gene. This involves gene targeting by homologous recombination to completely inactivate the target gene (often called gene 'knockout'). Different types of targeting

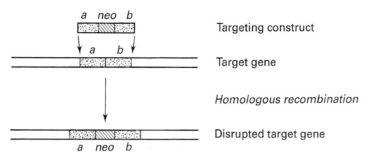

Figure 1.27 Gene targeting by homologous recombination. A transgenic 'knock-out' animal is created by replacing a segment of the target gene with a construct that includes a selectable marker gene, such as neo, a drug-resistance gene.

gene construct are used, but commonly they will consist of two regions of homology with the target normal gene that are separated by an intervening DNA segment (Fig. 1.27). This intervening segment is generally a drug-resistance gene that will both interrupt and mutate the target gene and also allow ES cells to be selected according to whether the construct has been integrated or not. This approach has been widely used to study the functions of candidate genes in tissue development and recently the role of tumour suppressor genes such as Rb and p53 (see page 19–20).

Targeted dominant negative receptor mutants

Finally, transgenic animals have recently been used to study effects of hormones or drugs on specific tissues in intact animals by interfering with normal receptor function. Dominant-negative receptors (see page 34) may occur in disease states or may be deliberately engineered: they are themselves inactive but have the effect of blocking the function of the normal receptors in a cell. Dominant-negative growth factor receptor cDNAs can be linked to a strong tissue-specific promoter in transgenes such that the transgenic animal will express the mutant receptor only in a specified cell type. In such a way, the role of keratinocyte growth factor (KGF) in skin development and wound healing has been deter-

mined using a construct linking the KGF receptor dominant-negative mutant to a skin-specific gene promoter, providing unique new information about skin differentiation and wound re-epithelialisation.

Analysis of abnormal DNA

A number of molecular techniques have been used to identify genetic abnormalities associated with disease. Here, a brief summary outlining the rationale for some of the standard approaches is given.

Southern blotting: gene deletions

In the simplest case, some diseases are known to be caused by the total absence of a known gene product, suggesting a single gene deletion. For example, in type 1A isolated growth hormone deficiency, growth hormone production is completely absent, and deletion of a large part of the growth hormone gene cluster in these patients was demonstrated directly by Southern blotting. Genomic DNA (obtained from peripheral blood leucocytes) was digested with an endonuclease that was known to yield a characteristic pattern of DNA fragments within the growth hormone gene. Then the digestion products were electrophoresed and transferred by Southern blotting onto a membrane for hybridisation with a radio-labelled growth hormone cDNA probe (see Fig. 1.28).

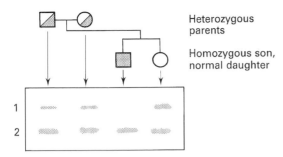

Heterozygous parents

Homozygous son, normal daughter

1

2

Figure 1.28 Deletion of the growth hormone gene shown by Southern blot analysis in type 1A isolated growth hormone deficiency. Both heterozygous parents show reduced intensity in band 1, which is completely absent in the homozygous son but normal in the unaffected daughter.

Southern blotting: restriction fragment length polymorphisms

In other conditions, a candidate gene has not been identified, and here Southern blotting has been used in a less direct way to determine disease associations with chromosomal locations and hence to progressively localise an unknown abnormal gene linked with the disorder. This technique uses natural inherited polymorphisms (variations) in DNA sequence among different individuals to track the segregation of disease in families with particular chromosomal markers. Polymorphic DNA sequences can create or destroy restriction endonuclease sites, resulting in characteristic fragment lengths when given pieces of genomic DNA are digested with certain endonucleases. These restriction fragment length polymorphisms (RFLPs) have no disease significance in themselves but are simply markers that can be identified by using a series of chromosomal probes. They may or may not be close to a disease locus. As RFLPs are polymorphic, this type of analysis requires a set of family members affected or unaffected by the disease in order to determine whether a particular locus really segregates with the disease through the generations. The principles are illustrated in Fig. 1.29. Once a sufficiently small region of chromosomal DNA has been localised, direct genetic analysis by sequencing becomes feasible and a disease gene can be firmly identified and characterised. RFLP analysis linked early-onset familial Alzheimer's disease with chromosome 21 in the area involved in *Down's* syndrome. Patients with *Down's* syndrome also develop Alzheimer's disease in middle age. RFLP analysis has also been used to detect fragile X syndrome.

Disease genes: mutation analysis

In many cases of human disease, a particular gene is known to be abnormal. This gene may be subject to mutational change (deletions or point mutations with single-base changes), giving either loss of function of the protein product or, in some cases, gain of function.

Analysis of DNA sequence is normally undertaken using genomic DNA (usually from leucocyte DNA) in cases of germ-line mutations (e.g. inherited diseases) or cDNAs from affected tissues in cases of somatic mutations acquired since conception (e.g. tumours). Mutational change may be heterozygous, affecting only one allele, or homozygous, affecting both alleles, and a number of different types of mutation are found. Point mutations (changes affecting a single base) include substitution of a base with an abnormal base, which may change the amino acid sequence or may encode a premature stop codon, which will terminate translation. Single-base deletions or insertions result in a frameshift, disrupting the reading frame of triplet codons so that a nonsense non-coding mRNA sequence is produced downstream of the mutation. Point mutations are the molecular defect in the β-thalassaemias. In some cases, several bases may be deleted, as in cystic fibrosis, where a deletion of three nucleotides results in loss of a phenylalanine residue in the ATP-binding domain of a transmembrane protein.

As mentioned above, some diseases are associated with expansion of repetitive DNA sequences, such as triplet repeats within coding regions or untranslated regions of disease genes, and these mutations may have general transcriptional repressive effects. For example, myotonic dystrophy results from an unstable trinucleotide repeat $(AGC)n$, with disease severity

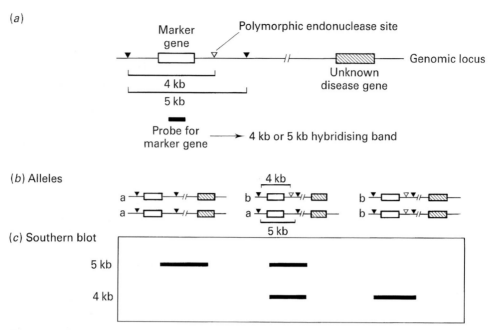

Figure 1.29 RFLP analysis. (*a*) Restriction endonuclease sites may be constant (▼) or be created by polymorphic variation in the DNA sequence (▽). (*b*) A probe for a marker gene will hybridise to variable fragment lengths of genomic DNA depending on the presence or absence of the restriction site. (*c*) The appearance of a Southern blot of the three potential combinations of alleles. A pedigree analysis within a family where a disease occurs will show whether the marker gene segregates with the disease phenotype.

parelleling the number of repeats. Larger-scale chromosomal deletions or rearrangements have more or less drastic effects on the coding genes, but in some cases can lead to one gene's coding sequence coming under the control of another gene's promoter, giving rise to abnormally regulated protein synthesis. An example is the Bcr–Abl hybrid oncogene caused by a translocation of chromosome 9 to 22 and responsible for chronic myeloid leukaemia (page 18).

Point mutations giving rise to amino acid substitutions may have a variety of effects. Some lead to loss of protein function: for example, mutations of tumour suppressor genes, such as p53, play a role in many different cancers. Others cause abnormal activation: for example, the $G_s\alpha$ subunit gene mutation *gsp* is a constitutive activator (that is, no longer regulated) of adenylate cyclase that is found

in various benign endocrine tumours. Some point mutations give rise to a profound change in phenotype even though they occur on only one allele, which implies that they over-ride the function of the normal protein, termed a '*dominant-negative*' effect.

Functional effects of mutations such as these have been investigated in two different ways: (1) by cloning the mutated sequence, the abnormal protein can be expressed in transfected cells and its transcriptional effects determined using promoter–reporter gene constructs and (2) transgenic mice can be produced in which the phenotypic effects of particular mutations can be analysed in more detail than may be possible in humans.

A variety of screening techniques have been developed to enable large numbers of clinical cases to be studied for mutations; in most cases, these techniques rely on PCR amplification of genomic DNA. Direct analysis of known mutation 'hot spots' can be made by hybridisation with wild-type (natural) or mutant sequences using specially made oligonucleotide probes. Other methods, such as *single-strand conformational polymorphism* (SSCP), screen for potential unknown mutations in larger regions of DNA by detecting small changes in electrophoretic mobility of mutant DNA strands compared with wild-type fragments.

Gene therapy

The amazing speed of molecular biology's advances since the early 1980s will be apparent from the preceding sections. It means that gene therapy has moved from being an exciting but speculative possibility to a practical reality in modern medicine. The scope for gene therapy is obvious and would include not only replacing defective or absent genes with normal ones but also engineering new genes to inhibit expression of deleterious disease genes. Techniques will vary depending on whether the therapeutic gene must be introduced into every cell (e.g. replacing a defective tumour suppressor gene in cancer) or whether less than 100% replacement will rectify the clinical phenotype (e.g. cystic fibrosis).

The essential problem of gene therapy is one of drug delivery: that of transporting a large, highly charged molecule to the nucleus. A series of strategies have been developed, mostly involving virus-based vectors but also including other approaches such as molecular conjugates (for example DNA–protein complexes), using ligands for cell targeting and using liposomes. Viral vectors include retroviruses, adenovirus and adeno-associated virus (AAV); these can be used to package the DNA construct and infect human cells so that the DNA is taken up into the nucleus.

Example: homozygous familial hypercholesterolaemia

A recent successful example of gene therapy is the experimental treatment of homozygous familial hypercholesterolaemia. This disease results from a mutation of the receptor for low-density lipoprotein (LDL), which prevents clearance of LDL from plasma. The heterozygous form of the disease is common, affecting 1 in 400 people in Britain, and it results in the early onset of ischaemic heart disease. The very severe homozygous form usually results in death from heart disease before 30 years of age. This severe, single-gene disease was, therefore, a good candidate for gene therapy, and early successes have been reported.

Gene therapy here has involved resection of a portion of the patient's liver, using the patient's hepatocytes to generate primary cell cultures that are then infected with retrovirus containing the LDL receptor cDNA. Virus particles are removed, and the transfected cells are reintroduced into the patient via a catheter in the hepatic portal vein to allow seeding in the host liver. After pilot studies in rabbits and then primates to establish feasibility and safety, a number of patients have been treated, with clinically useful although only partial reductions in circulating LDL-cholesterol for over a year.

Antisense gene therapy

A number of candidate diseases have now been proposed for development of 'replacement' gene therapy approaches, but the more challenging cases will be those that require interference with endogenous gene function. A number of experimental examples have suggested that this too is feasible and practicable. 'Antisense therapeutics' is being developed on the basis that antisense RNA will bind (by complementary base pairing) to mRNA and prevent its translation into protein or in some cases may generate a triple helix with double-stranded DNA to prevent transcription. One of several exciting recent examples of experimental uses of this therapy is the suppression of Philadelphia chromosome–positive human leukaemia cells in immunodeficient mice by systemic administration of a 26-mer antisense to the B2A2 breakpoint junction of the *bcr–abl* fusion gene.

A variety of modified antisense molecules have been developed, including modified oligonucleotides that are resistant to ribonuclease digestion, and 'peptide nucleic acids' in which the entire deoxyribose phosphate backbone is replaced by a polyamine backbone. Ribozymes are naturally occurring 'RNA enzymes' that can be modified to cleave specific RNA sequences; these have been targeted against oncogenes such as *ras* and also against the human immunodeficiency virus (HIV).

Further examples of gene therapy approaches are being developed. For example, there is *in vitro* evidence that it is possible to correct a malignant phenotype by insertion of normal tumour suppressor genes, and trials are in progress in which the normal Rb gene is inserted intravesically in bladder cancer, and in which bronchoscopic application of the normal p53 gene is made in lung cancer. More common diseases may also be susceptible to these new therapies: in the case of vascular disease, excessive smooth muscle cell proliferation can be reduced with locally applied gene therapy (for example antisense c-*myb* DNA) using carefully targeted intra-arterial catheters; by comparison, vascular endothelial growth factor (VEGF) cDNA can be applied locally to induce angiogenesis in ischaemic limbs. For many of these new applications, gene therapy may prove to be both cheaper and more effective than alternative treatments with recombinant proteins.

Cell biology: methods of investigation

Cell culture

Detailed analysis of the principles of cell biology became possible with the advent of techniques for growing individual cell types in isolation from the whole animal, a technique known as cell culture (see Fig. 1.30).

Primary culture

In its simplest form, primary culture entails preparing a suspension of cells from a tissue and using

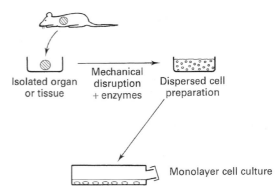

Figure 1.30 Primary cell culture. A suspension of isolated cells is prepared and forms a monolayer that is maintained in nutrient culture media.

enzymes to break down the intercellular matrix. The isolated cells can then be maintained *in vitro* as a primary culture using a nutrient growth medium of essential amino acids, sugars, vitamins and salts, usually supplemented with animal sera to provide essential growth factors. Primary cultures can readily be maintained for several weeks, and certain cell types will proliferate, allowing much longer-term cultures to be established. Cells in primary culture re-establish cell–cell interconnections, and they have the advantage of being closely representative of the cells present in the intact tissue *in vivo*. However, such cultures often include several different cell types, and for this reason clonal cell lines may be preferred.

Clonal cell lines

Clonal cell lines are cell cultures that represent the progeny of a single cell and, in general, these cells are characterised by unlimited proliferative potential, defined as being capable of subcultivation at least 70 times. Such cell lines may be derived by selecting clones that arise in primary cultures under the influence of hormones or growth stimuli or, for some tumour cell lines, by alternate culture and transplantation in animals. They have the advantage that they contain a single cell type that is immortalised and able to survive indefinitely in culture conditions, avoiding the need to obtain tissue repeatedly from living animals. They can grow as monolayers, adherent to a plastic substratum or, in the case of 'anchorage-independent' cells such as haemopoietic cells or transformed or malignant cells, as suspension cultures. However clonal cell lines may have some disadvantages: the cells may be 'transformed', implying some genetic alteration that allows unrestrained growth, and they may lose certain differentiated characteristics, acquiring abnormal morphology and karyotype. Clonal cell lines can be modified by incorporation of transgenes. Exogenous genes may be introduced into a cell by a variety of transfection procedures and are expressed transiently for a few days. In a very small proportion of cells, the transgene is incorporated into the host genomic DNA, and these transgenic cells can be selectively propagated if the incorporated DNA includes a suitable marker, such as an antibiotic resistance gene. In this way, stable transfectant cells can be generated that express a gene product such as an enzyme or a secreted protein, and such cells can be used for many applications. In particular, modified cell lines expressing receptors, enzymes or reporter genes have increasingly been used as the basis for high-throughput screening procedures by pharmaceutical companies seeking novel compounds for drug development.

Immortalisation of cells

Immortalisation of cells can be valuable as a way of generating new cell lines from primary cell cultures. A standard approach has been to use the SV40 virus, whose large T antigen can be transfected into quiescent non-proliferating cells to induce growth. Temperature-sensitive mutants of SV40 have become popular, such that large T antigen will be expressed at 33°C but not at 37°C: thus the cells can be induced to proliferate at the lower temperature but become quiescent (and potentially express their differentiated characteristics) at 37°C.

A huge range of very well characterised cell lines from human and animal tissues is now available, and these have provided a fundamental resource for the cell biological and molecular biological studies outlined earlier. Cell culture requires special dedicated facilities, including humidified 37°C incubators, laminar flow hoods, and meticulous technical care to minimise contamination by bacteria and fungi. Nonetheless, it has come to be centrally important in many different disciplines, including the study of the cell cycle itself, the control of tumour growth, regulation of gene expression and developmental biology.

Protein detection

Antibody production: monoclonal antibodies

Proteins can be identified in tissue extracts on the basis of their chemical properties, using gel electrophoresis, but much modern protein detection relies on their immunological properties. Thus, proteins can be detected by their ability to react with highly specific antibodies that have been labelled with radioactivity or colour-generating reagents.

Antibodies can be raised in an animal in response to injected foreign protein, and the animal's serum may then be purified to yield the immunoglobulin fraction. These antisera are *polyclonal* in that they contain many different antibodies of differing specificity and affinity for different parts of the injected protein. Another disadvantage is that antibody production is limited to the lifetime of the immune animal. Nonetheless, their properties have been exploited to form the basis of much of the protein detection system that has developed since the early 1970s.

An alternative approach is to produce monoclonal antibodies. These are antibodies of single specificity secreted by hybrid cell lines *in vitro*. The mice immunised with the foreign protein are used as the source of antibody-producing splenocytes that are fused with myeloma cell lines to confer immortality on the resultant hybrid cells. The hybridoma cells are cloned to separate different antibody-secreting cells, which are then selected on the basis of their production of antibody reactive with the target protein. The technique of monoclonal antibody production was a major advance in immunology, allowing almost limitless production of individual well-characterised antibodies from clonal cells grown in suspension culture.

Immunocytochemistry

The proteins expressed within or on the surface of intact cells can be identified immunologically using either monoclonal or polyclonal antibodies coupled to a visualisation system. This approach is particularly applicable to tissues from a whole animal but can equally be applied to cultured cells. Tissues are fixed, sectioned and processed for microscopic analysis as for routine histology, but with special steps taken to allow adequate penetration of antibody into the section. Antibodies may be coupled to detection reagents such as fluorescent dyes (e.g. fluorescein or rhodamine) without destroying their specificity, and these conjugates are able to bind to antigen present in a tissue section. Fluorescent dyes require the use of a fluorescence microscope but have a particular advantage over other detection systems in that more than one fluorochrome may be simultaneously detectable in the same cell: thus, two or more specific antibodies may be linked to different fluorochromes, and exposure of the same tissue to light of different excitation wavelengths will produce different colours, allowing studies of co-localisation of different peptides.

Flow cytometry and fluorescence activated cell sorting

Antibody binding to cells can have a number of applications apart from direct visualisation of protein expression. The amount of fluorescent antibody bound to each cell can be quantified by *flow cytometry*. Cells stained with fluorescent antibody can be dispersed and made to flow past a laser beam of a chosen wavelength: a first light detector is arranged to measure the amount of fluorescent light emitted, while a second light detector measures cell size by 'forward light scatter'. This technique generates a

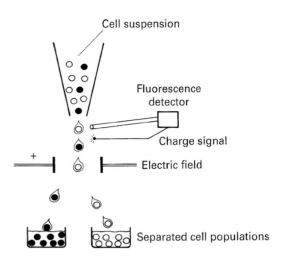

Figure 1.31 Fluorescence activated cell sorting. A suspension of individually dispersed cells, some labelled with fluorescent dye, is separated by charging the fluorescent cells and diverting these charged cells with an electric field.

two-dimensional plot of antigen expression against cell size, giving quantitative data about different cell populations within a whole tissue.

Cells can be specifically selected, using fluorescent antibodies, according to the antigen expressed on the cell surface in a technique termed *fluorescence activated cell sorting* (FACS). A dispersed preparation of single cells can be arranged to flow in a stream as for flow cytometry: the stream is broken into droplets each containing one cell, which are charged according to whether or not they give a fluorescent signal. The charged droplets are diverted by an electric field so that these cells can be separately collected, resulting in a sorted subpopulation of cells (Fig. 1.31).

Immunoassay techniques

Proteins (and other small molecules) can be detected immunologically in complex biological fluids or cell extracts using a series of different immunoassay techniques. These assay methods have amazing sensitivity and specificity and rely on quantifiable

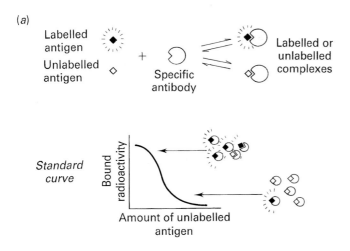

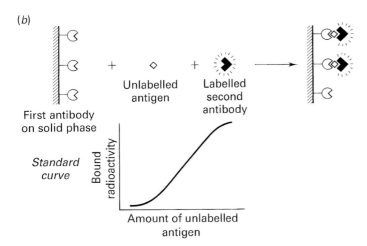

Figure 1.32 Immunoassay techniques. (*a*) In immunoassays, competition between labelled and unlabelled antigen for limited amounts of antibody result in varying amounts of radioactivity in the antigen–antibody complexes formed. (*b*) In immunometric assays, labelled second antibody is only able to the solid phase via the antigen. As a result, bound radioactivity is proportional to the amount of antigen present.

interactions between the protein antigen and the antibody that has been conjugated with a label. A series of labels is now available, from the traditional ^{125}I radioactive label to enzyme-linked reactions and chemiluminescent reagents that avoid the use of radioactivity. Two classical techniques, immunoas-

say and immunometric assay, are illustrated in Fig. 1.32 and described below.

Immunoassay

The principle involved in immunoassay is the competition between radioactively labelled antigen and the unlabelled antigen in a biological fluid for a fixed and limited amount of antibody. Various methods can be used to separate complexes of antigen–antibody from excess labelled protein, and the amount of label in the complexes is then inversely proportional to the amount of unlabelled protein, allowing a calculation to be made of its concentration. This technique was first developed in the 1960s and is still routinely used to detect very small quantities of protein down to the picomolar range (10^{-12} mol/l).

Immunometric assays

These assays have proved even more sensitive and robust than immunoassay and have been widely developed as commercial kits for rapid measurement of antigens, including peptide (and steroid) hormones, immunoglobulins and drugs. Essentially, a first monoclonal antibody is coated onto a solid phase such as plastic, the unknown antigen solution is added and allowed to bind and, after washing, the amount of antigen bound to the solid-phase first antibody can be estimated by adding an excess of labelled second antibody. In this case, the more antigen that is present, the more labelled second antibody will be bound to the solid phase. With high-affinity monoclonal antibodies that can recognise different parts of a protein molecule, two-site immunometric assay has become highly specific and sensitive, and many automated assays can be performed simultaneously in as little as 1 h in diagnostic laboratories.

Future perspectives

The explosion of knowledge of cell and molecular biology since the early 1970s has at times seemed abstruse and unconnected with clinical practice, yet already the practice of medicine, both diagnostic and therapeutic, has been transformed by this knowledge. Therapeutic agents are now produced by recombinant DNA techniques, including insulin, growth hormone, erythropoietin and coag-

ulation factor VIII, avoiding the risks and limitations of extracting these substances from human tissues. Recombinant vaccines are also becoming available, and drug design is able to look to new targets such as transcription factors. Gene therapy is already practicable for a number of diseases and is likely to make a major impact in the developed world very soon. For the practice of medicine in the Third World, too, molecular biology is now relevant to a series of issues: not only are the techniques becoming cheaper and more robust for diagnostic purposes but the more immediate medical priorities of food supply and vaccine development are becoming major targets for the new technology.

Summary

This chapter has reviewed key elements of molecular and cell biology that are relevant to our current understanding of some mechanisms of human disease. The aim has been to describe normal cell function, with some illustrations from specific diseases; later chapters offer fuller accounts of pathogenetic mechanisms of different types of disease.

Analysis of gene structure has led to a clear understanding of the mechanism of gene transcription and to the identification of many different transcription factors. In some cases these factors are actually hormone receptors, whereas in others they are nuclear proteins activated by extracellular stimuli. Mutations in these proteins may lead to loss of function and lack of target-gene expression; for example, the hypopituitarism seen with mutations in the pituitary-specific factor Pit-1; on the other hand, mutations in steroid and thyroid hormone receptors cause typical hormone resistance syndromes.

Cell membrane receptors are linked to intracellular signalling systems, which are made up of chains of cellular proteins. The complexity of the signalling systems is important in that it enables cells to integrate many different signals from the environment. Many of these proteins may be susceptible to mutation, with loss of function or increased function, and the normal cellular proteins have been identified as the proto-oncogene counterparts to viral oncogenic proteins that commonly cause cancer.

The techniques of DNA and RNA manipulation and gene transfer have been fundamental to the dissection of normal and abnormal cellular function, but they have also been developed to the point where gene therapy is being applied to human diseases that are otherwise often untreatable, such as homozygous familial hypercholesterolaemia and some cancers.

FURTHER READING

Lachman, D. S. (ed.). (2005). *Gene Regulation*, 5th edn. London: Routledge.

Gaucher's disease: a model disorder for therapeutic exploration of the lysosome

Timothy M. Cox

Gaucher's disease is a very rare condition but it is the most frequent of a large group of inherited disorders affecting a single intracellular organelle – the lysosome. This organelle was discovered by the Nobel Prize–winning biochemist and physician Christian de Duve. He postulated the existence of a previously unknown intracellular compartment containing a rich complement of hydrolases, which have an optimal activity at acid pH. Gaucher disease, a multi-sytem disorder, is the first lysosomal disorder for which a definitive treatment has been developed. The success of targetted enzyme therapy for functional complementation of the defective organelles in Gaucher's disease has allowed the growth of a major international biotechnology company and stimulated competitive pharmaceutical investment for the innovative treatment of 'ultra-orphan' disorders – including other lysosomal diseases.

Lysosomes

Lysosomes are responsible for the continuous breakdown and recycling of membrane components and the degradation of macromolecular substrates derived either by autophagy of other organelles within the cell or from external sources. *Receptor-mediated endocytosis* involving coated pits delivers ligands and receptors to the acidic lysosomal compartment for breakdown; the specialized lysosomes of *macrophages* fuse with the phagosome after engulfment of particulate material, including microbes, to form *phagolysosomes*. After recognition at the macrophage surface, the material is rapidly degraded by acidification, proteolysis and the influx of degradative molecules, including nitric oxide and superoxide ions, into phagolysosomes that complete the breakdown of the entire ingested structure.

Lysosomal storage diseases

Henri-Géry Hers, a colleague of de Duve in the University of Louvain, Belgium, was the first to recognize the lysosomal storage diseases. She and colleagues noted that unitary defects in lysosomal acid hydrolases led to the accumulation of macromolecules within cells and distention of the organelles with undigested substrate.

At least 50 lysosomal storage diseases have been identified, most of which result from hereditary deficiencies in the activity of a specific acid hydrolase (Table 2.1). In some, such as cystinosis and Salla disease, defective transport of hydrolytic products out of the lysosome is responsible for pathological storage within the organellar space. Certain lysosomal enzymes require the presence of one or more activator proteins, such as the sphingolipid activator proteins saposins A to D, responsible for the activation of particular hydrolases towards their natural substrates. Mutations in these activators or the gene encoding their precursor polypeptide cause storage diseases in which several substrates usually accumulate. In a few unusual lysosomal storage disorders, failure of activation or stabilization

Table 2.1 Lysosomal diseases

Name	Primary defect	Principal storage
Generalised defects		
I-cell disease (mucolipidosis II)	N-acetylglucosamine-1-phosphotransferase (with hypersecretion of numerous lysosomal hydrolases)	Lipids, oligosaccharides Mucopolysaccharides
Pseudo–Hurler polydystrophy (mucolipidosis III)	N-acetylglucosamine-1-phosphotransferase (with hypersecretion of numerous lysosomal hydrolases Failure to modify key cysteine residue in common active site of sulphatase enzymes	Lipids, oligosaccharides, Mucopolysaccharides
Multiple sulphatase deficiency (Austin's disease)	Arylsulphatases A,B & C	Mucopolysaccharides, sulphatide and other sulphated lipids including steroid sulphates.
Sphingolipid activator protein (saposin) deficiency		
Sap precursor	Absent saposins A-D	Ceramide,glucosylceramide galactosyl ceramide,sulphatide gangliosides
Sap-A	Impaired glucosyl and galactosylceramidase	Glucosyl and galactosyl ceramidase
Sap-B	Impaired arylsulphatase A, sphingomyelinase, β-galactosidase	Predominantly sulphatide MLD*
Sap-C	Impaired glucosylceramidase	Gaucher-like storage
GM$_2$ activator	Impaired hexosaminidase A activity	GM$_2$ GA2 gangliosides
Galactosialidosis	Protective protein deficiency causing combined degradation of β-galactosidase and neuraminidase	Sialyloligosaccharides
Chediak-Higashi syndrome	Impaired function of lysosomal trafficking regulator,LYST	Defective targeting of secretory lysosomal proteins including melanosome proteins; giant granules in leukocytes
Hermansky-Pudlak syndrome	HPS 1-β-3A subunit of adaptin	Defective platelets (no dense granules), melanosomes, lysosomes contain ceroid storage material
Transport defects		
Cystinosis	Cystine transporter (integral lysosomal membrane protein)	Reduced cystine efflux
Niemann-Pick diseases type C1 and C2 (distinct complementation groups)	Lysosomal membrane proteins NPC1, NPC2	Impaired cholesterol and sphingolipid trafficking
Salla disease	Sialic acid transporter, sialin (AST)	Free sialic acid
Cobalamin deficiency *(Cb1F)*	Unknown cobalamin transporter	Reduced free cobalamin efflux

(Cont.)

Table 2.1 (Cont.)

Name	Primary defect	Principal storage
Sphingolipidoses		
GM$_1$ gangliosidosis (see Morquio B)	β-galactosidase	Ganglioside GM$_1$ and asialoganglioside A.
GM$_2$ Gangliosidoses		
(a) Tay-Sachs disease	β-hexosaminidase A	GM$_2$ gangliosides
(b) Sandhoff disease	β-hexosaminidase A and B	GM$_2$ gangliosides oligosaccharides
Anderson-Fabry disease	α-galactosidase A	Trihexosylceramide
Gaucher's disease	Glucocerebrosidase	Glucosylceramide
Niemann-Pick disease A and B	Acid sphingomyelinase	Sphingomyelin
Krabbe's disease	β-galactocerebrosidase	Psychosine, galactosylceramide
Metachromatic leukodystrophy	Arylsulphatase A	Sulphatide
***Mucopolysaccharidoses (*MPS)**		
MPS I (Hurler)	α-L-iduronidase	Dermatan sulphate, heparan sulphate
MPS I S (Scheie)	α-L-iduronidase	Dermatan sulphate, heparin sulphate
MPS I H/S (Hurler-Scheie)	α-L-iduronidase	Dermatan sulphate, heparin sulphate
MPS II (Hunter)	Iduronate sulphatase	Dermatan and heparin sulphate
MPS IIIA Sanfilippo A	Heparan N-sulphate	Heparan sulphate
MPS IIIB Sanfilippo B	α-N-acetylglucosaminidase	Heparan sulphate
MPS IIIC Sanfilippo C	Acetyl CoA: α-glucoaminide acetyl transferase	Heparan sulphate
MPS IIID Sanfilippo D	N-acetylglucosamine 6-sulphatase	Heparan sulphate
MPS IVA Morquio A	Galactose 6-sulphatase	Keratan sulphate, chondroitin 6-sulphate
MPS IVB Morquio B (see GM$_1$ gangliosidosis)	β-galactosidase	Keratan sulphate β-galactosyl oligosaccharides
MPS VI Maroteaux-Lamy	Arylsulphatase B	Dermatan sulphate
MPS VII Sly	β-glucuronidase	Dermatan sulphate Heparan sulphate Chondroitin 4- and 6-sulphates
Glycoproteinoses		
Schindler disease	α-N-acetylgalactosaminidase	N-acetylgalactosaminyl peptides and oligosaccharides
α-Mannosidosis	α-mannosidase	Oligosaccharides
β-Mannosidosis	β-mannosidase	β-mannosyl glycoconjugate
Fucosidosis	α-fucosidase	Glycopeptides, oligosaccharides
Sialidosis	Neuraminidase	Sialylated oligosaccharides
Aspartylglucosaminuria	Aspartylglucosaminidase	Aspartylglucosamine

Table 2.1 (Cont.)

Name	Primary defect	Principal storage
Lipid disorders		
Farber's disease	Acid ceramidase	Ceramide
Cholesterol ester storage disease	Acid lipase	Cholesterol, cholesterol esters)
Wolman's disease	Acid lipase	Cholesterol, cholesteryl esters)
Glycogen storage diseases (GSD)		
Pompe's disease [GSD II (A)] (adult, juvenile and infantile)	Acid maltase (acid α- 1,4 glucosidase)	Glycogen
Danon's disease [GSDII (B)]	Lysosomal membrane Glycoprotein 2	Glycogen and other storage material.
Miscellaneous defects		
Neuronal ceroid lipofuscinosis (CLN)		
(Batten's disease)		
CLN1	Palmitoyl-protein thioesterase	Ceroid (autofluorescent lysosomal storage
CLN2	Tripeptidyl-peptidase I	of cytochrome C peptide and other
CLN3	Lysosomal pH control	polypeptide and lipid remnants)
CLN8	Cathepsin D	
Papillon-Lefèvre syndrome(keratopalmar periodontitis)	Cathepsin C deficiency	No storage –neutrophil phagocytic defect
Pyknodysostosis	Cathepsin K	Type I collagen fragments

of a complement of organellar enzymes impairs several lysosomal activities. Multiple sulphatase deficiency, resulting from defective modification of an active-site cysteine residue common to the catalytic domains of all eukaryotic sulphatases, is an example of such a complex disorder.

A further category of lysosomal storage disorders results from a failure of delivery of nascent lysosomal proteins to the organelle after their biosynthesis on the rough endoplasmic reticulum. It turns out that many lysosomal enzymes require an appropriate "address," which is acquired co-translationally during biosynthesis and determines their intracellular sorting to lysosomal spaces. This signal in many instances turns out to be a mannose 6-phosphate residue on lysosomal glycoproteins; it is acquired in the *trans*-Golgi network. Specific receptors for mannose 6-phosphate in intermediate endosomes allow them to take up newly formed lysosomal proteins into mature lysosomes. This mechanism of intra-

cellular delivery and sorting of lysosomal proteins in important for two reasons: first, deficiencies in the targeting and receptor process lead to a deficient complement of multiple hydrolases within the lysosomes and, second, the targeting process itself can be harnessed to deliver therapeutic proteins to the lysosomes of tissues in patients who lack specific hydrolytic activities and suffer from the lysosomal storage disorders.

Access to the lysosomal space

Christian de Duve, a qualified doctor, is one of the founding fathers of cell biology – a science that is increasingly applied to medicine – and now dignified by the modern term molecular cell biology. Having discovered lysosomes as a biochemist before they were identified by electron microscopy, de Duve realized that their particular features would allow access from the fluid phase outside the cells.

He realized that they were involved in membrane cycling, and it has indeed been shown that lysosomes interact constantly with internalized membrane during receptor-mediated endocytosis.

De Duve's predictions were confirmed by elegant culture experiments conducted by Elisabeth Neufeld and colleagues at the National Institutes of Health. At the time, she was investigating storage of glycosaminoglycans in cultured fibroblasts obtained from patients with the mucopolysaccharidoses,(MPS), a class of diseases that has unexpectedly proved to be informative about lysosomal biology. The initial experiments were carried out using cells obtained from patients with genetically distinct mucopolysaccharide storage disorders in the hope that it would be possible to characterise and identify metabolic abnormalities in fibroblasts cultured from easily obtained skin biopsy specimens.

After culturing fibroblasts from patients in the presence of radioactive sulphate, it was shown that the rate of degradation, rather than the rate of synthesis or secretion of radiolabelled glycosaminoglycans, was markedly reduced. The labeled glycosaminoglycans showed prolonged turnover rates. However, when Neufeld and colleagues co-cultured fibroblasts obtained from patients with distinct mucopolysaccharidoses (Hurler's disease, MPS 1, now known to be caused by α-L-iduronidase deficiency, and the X-linked Hunter's disease, MPS 2, due to deficiency of iduronate sulphatase), the biochemical abnormalities and accumulation of glycosaminoglycans reverted. Pulse-labelling studies showed that the rate of breakdown of the glycosaminoglycans, which that accumulate in these disorders, was restored to normal.

Lysosomal complementation and biogenesis

Further intensive investigations showed that specific "corrective factors" were released by cultured fibroblasts into the medium, where they could be taken up to complement the enzymatic defect in cells lacking the capacity to degrade particular glycosaminoglycans. The corrective factors ultimately were shown to be high-molecular-weight forms of the enzymes whose activities were found to be lacking in the individual disorder; these proteins were secreted into the medium and taken up by a receptor-mediated pathway involving a mannose 6-phosphate–containing carbohydrate component, thus named the lysosomal 'recognition marker'. Functional complementation has been demonstrated in metachromatic leucodystrophy, Wolman's disease, β-glucuronidase deficiency, Sandhoff disease, fucosidosis as well as acid maltase deficiency, the first lysosomal defect to be identified by H.-G. Hers – Pompe's disease (glycogenosis type II.).

The capacity to correct the enzyme defects in the lysosomes of cells obtained from patients with storage disorders immediately raised the possibility that enzyme replacement could be used therapeutically. However, despite the fact that functional complementation in cells cultured from several categories of lysosomal storage diseases, this is by no means a universal phenomenon. Indeed, Gaucher's disease fibroblasts do not take up a complementing enzymatic activity from the medium even when co-cultured with fibroblasts obtained from healthy individuals. Glucocerebrosidase, the deficient enzyme in Gaucher's disease, appears to be loosely bound to proteins in the inner lysosomal membrane and is not normally secreted.

Inherited defects in the lysosomal targetting mechanism

The importance of the lysosomal recognition marker has been further demonstrated in patients suffering from the very rare but distinctive storage disorders that clarified the mechanism for intracellular sorting of newly synthesized lysosomal enzymes and the mechanism of enzymatic complementation of lysosomal defects. Patients with *I-cell disease* show diverse clinical features of several lysosomal storage disorders (see below). Examination of their cultured I-cell fibroblasts and indeed cells obtained by biopsy of patients with this disorder reveals characteristic inclusion bodies. Although the disorder shares features of the mucopolysaccharidoses, abundant plasma activities of several glycosamino-glycan-degrading enzymes are found in the plasma of patients with I-cell disease. Excretion of glycosaminoglycans in the urine is usually normal. When fibroblasts from patients with I-cell disease are cultured, they take up and retain lysosomal enzymes that have been released into the medium by healthy fibroblasts. However, not only are the cells obtained from I-cell patients themselves deficient in many lysosomal enzyme activities but the enzymes they release into culture media cannot be taken up by fibroblasts from patients with other lysosomal defects or by fibroblasts cultured from healthy persons.

Later studies showed that the high-molecular-weight glycoisoforms of lysosomal enzymes that serve as the respective corrective factors could be biosynthetically labelled with radioactive phosphorus. The proteins are phosphorylated specifically at the 6 position of mannose residues at exposed positions of their glycan moieties. In I-cell disease, inherited defects in the specific enzymatic pathway for the biosynthesis of mannose 6-phosphate–linked lysosomal glycoproteins leads to a failure of intracellular lysosomal targeting and a deficiency of many enzymes within the lysosome compartment. Thus, instead of finding their way to their destination within the lysosomes, the enzymes leak into the fluid phase and their activities may be detected abundantly in the plasma.

Nascent lysosomal enzymes carrying the mannose 6-phosphate residues bind to two specific membrane receptors for this sugar. One, a large protein, also serves as a receptor for insulin-like growth factor, which binds at a site independent from the mannose 6-phosphate–binding domain; the other, smaller membrane receptor appears to be more specific for mannose 6-phosphate–containing proteins. Lysosomal proteins harbouring mannose 6-phosphate residues bind to the receptor on the endolysosomal compartment of the trans-Golgi network, allowing the nascent proteins to be directed preferentially to the lysosomal pathway. Mild acidification facilitates dissociation of the processed hydrolases from the mannose 6-phosphate receptor and thus promotes vectorial delivery to the lysosome.

Relevance to therapeutic lysosomal complementation

The membrane-bound mannose 6-phosphate receptors recycled to the trans-Golgi and the residual fraction of 10% to 20% is expressed on the plasma membrane at the cell surface, where it participates in receptor-mediated endocytosis of secreted enzymes. This process allows lysosomal enzymes to be transferred by a secretion–capture mechanism that permits local complementation of lysosomal enzyme deficiency. It is this process that allows for the cross-correction of enzymatic deficiencies of soluble lysosomal enzymes delivered by means of the mannose 6-phosphate receptor and apparently released at the cell surface as a result of a universally 'leaky' intracellular sorting mechanism.

It should be emphasised that the M6P mechanism cannot be used for the delivery of therapeutic proteins to the phagolysosomal compartment of macrophages, and it is these cells that are the pathological focus of Gaucher's disease.

Gaucher's disease: a special lysosomal disorder

The estimated frequency of Gaucher's disease in studies from the Netherlands and Australia is approximately 1 in 150 000 to 1 in 60 000 live births (Table 2.2). The predicted frequency of the condition in the Ashkenazi Jewish population is considerably higher; overall, it is estimated that there are 30 000 to 60 000 patients with the condition worldwide, and about 6000 affected individuals in the so-called developed countries. Gaucher's disease has risen to prominence not only because it is one of the most frequent lysosomal disorders but because it is the first so far to be treated definitively. Enzyme replacement therapy for Gaucher's disease has proved to be a highly successful pharmaceutical venture, noted both for its clinical efficacy and its commercial triumph in the 'niche' market of orphan diseases (i.e. those with a prevalence of less than 200 000 US citizens or affecting less than 1 in 2000 Europeans).

Table 2.2 Lysosomal storage diseases

Disease	Incidence	Prevalence
Cystinosis	1:231 000	1:192 000
Anderson-Fabry	1:117 000	1:117 000
Gaucher's	1:59 000	1:57 000
GM1 gangliosidosis	1:422 000	1:384 000
Krabbe disease	1:201 000	1:141 000
α-Mannosidosis	1:1 056 000	1:1 056 000
Metachromatic leucodystrophy	1:121 000	1:92 000
MPS I	1:111 000	1:88 000
MPS II	1:162 000	1:136 000
Niemann-Pick A and B	1:264 000	1:248 000
Niemann-Pick C	1:211 000	1:211 000
Pompe	1:201 000	1:146 000
Sandhoff	1:422 000	1:384 000
Tay-Sachs	1:222 000	1:201 000
Wolman's	1:704 000	1:528 000
All lysosomal diseases	1/9 000	1/7 700

Source: Meikle, P. J., Hopwood, J. J., Clague, A. E. *et al.*, (1999). Prevalence of lysosomal storage disorders. *Journal of the American Medical Association* **281**, 249–54.

Enzyme replacement therapy for Gaucher's disease first emerged with a licensed preparation of the human enzyme glucocerebrosidase extracted from human placental tissue. Latterly the corrective protein is obtained from genetically engineered rodent cells as a recombinant human product, imiglucerase (Cerezyme™), which is administered intravenously. Imiglucerase has been a signal success for modern biotechnology in medicine and is noteworthy as a highly specialized therapeutic protein for use in a niche clinical market. Cerezyme, the product of the Genzyme Corporation, was licensed under the aegis of the US Orphan Drugs legislation but is now a global best seller in this category of so-called ultra-orphan therapeutics – about 4500 patients receive the drug worldwide. There are about 200 patients receiving the drug in the United Kingdom. Cerezyme is the single largest source of revenue for Genzyme, and the predicted annual sales will exceed $1.3 billion in 2007.

Definition

Gaucher's disease results from a functional deficiency of the lysosomal acid β-glucosidase glucocerebrosidase, otherwise known as glucosylceramidase (E. C. 3.2.1.45). The enzymatic deficiency leads to the accumulation of N-acylsphingosyl-1- 0-β-D-glucoside and other minor glycolipid metabolites, including the lysosphingolipid glucosylsphingosine (Fig. 2.1). The accumulated glycosphingolipids represent metabolic intermediates derived from the cellular turnover of membrane lipid macromolecules of the ganglioside and globoside classes.

Gaucher's disease is a multi-system disorder principally affecting cells of the mononuclear phagocyte system (macrophages) and classified in the catalogue of *Mendelian Inheritance in Man* (MIM) as recessive traits distinguished in categories 1 to 3 as 23080, 23091 and 23100. Rare variant forms of the condition also result from deficiency of the sphingolipid activator protein saposin C, which gives rise to a lethal clinical phenotype resembling Gaucher's disease with combined visceral and neuronopathic manifestations (Table 2.3).

Pathology of Gaucher's disease

Type 1 Gaucher's disease is the disorder first described in a young woman with hepatosplenomegaly by Phillipe Gaucher in his doctoral thesis accepted by the University of Paris in 1882 (Fig. 2.2). The unique histopathological features of the disorder were originally thought to represent a neoplastic process, as the title of Gaucher's dissertation indicates: '*L'épithelioma primitif de la rate sans leukemie*'. Beautiful camera obscura engravings of Gaucher's microscopic sections reveal large mononuclear cells filling the sinusoidal spaces of the spleen, which have come to be known as the eponymous Gaucher's cells; in reality, they are disordered macrophages which are hypertrophied and contain greatly increased glycolipid within distended vacuoles formed by fusion of engorged lysosomes. Electron microscopy reveals a striated appearance to

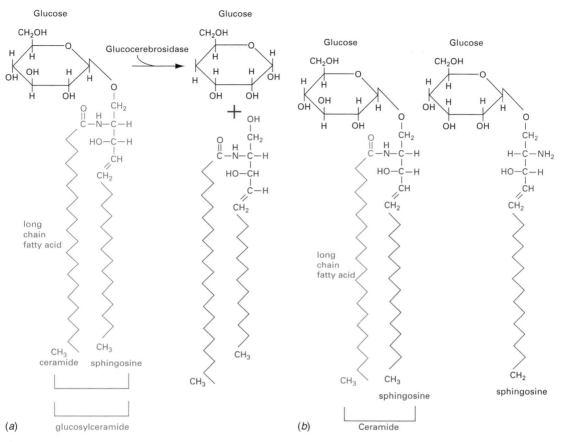

Figure 2.1 (*a*) Enzymatic defect and (*b*) Substrates accumulating in Gaucher's disease.

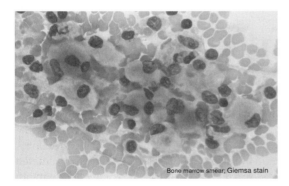

Figure 2.2 Gaucher Cells – note the large abnormal Macrophages in marrow aspirate stained by the Giemsa method. (See colour plate section.)

this intracellular storage material, which results from the head-to-tail fusion of amphipathic glucosylceramide (glucocerebroside) molecules.

The engorged macrophages represent the pathological focus of Gaucher's disease: they are found in all tissues that harbour histiocytes, principally the bone marrow, liver, spleen, lung and, occasionally, the Virchow-Robin spaces of the brain and in the renal glomerulus. In untreated Gaucher's disease, storage cells replace the normal complement of macrophages in the parenchymal organs (e.g. Kupffer cells) and are associated with local injury, including cell death, ischaemic necrosis, lymphocytic infiltration, and fibrotic scarring. The

Table 2.3 Clinical sub-types of Gaucher's disease

Manifestation	Type 1	Type 2	Type 3A	Type 3B	Type 3C	Collodion infants
Age of onset	> 1 year	< 1 year	> 10 years	< 5 years	2–20 years	At birth
Hepatosplenomegaly	++	±	±	+++	+	±
Bone disease	++	−	−	+++	−	+++
Cardiac valvular disease	−	−	−	−	+++	−
Progressive brain disease	−	+++	+	±	±	+
Oculomotor apraxia	−	+	+	+	+	?
Corneal opacities	−	?	−	−	+	?
Icthyosis	−	−	−	−	−	+++
Age at death	∼ 60 years	< 3years	< 20 years	< 30 years	< 20 years	< 1 month

viscera become greatly enlarged, especially the spleen, which may weigh up to 8 kg, compared with the normal of up to 140 g (Fig. 2.3). Symptomatic hypersplenism due to sequestration of all three formed elements of the blood within the hypertrophied viscus, whose sinuses are replaced by infiltrating macrophages, is frequent. Foci of extramedullary haematopoiesis are common in the liver and spleen; these may form macroscopic nodules throughout the parenchymal organs. Replacement of normal haematopoietic marrow and fat also contributes to cytopenias and is associated with episodic avascular necrosis principally occurring at the epiphyses of long bones as well as the vertebrae and pelvic bones.

The process by which necrosis of bone develops is unknown, but it is a common feature of Gaucher's disease in children and adults and contributes greatly to the burden of illness experienced in this condition. Local injury in the liver may, in about 5% of patients with type 1 Gaucher's disease, cause extensive scarring and portal hypertension. In a few patients with severe Gaucher's disease, Gaucher's cells replace normal alveolar macrophages and infiltrate the air spaces of the lung, impeding gas exchange and usually heraldings the terminal phase of the illness.

Gaucher's cells express classical markers of the monocytic myeloid cells that form histiocytes, or fixed tissue macrophages. In neuronopathic Gaucher's disease, these pathological cells may be found in the perivascular Vichow-Robin spaces adjacent to the meninges and also sporadically within deep layers of the cerebral cortex and cerebellum. Mid-brain, brainstem and cerebellar nuclei also show neuronal cell loss and neuronophagia by activated microglia associated with reactive astrogliosis (brain scarring). These features are restricted to the neuronopathic variants of Gaucher's disease, in which a profound deficiency of lysosomal sphingolipid breakdown leads to the buildup of toxic macromolecules that originate from the high *in situ* turnover of membrane gangliosides in neural cells.

Biochemical genetics of Gaucher's disease

Patients with Gaucher's disease inherit two mutant alleles of the human glucocerebrosidase gene, which maps to chromosome 1q21. Clinical disease is inherited as a typical autosomal recessive trait. Occasional families with generation-to-generation

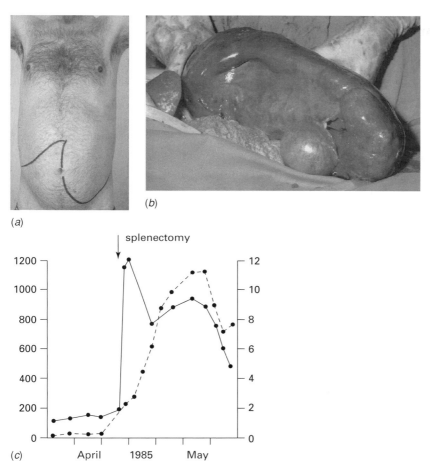

Figure 2.3 (*a*) Massive hepatosplenomegaly in a young man with Gaucher's disease and haemorrhage. Treatment before 1991: (*b*) splenectomy specimen; (*c*) effect of splenectomy on leucocyte and platelet counts. (See colour plate section.)

transmission of disease occur, especially in Ashkenazi Jewish populations, in which several mutant alleles of the human glucocerebrosidase gene occur with polymorphic frequency (greater than 1%); homozygosity or compound heterozygosity for these mutations occurs in approximately 1 in 850 Ashkenazi Jews.

More than 150 mutations associated with Gaucher's disease have been described in the human glucocerebrosidase gene. These genetic defects vary from single or multiple point mutations to deletions; not all mutations have been causally associated with glucocerebrosidase deficiency, but several alleles occur with high frequency in Gaucher's disease and are sufficiently widespread to be useful for direct diagnosis. Two point mutations, conveniently referred to by their effects on the amino acid sequence of human glucocerebrosidase polypeptide, are informative about disease severity. The N370S mutations (Asn^{370}->Ser) occurs with a high frequency in the Ashkenazim but is found in non-Jewish populations worldwide; the L444P mutation (Leu[444]->Pro) is predominantly non-Jewish but occurs with a particularly high frequency in a community isolate of type 3 Gaucher's patients in the northern Swedish regions of Norrbotten and Vesterbotten.

Homozygotes for N370S show an astonishing variability in the severity of disease; indeed, among Jews, perhaps 40% of N370S homozygotes in the population remain healthy or apparently asymptomatic throughout life. Monozygotic twins in their eighties who are discordant for clinical evidence of Gaucher's disease have been described. On the other hand, full-blown Gaucher's disease, with disabling complications, frequently occurs in N370S homozygotes. *In vitro* expression studies have shown that the N370S enzyme has normal or near normal catalytic activity, and it appears that cells with this mutant protein are principally deficient in glucosylceramide-degrading activity because of deficient co-translational processing of the newly synthesized enzyme. In contrast, the specific activity of the L444P mutant protein is markedly impaired and the enzyme is also unstable: the enzyme contributes very little residual cleavage activity in cells homozygous for this allele. Although L444P homozygotes tend to show severe clinical features of Gaucher's disease, this genotype has been found in patients with all three principal sub-types of the disease, again indicating the striking clinical diversity of this condition. From these studies (and apart from the special case of the rare D409H [Asp[409]->His] mutation), only limited prognostic information can be obtained from human glucocerebrosidase genotyping. It can, however, be stated with confidence that possession of at least one N370S allele precludes the development of neuronopathic Gaucher's disease.

Diagnosis

Patients with Gaucher's disease have acid glucocerebrosidase activities that are generally less than 10% of normal control values. The enzyme is deficient in all cells, but primary fibroblasts cultured from skin biopsies or acid β-glucosidase activities determined in leucocytes obtained from peripheral blood are simple and convenient sources for confirmatory testing of the suspected diagnosis. Biochemical assays employ a simple fluorogenic substrate analogue and are sufficiently sensitive to provide diagnostic information using small samples of biopsy material or peripheral blood. In the extremely rare patients with atypical Gaucher disease and neurological manifestations due defective activation by saposin C, acid β-glucosidase activity determined by use of flurogenic artificial substrates may be normal; under these circumstances, the enzymatic defect can be identified by using the natural substrate [usually as glucocerebroside, in which the glucose moiety is labelled with radioactive carbon (^{14}C)].

Family screening

The wide range of acid β-glucosidase deficiency observed in obligate heterozygous carriers of Gaucher's disease renders enzymatic screening of families impractical. Mutation studies using molecular analysis of the human glucocerebrosidase gene are often informative in combination with enzymatic measurement for the identification of heterozygotes and homozygotes in at-risk pedigrees who request predictive genetic testing. The frequency of the N370S allele and others, such as the frameshift 84gg insertion, in Ashkenazi families that are aware of the high risk of disease transmission is often sufficiently great to simplify diagnostic DNA analysis for Gaucher's disease in at-risk communities.

Clinical manifestations

Several clinical sub-categories of Gaucher's disease are recognized, giving rise to distinct syndromes. In type 1 (chronic non-neuronopathic) Gaucher's disease, anaemia, thrombocytopenia, leucopenia, hepatosplenomegaly, pulmonary disease and bone disease occur; the symptoms often develop in

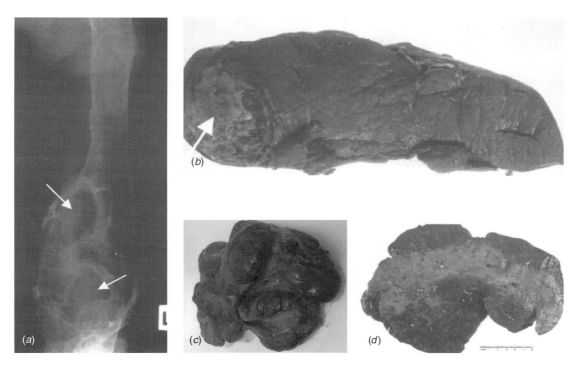

Figure 2.4 Irreversible sequelae of Gaucher's disease: (*a*) Lytic lesion lower femur in young woman splenectomised in childhood; (*b*) splenectomy specimen sectioned to show fresh splenic infarct; (*c*) cirrhotic liver in 47-year-old Gaucher patient; (*d*) liver explant showing lobar fibrosis in man with Gaucher's disease requiring hepatic allotransplantation for cirrhosis and hepatogenous cyanosis – with regular infusions of enzyme therapy, this individual remains well, 10 years later.

childhood, but in some patients the onset occurs in mature adult life. Although bone disease (Fig. 2.4 and 2.5) and systemic manifestations may be prominent, a key feature of type 1 Gaucher's disease is the absence of primary central nervous system disease, and this is by far the most common clinical variant. Patients with neurological Gaucher's disease have been classified as type 2 Gaucher's disease (acute neuronopathic), in which there is an early onset of neurological features with bulbar paresis, cranial nerve palsies, opisthotonus, spastic paresis with variable hepatosplenomegaly and, usually, mild haematological abnormalities. This acute neuronopathic form of Gaucher's disease is fatal before the age of 2 years as a result of malnutrition and aspiration pneumonia due to recurrent seizures and the evolution of a decerebrate state.

Patients with chronic neuronopathic Gaucher's disease are categorized as type 3 Gaucher's disease. Operationally this may be described as neuronopathic Gaucher's disease that is not type 2 and in practice represents a highly heterogeneous multisystem disorder including neurological deficits.

Patients with the so-called type 3A Gaucher's disease develop progressive neurological failure with cognitive impairment, tonic–clonic epilepsy, horizontal supranuclear gaze palsies, ataxia and myoclonic attacks; organomegaly is usually mild and the patients succumb to progressive injury to the brainstem or uncontrollable seizures. Patients with type 3B Gaucher's disease usually have a static but overt supranuclear gaze palsy usually of horizontal but occasionally of vertical type; in contrast to type A disease, they have marked visceral manifestations

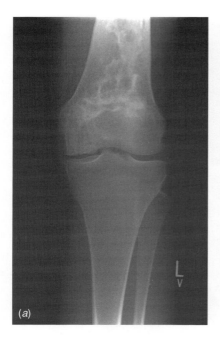 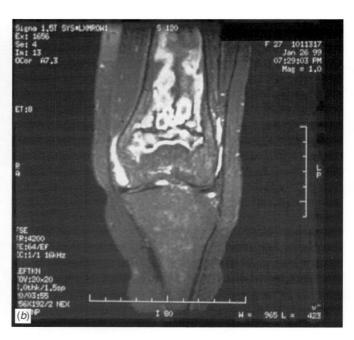

Figure 2.5 (*a*) Plain radiograph; (*b*) T2 weighted MRI of lower femur and upper tibia of 32-year-old woman with acute avascular necrosis ; note geographical proton signal in marrow space near epiphysis.

with severe hepatosplenomegaly, anaemia, portal hypertension and extensive osseous manifestations including vertebral necrosis and gibbus formation at the upper thoracic level. Type 3B patients usually die as a result of pulmonary infiltration, uncontrollable haemorrhage, or hepatic disease.

A further type of chronic neuronopathic Gaucher's disease (so-called type 3C) has been associated hitherto only with homozygosity for the rare missense mutation D409H in the glucocerebrosidase gene. In this syndrome, reported principally from Arab patients, Spain and the Balkans as well as Japan, there is a non-progressive oculomotor apraxia with moderate splenic enlargement. Hepatomegaly and skeletal manifestations may not be prominent, but clinical inspection reveals bilateral corneal opacification. The heart is characteristically affected with progressive thickening and calcification of mitral and aortic valves, associated with mitral regurgitation,

mild aortic insufficiency, or severe aortic stenosis. Heavy calcification of the valve leaflets and coronary arteries has been observed. Some patients have died suddenly as a result of cardiac tachyarrythmias before surgery for aortic valve disease. Cranial computed tomography (CT) scans show dilatation of the lateral ventricles with brachycephaly. Clinically, type 3C disease resembles an intermediate syndrome between a glycosphingolipidosis and a mucopolysaccharidosis; the condition responds incompletely if at all to enzyme replacement therapy.

Neonatal Gaucher's disease presenting with premature labour or in the neonatal period has been reported in association with severe congenital ichthyosis. At birth, massive enlargement of the liver and spleen has been seen in many fetuses in association with acute neuronopathic features and arthrogryphosis. These infants usually die as a result of dehydration in association with an unusual translucency and texture of the skin ('collodion' infants). In these patients, free ceramides (the products of glucocerebrosidase) are absent; this impairs the aqueous permeability barrier that forms part of the structural integrity of the integument. In this respect collodion babies closely resemble knockout mice homozygous for a disrupted glucocerebrosidase gene: in all instances these infants have been shown to inherit two inactivating mutations in the glucocerebrosidase gene on chromosome 1q.

Other rare manifestations of Gaucher's disease

Gaucher's cells have been identified histologically in the mesangium of the renal glomeruli in patients with proteinuria, which appears very occasionally sufficiently severe to cause the nephrotic syndrome. Rare infiltrates have been reported in association with pericardial calcification and calcification in the pericardial membrane. At least one patient has been reported with profuse lower intestinal bleeding in association with mucosal infiltration of the colon by Gaucher's cells. Most of these manifestations appear to be pathological curiosities often occurring in severe end-stage systemic disease.

Parkinsonian manifestations

There have now been several case reports of the occurrence of Parkinson's disease in patients with type 1 Gaucher's disease. The mean onset of the Parkinson syndrome, which progresses rapidly, is between the fourth and sixth decades of life and is thus apparently earlier than the mean onset of Parkinson's disease uncomplicated by Gaucher's disease (which generally occurs at about 60 years of age). The unusual feature of the Parkinson syndrome is its apparent resistance to conventional anti-parkinsonian medications. Its cause and the associated pathological features are quite unknown; as yet, no neuropathological description of the condition has been provided from autopsy studies. The formal possibility exists that parkinsonism in association with Gaucher's disease in fact represents a bona

fide manifestation of neuronopathic disease occurring late in life and not being declared at birth, as is usually the case with the neuronopathic variants of Gaucher's disease now referred to as type 2 and type 3.

Metabolic abnormalities in Gaucher's disease

Infiltration of the tissues of Gaucher's patients by storage cells, principally of the macrophage series, is associated with local pathological injury, including necrosis, infarction and proliferative responses accompanied by fibrotic scarring. In the affected tissues there is a greatly increased concentration of free glucosylceramide, which has been found in the bone marrow and visceral organs as well as the brain. Accompanying the lysosomal proliferation is a several-fold increase in the activity of unrelated acid hydrolases, such as β-hexosaminidase and tartrate-resistant acid phosphatase.

A striking feature, however, of the pathological process in the viscera is the disparity between the enlargement of the organ caused by the proliferative response to Gaucher's cell infiltration and the absolute quantity of glycolipid that is stored. Most of the additional size of the organ (in the case of the spleen, up to 80-fold greater than normal), is accounted for by inflammatory cells and increased tissue water, which results from their presence, rather than to the mass of the accumulated glycosphingolipid. In summary, the glycosphingolipid clearly provokes a dramatic pathological response accompanied by cellular infiltration and local pathological injury; the accumulated sphingolipid itself contributes but a minute fraction (less than 3%) of the increased mass of the visceral organs, such as the liver and spleen, which are so characteristically enlarged in Gaucher's disease.

In the plasma, a slight increase, approximately two-fold, of glucosylceramide concentrations is seen in patients with Gaucher's disease; in some patients, the plasma concentration of this lipid is within the normal range. However, there are many other marked abnormalities of the plasma in patients with established Gaucher's disease. These include reduced low- and high-density lipoprotein concentrations, raised apolipoprotein E, elevated serum concentrations of ferritin (in the absence of other signs of iron excess), increased vitamin B12 binding capacity due to increased transcobalamin II, and increased angiotensin converting enzyme.

Secondary release of lysosomal enzymes

Lysosomal enzymes, β-hexosaminidase A and B, tartrate-resistant acid phosphatase, lysozyme and chitotriosidase (a chitinase) are greatly elevated (in the case of chitotriosidase, up to a thousand-fold above the normal range). These analytes are therefore of value in following the course of Gaucher's disease and especially in its response to specific treatments. Thus the over-expressed lysosomal enzymes serve as surrogate markers of disease activity and can be conveniently measured in plasma or serum derived from routine samples of blood. Chitotriosidase in particular appears to be very stable on storage, and longitudinal studies of its activity conducted in thousands of patients have confirmed its utility as an independent plasma analyte for the monitoring of treatment responses and as a broad indicator of disease severity. Other abnormalities of the plasma include altered clotting and fibrinolytic factors, including deficiencies of factors V, VIII and IX. These may improve after splenectomy or after enzyme replacement therapy, suggesting that they are related to low-grade intravascular coagulation in untreated Gaucher's disease.

B-cell proliferative responses

Active Gaucher's disease is associated with a polyclonal hypergammaglobulinaemia and, in many patients over the age of 50 years, with a high frequency of monoclonal and oligoclonal gammopathies. Several reports of amyloidosis have been provided in patients with Gaucher's disease, which provide further evidence that chronic B-cell stimulation occurs in this condition. The most severe lymphoproliferative complications of Gaucher's dis-

ease, however, are those associated with malignant responses: multiple myeloma and B-cell lymphoma/leukaemia are the most common neoplasms reported. Hodgkin's disease and acute myeloid leukaemia have also been reported sporadically. In any event, the lymphoproliferative disorders of B-cell type that accompany Gaucher's disease strongly suggest that the abnormal storage material within macrophages leads to a chronic stimulation of B lymphocytes and their progenitors. This, associated with acute-phase responses, may be attributed in part to the increased concentrations of the cytokine interleukin 6, which has been found in the plasma of patients with Gaucher's disease.

Course of Gaucher's disease

Such is the diversity and clinical heterogeneity of Gaucher's disease, that it has proved very difficult to predict its course. Patients homozygous for the N370S mutation, which is widespread in the Ashkenazi Jewish population, may have disease that remains asymptomatic to the ninth decade of life or suffer the early onset of disabling avascular necrosis of bone or pancytopaenia. Indeed, the author's group has reported monozygotic twins homozygous for this mutation who lived together all their lives but in whom the disease was highly discordant: one of the pair had required splenectomy for life-threatening bleeding and developed bone disease; the other remained asymptomatic and without clinically detectable disease to the age of 84 years. Some associative evidence of the triggering effect of environmental co-factors such as viral infections (especially Epstein-Barr virus) suggests that genetic predisposition is not sufficient to guarantee disease expression in many patients. On the other hand, many patients with Gaucher's disease suffer progressive skeletal deformity and increasing neurological deficit after an early onset of disease in infancy or childhood and with greatly shortened lives. In a large series of patients in the era before the appearance of enzyme replacement therapy, the mean age of death of patients with type 1 disease was about 60 years, which is significantly lower that of the general population; a large proportion of the deaths due to the disease were associated with infection and with malignancy, especially B-cell malignancy (see above). Rarer patients with neuronopathic disease die in childhood, adolescence, or early adult life; even those with non-progressive neurological manifestations usually have severe systemic disease from which survival beyond the age of 35 years is unusual. All patients with acute neuronopathic disease die in infancy or very early childhood.

With increasing awareness of Gaucher's disease and identification of patients with milder symptoms as a result of pedigree study, a more general view of the evolution of type 1 Gaucher's disease has emerged. Most patients with symptomatic disease in childhood show slow but significant progression throughout life, with reduced quality of life and often episodes of disabling osseous disease. It is generally held that the earlier in life that the disease manifests itself, the more rapidly it progresses. Splenectomy, in the past carried out to relieve pressure symptoms caused by the markedly enlarged viscus or life-threatening cytopaenias, is associated with an adverse outcome from infections. Splenectomy appears also to be associated with, and possibly causally linked, to the severity of osteonecrosis. In patients with chronic neuronopathic Gaucher's disease (type 3 disease), splenectomy is known to have an adverse event on outcome, since the procedure is associated with accelerated neurological injury. The pulmonary manifestations of Gaucher's disease (parenchymal infiltration of lung spaces by Gaucher's cells and/or pulmonary hypertension) carries a bad prognosis and responds incompletely to enzyme replacement therapy.

Another severe prognostic sign in Gaucher's disease is the onset of hepatic fibrosis; this is associated with portal hypertension and an unusual histological picture resembling cirrhosis or the hepar lobatum previously documented in congenital hepatic syphilis. Clearly, portal hypertension is irreversible, and the severe hepatic injury associated with Gaucher's disease usually progresses to hepatic failure or fatal variceal haemorrhage.

Studies in Europe and particularly The Netherlands indicate that once a patient with the common variant of Gaucher's disease, type 1 Gaucher's disease, becomes symptomatic, he or she slowly deteriorates, with decreasing blood counts and increasing splenic enlargement punctuated by episodes of bone collapse related to osteonecrosis and, in some cases demineralization of the bone, leading to manifest osteoporosis with a high risk of fragility fractures. Although many such patients survive to middle age and beyond, their quality of life is severely impaired by active disease and the sustained inflammatory response with which it is associated.

Treatment of Gaucher's disease

Supportive therapy

Gaucher's disease is a multisystem disorder and in the untreated state patients require analgesia for pain, usually due to bone infarction and/or fragility fractures; joint replacement surgery is often needed. Hypersplenism, with or without haematopoietic marrow failure, reduces the concentration of all the cellular blood components and may require transfusion of blood products – especially at times of surgery or during obstetric delivery. In the recent past, splenectomy was frequently carried out to relieve pancytopenia, but this is associated with the danger of overwhelming protozoal and bacterial infection – and, it is now believed, a greatly increased frequency of bone infarction crises (avascular necrosis). In some patients with cirrhosis and liver failure, allogeneic liver transplantation has been carried out successfully. Pulmonary hypertension, a rare but dreaded complication of the disease, may require administration of prostacycline derivatives and antagonists of endothelin and phosphodiesterase 5, such as bosentan and sildenafil.

Bone marrow transplantation

As a disorder principally of the macrophage system of mononuclear phagocytes, which are of haematopoietic origin, Gaucher's disease can be treated by allogeneic bone marrow transplantation; indeed, the disorder was in the early group of inborn errors of metabolism in infants and children in whom this approach was first explored. In those individuals who survived the procedure and avoided chronic graft-versus-host disease, outcomes were spectacularly successful, with reduced liver and spleen volumes and improved blood counts. In those patients with complete engraftment and donor chimerism, further progression of visceral disease and the skeletal manifestations was arrested; normal growth patterns and general health were restored. These outcomes provide compelling evidence that the principal non-neurological manifestations of Gaucher disease are the consequence of abnormal tissue macrophages that originate from the haematopoietic stem cells in the host. Unfortunately, bone marrow transplantation is not a realistic option for most patients with Gaucher's disease – or even severely affected children with the early onset of a rapidly progressive disorder. Not only are HLA-matched related donors often not available but the mortality of all forms of allogeneic marrow transplantation renders decision making a fraught and faulted process, particularly because the course of Gaucher's disease is so difficult to predict with confidence in any individual patient.

Development of enzyme replacement therapy

As indicated in the introduction, Gaucher's disease, the most frequent of the lysosomal storage disorders, provides a striking example of the marriage between laboratory science, clinical research and pharmaceutical development within the realm of biotechnology. Soon after the demonstration of the enzymatic defect in the 1960s by Roscoe Brady and colleagues, the US National Institutes of Health (NIH) set out to prepare a sufficient quantity of human glucocerebrosidase for the purposes of enzyme replacement therapy. They later realized that glucocerebrosidase was a lysosomal enzyme, and Christian de Duve himself had indicated, in his early descriptions of the lysosome, that functional defects within it would be susceptible to comple-

mentation from the fluid phase. At the time, Gilbert Ashwell and colleagues, also at the NIH, had been studying the hepatic uptake of plasma glycoproteins mediated by the asialoglycoprotein and cognate receptors; these were identified after modification of glycans present on the protein ligands using chemical methods and enzymatic digestion with specific glycosidases. By the early 1970s, Peter Pentchev in the Brady group had purified glucocerebrosidase from human placenta: its administration to two patients with Gaucher's disease showed that the enzyme was able to reduce the tissue concentrations of glucocerebroside measured by hepatic biopsy. At the same time, blood glucocerebroside concentrations decreased over a few days and remained low for several months, only to return slowly to the previous high values.

Despite increasing the amount of enzyme available for administration, reduction in hepatic glucocerebroside concentrations after infusions in Gaucher's patients proved to be very inconsistent. Further studies indicated that the uptake of the exogenous glucocerebrosidase was principally in the parenchymal rather than the macrophage (Kupffer) cells in the liver tissue. With this understanding, there was a need to target macrophages within spleen, bone marrow and liver, and with the discovery by Achord and Sly that macrophages, and by Stahl that human alveolar macrophages possess a specific lectin-like receptor (the mannose receptor) that binds mannosylated glycoconjugates on their surface, an analysis of the four oligosaccharide chains on human placental glucocerebrosidase was undertaken. Most of the chains on placental glucocerebrosidase were of the complex type and terminated in sialic acid. To reveal terminal mannose residues for uptake by the mannose receptor of macrophages (and endothelial cells), sequential enzymatic removal of sialic acid, galactose and N-acetylglucosamine residues was undertaken using exoglycosidases purified from plant sources, including the Jack bean.

Scott Furbish, working with John Barranger in the Brady group at the NIH, found that modification of human placental glucocerebrosidase, to reveal terminal mannose residues on its four oligosaccha-ride chains, greatly enhanced its uptake by Kupffer cells (macrophages). This finding formed the basis of a further clinical study in eight patients with type 1 Gaucher's disease who received weekly injections of the modified placental enzyme starting in 1981 with enzyme supplied by the newly formed Genzyme Cor-poration. Only one of the enzyme recipients (a child) in this trial showed a clear therapeutic response after enrollment in 1983, with improved blood counts and improved energy. On stopping the infusions, his haemoglobin and platelet count returned to pre-infusion levels. It was clear that this individual, Brian Berman, who had experienced a salutary therapeu-tic effect and was only 4 years old at the time, had received more enzyme on a body-weight basis than others in the trial,. Since completion of the trial, he has received 30 units of human glucocerebrosidase in its modified form each week, with restoration of his haemoglobin and platelet counts to the normal range and a substantial reduction in the size of his spleen. It is now 24 years after the first successful treatment of this disease with modified human pla-cental glucocerebrosidase in Mr.Berman: he is well, has married and fathered children of his own, and remains largely disease-free.

Later, Henry Blair, Genzyme's scientific founder, and Henry Termeer, its new chief executive officer, made a number of courageous decisions to risk the future of their company on developing enzyme treat-ment for Gaucher's disease. In 1987, a trial involv-ing 12 patients with type 1 Gaucher's disease using human placental glucocerebrosidase in an open-label study for 6 months was undertaken: a dose of 60 units per kilogram of body weight was infused every 2 weeks. This trial, which cost about $3 million, was financed by donations from numerous investors and by donations from members of the National Gaucher Foundation (NGF). This organization, established in 1984, was founded by Dr. Robin Berman, the mother of Brian, as a non-profit, tax-exempt organization dedicated to supporting and promoting research into the causes of and a cure for Gaucher's disease; the NGF was critical to the fund-raising initiative. In the event, all the participants in the trial, which was conducted at the NIH, showed beneficial responses to the enzyme infusion.

The drug, later known as alglucerase (Ceredase), was licensed in 1991 using the special regulations that had been newly applied for the treatment of orphan diseases under special conditions. It is, how-ever, salutary to consider the odds against this com-mercial venture in the early days of the US orphan drug legislation: there was no animal model of the disease in which to test the potential medication; the population of patients was extremely small – and, for the original investors, only one patient had shown a beneficial effect. In 1987, at a time when the HIV/AIDS epidemic was under way and where human tissues were known to be the source of HIV-1 in blood products as well as the agent of Creutzfeld-Jacob disease in corneal grafts and growth hormone preparations, confidence – amounting to near reck-lessness – was needed to support the therapeutic development of a product requiring glucocerebrosi-dase purified from more than 20 000 human placen-tae to treat a single Gaucher's patient for ae year.

Since these early days, numerous patients world-wide have been treated with varying doses of man-nose-terminated human glucocerebrosidase, with therapeutic benefit. The patients report enhanced quality of life, a reduction in fatigue, improvement in blood counts, regression of hepatosplenomegaly, and a decreased frequency of sporadic bone infarc-tion crises.

A few years after the licensing of alglucerase, which was prepared on an industrial scale from placen-tae collected from international sources, a recombi-nant human preparation was introduced after many years of development with the launch of the Gen-zyme Corporation's protein production facility in Alston, Massachusetts. Recombinant human glu-cocerebrosidase is expressed *in vitro* in Chinese hamster ovary cells and then further modified by enzymatic deglycosylation to expose, as before, core mannose residues that allow the exogenous enzyme to behave as a ligand for macrophage mannose receptors. Although this engineered drug, imiglucerase (Cerezyme) is very expensive and full doses of 60 units per kilogram of body weight every

2 weeks may cost in excess of $300 000 per year for an adult, the drug is used at (varying dosages) for patients with Gaucher's disease all over the world. The principal indication for treatment with mannose-terminated glucocerebrosidase – imiglucerase (Cerezyme) – is symptomatic type 1 Gaucher's disease; the drug has proved to be beneficial for patients with more severe disease, including those with chronic neuronopathic features.

Suppression of systemic disease in patients with the neuronopathic variant, type 3, is associated with improved mobility and in some cases neurological stabilization or improvement of cognitive skills. This has occurred surprisingly in the face of evidence that a large protein such as glucocerebrosidase would not be expected to penetrate the blood–brain barrier. The salutary effects of enzyme therapy on cognition and performance may reflect the benefit of improved general health and vitality. However, it may also reflect decreased circulating plasma glucosylceramide concentrations, which might improve type 3 Gaucher's disease directly because uptake of this glycolipid from plasma by macrophages may give rise to adventitial Gaucher's cells accumulating at perivascular sites such as the Virchow-Robin space.

In patients with Gaucher's disease who receive enzyme replacement therapy with mannose-terminated human glucocerebrosidase (they nearly all now receive the purified recombinant enzyme imiglucerase), objective measures of disease improvement include a reduction in liver and spleen volumes; increased haemoglobin, white cell and platelet counts; and a decrease in the surrogate biomarkers of disease activity (Fig. 2.6). The latter include plasma acid phosphatase, β-hexosaminidase and especially chitotriosidase activities. Biopsy samples – which are not routinely carried out – have clearly also demonstrated a reduction in the number of Gaucher cells infiltrating bone marrow and liver tissue.

Nearly 4500 patients worldwide now receive imiglucerase (Cerezyme) the commercial success of which has raised the profile of the Genzyme Cor-

poration: it is now the world's third largest biotechnology company with an annual turnover of more than $3.2 billion. Competitors of Genzyme, Shire Human Genetic Therapies (formerly Transkayotic Therapies) and Protalix, an emerging biotechnology company based in Israel, are developing their own recombinant products for Gaucher's disease. Shire is currently producing mannose-terminated human glucocerebrosidase by activating the endogenous gene in human fibroblasts cultured in the presence of kifunensine, an inhibitor of an endogenous glycoprocessing mannosidase; this agent, gene-activated glucocerebrosidase (GA-GCB), is undergoing phase 3 clinical trials. The preparation from Protalix, prGCD, which is produced in genetically engineered cultured carrot cells and with a different carbohydrate composition, has a longer plasma half-life that the other preparations. The new agents have strong therapeutic activity and the clinical data so far obtained are very encouraging. However, it is not clear whether, in the absence of a compelling clinical difference in efficacy, these agents which seek to compete with Cerezyme but are 'biosimilars' will prove to be successful and viewed as sufficiently distinctive to gain the necessary marketing exclusivity as registered orphan products. The huge cost of treating an individual Gaucher's patient with Cerezyme ($100 000 to 300 000 annually) prohibits availability of the agent for most patients in all but the richest countries; it is thus likely that unless there is an economic reason to switch to another agent, Genzyme's competitors will struggle to succeed in the international markets. Because GA-GCB and prGCD are experimental therapeutic molecules with structures that differ significantly from imiglucerase, these cannot be considered as genuine generic drugs. As a consequence, their manufacturers will also face the exorbitant costs of clinical trials, pharmaceutical and marketing development. With this in mind, a significant price discount (doubtless with an accompanying price war) will be very difficult to mount: were it to be successful, however, the competition will have improved the availability of treatment for many Gaucher's patients who are

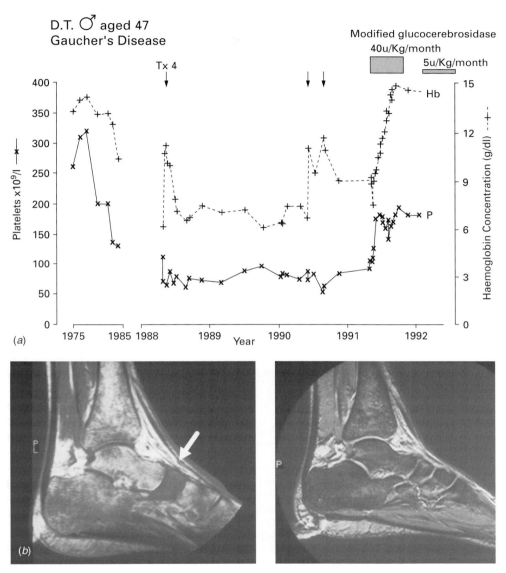

Figure 2.6 Effect of macrophage-targeted enzyme replacement therapy in 47-year-old man splenectomised at 16 years for Gaucher's disease. He had active marrow disease in the extremities and avascular necrosis of the small bones in his feet, rendering him unable to walk; he was also transfusion-dependent with anaemia and thrombocytopenia due to bone marrow failure. The haematological disease, (a), and bone pain visualised in the extremities by T1WI MRI, (b), responded rapidly to infusions of mannose-terminated human placental glucocerebrosidase (alglucerase, Ceredase™); the patient remains well and fully mobile, with normal blood counts and little biochemical or radiological evidence of disease while receiving regular infusions of recombinant human mannose-terminated glucocerebrosidase (imiglucerase, Cerezyme™), more than 16 years later. [From Mistry, P. K. *et al.* (1992). *Quarterly Journal of Medicine.*]

currently denied access to it on the grounds of cost. Commercial competition on this scale was never envisaged in relation to ultra-orphan drug development, but in just a few years, it has galvanized the entire field.

Another corollary of the emergence of successful treatment for Gaucher's disease, has been further pharmaceutical investment in other glycosylated lysosomal enzymes for the treatment of other storage diseases. In these instances, expression of therapeutic proteins harbouring several surface mannose-6 phosphate residues (as opposed to terminal mannose residues) has been important in order to target the lysosomal mannose 6-phosphate receptors. α-galactosidase A (Fabry's disease), L-iduronidase (Hurler's disease, MPS 1), iduronate sulphatase (Hunter's disease, MPS 2), arylsulphatase B (Maroteaux-Lamy disease, MPS 6) and acid maltase (Pompe's disease, glygogenosis type IIa) are now licenced; acid sphingomyelinase for Niemann-Pick disease type B is also under active pharmaceutical development. (Table 2.4). In relation to Gaucher's disease, immunological and sensitivity reactions to the infusions are rare; this is probably explained by the observation that most patients with the con-

dition harbour mutations that allow expression of residual glucocerebrosidase, thereby exposing the individual to polypeptide antigens that are shared between the mutant and the wild-type human glucocerebrosidase proteins. Further information about the effects of infusions of other recombinant lysosomal glycoproteins on the immune system and the effects on therapeutic efficiency will be important and is awaited.

Other stratagems for treating Gaucher's disease

Enzyme replacement therapy for Gaucher's disease has proved to be highly effective and has presaged the development of several glycoprotein products with appropriate safety and stability profiles for application in other lysosomal storage diseases. However, the production and, to some extent, the delivery of therapeutic proteins is an imprecise science, and patients with severe neuronopathic manifestations of Gaucher's disease typically have brain injury that persists despite correction of florid systemic disease by enzyme replacement.

Table 2.4 Enzyme replacement for lysosomal storage diseases

Disease	Enzyme (source)	Licenced name
Gaucher's	Alglucerase (human placenta)	Ceredase*
	Imiglucerase (CHO cells[†])	Cerezyme
Fabry's	Algalsidase-α (human fibroblasts)	Replagal
	Algalsidase-β (CHO cells[†])	Fabrazyme
Hurler/Hurler-Scheie (MPS 1)	Iduronidase (CHO cells[†])	Aldurazyme
Hunter's syndrome (MPS II)	Iduronidate sulphatase (human fibroblasts)	Elaprase
Pompe's (Acid α-glucosidase) rabbits	Acid maltase (CHO cells[†]; transgenic	Myozyme
Maroteaux-Lamy(MPS VI)	Arylsulphatase B (CHO cells[†])	Naglazyme
Niemann-Pick type B	Acid sphingomyelinase (CHO cells[†])	?

*Now largely outmoded by imiglucerase (Cerezyme).

[†]Recombinant human product expressed in Chinese hamster ovary cells.

Substrate reduction therapy

Radin developed an alternative concept for the treatment of the glycolipid storage diseases based on the relationship between the synthetic and breakdown pathways for glycosphingolipids. Glucocerebroside is formed from ceramide by the action of the rate-limiting enzyme glucosylceramide transferase, which is UDP-dependent. The transferase enzyme is located on the cytoplasmic side of the Golgi complex and the glucosylceramide that is formed passes by an unknown mechanism to the luminal side of the Golgi apparatus. Glucocerebroside serves as the precursor for numerous glycosphingolipids but its formation is distinct from the *galactosylceramide synthase*, which is responsible for the biosynthesis of the class of complex *galactosphingolipids*. Norman Radin postulated that small reduction in the rate of biosynthesis of glucocerebroside would improve the lysosomal storage of glucocerebroside by allowing residual glucocerebrosidase activity, which is present in nearly all patients with Gaucher's disease, to break down the accumulated glycosphingolipid.

Radin and colleagues set out to identify inhibitors of ceramide UDP–glucosyl transferase and identified several molecules including a reversible inhibitor, 1-phenyl-2-decanoylamino-3-morpholino-propanol (PDMP), which are high-affinity inhibitors of the enzyme. Further modifications of the PDMP parent compound have led to the identification of potent analogues with specific inhibitory effects on glucosylceramide synthase. The most potent of these analogues belong to the so-called P4 series, in which low nanomolar concentrations significantly decrease glucosylceramide concentrations in cultured cells. These PDMP homologues are very active *in vivo* and are currently undergoing evaluation for therapeutic use in the glycolipid storage diseases such as Fabry's disease, both GM_1 and GM_2 gangliosidoses, and Gaucher's disease, in which accumulation of glucosylceramide (glucocerebroside), or its more complex ganglioside derivatives, is impaired. Genzyme has developed several structural homologues of these morpholino compounds and

one, GENZ 112638 [(1R, 2R) – octanoic acid [2 -(2′, 3′- dihydrobenzo [1,4] dioxin-6′-yl)-2-hydroxy-1 pyrrolidin-1-yl-methyl-ethyl]-amide, supplied as the L-tartaric acid salt, is an orally active ceramide analogue currently in late phase II multi-centre clinical trials in patients with Gaucher's disease. This compound, which is a highly selective inhibitor of UDP-glucosylceramide synthase, is also potent: the IC_{50} as determined *in vitro* is approximately 25nM.

Iminosugars as substrate-reducing agents

The concept of substrate depletion to prevent the accumulation of glycosphingolipids by inhibiting their biosynthesis has been developed clinically using another set of compounds, the iminosugars. These derivatives of natural plant chemicals have been found selectively to inhibit the glucosyltransferase step without affecting glucocerebrosidase and acid glucosidases. The first of these sugars, N-butyldeoxynojiirimycin (Fig. 2.7), had previously been used in clinical trials in an attempt to arrest proliferation of the human immunodeficiency virus. The iminosugar was not found to have major human toxicity but failed to have any beneficial effect on the outcome of HIV infection. N-butyldeoxynojirimycin inhibits viral α-glucosidase, but Frances Platt and Terry Butters of the University of Oxford have discovered that it also has a selective effect on the UDP-ceramide glu-

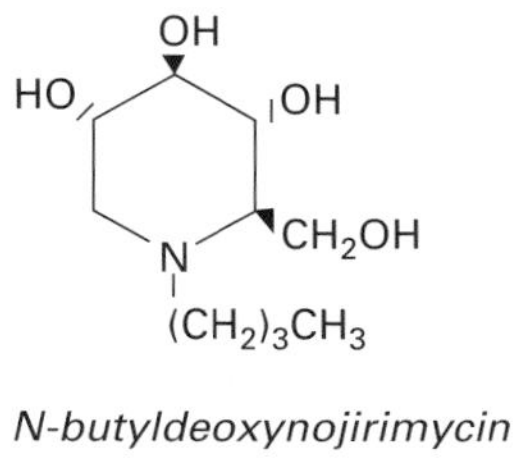

N-butyldeoxynojirimycin

Figure 2.7 Molecular structure of *N*-butyldeoxynojirimycin (miglustat) – an iminosugar licensed for the oral treatment of patients with mild to modreate Gaucher's disease unsuitable for enzyme replacement therapy.

cosyltransferase reaction. A further analogue, N-butyldeoxygalactonojirimycin (NB-DGJ) is found to have almost entirely selective activity against this initial glucosyltransferase step in the biosynthesis of glycolipids, with virtually no unwanted activity against glucosidases.

The administration of these simple iminosugars to genetically modified animals representing experimental models of the debilitating glycosphingolipidoses including the GM_2 gangliosidoses (Tay-Sachs disease and Sandhoff disease caused by deficiency of β-hexosaminidase A) showed reduced glycolipid storage with partial delay or arrest of the progression of injury and a small but significant prolongation of life expectancy.

Clinical trials of substrate-reduction therapy

The pharmacokinetics of NB-DNJ show that the drug, which achieves maximum plasma concentrations 2 to $2^1/_2$ h after the dosing, does not bind appreciably to plasma proteins. Its average half-life is 6 to 7 h with excretion of about 50% unchanged in the urine.

In an open-label trial comprising patients with Gaucher's disease, there was evidence of efficacy shown by a decrease in liver and spleen volumes, an increase in platelet count and haemoglobin concentration, and a significant decrease in chitotriosidase activity. These activities have continued during extension studies now up to 3 years after the inception of the study. The therapeutic effect is progressive on exposure to 100 mg three times daily in adult patients. A decrease in white blood cell glycolipid concentrations, indicating a reduction in the amount of speculating glycolipid delivered to macrophages, occurred as expected. Also as predicted, the therapeutic effect of substrate deprivation in Gaucher's disease was slow in onset because reduced storage in the macrophages is contingent upon the delivery of less membrane glycolipids from the breakdown of circulating blood cells, (principally leucocytes).

On the basis of the results of the pivotal study and its extension, a modest sustained effect on patients

with mild-to-moderate type 1 Gaucher's disease was established. At the time of writing, an effect of the drug in the maintenance of disease remission after enzyme replacement therapy is yet to be defined. There were no deaths reported in the three Gaucher studies in 80 patients with type 1 Gaucher's disease, but a number of unwanted effects occurred: diarrhea was reported in the majority of patients at the outset of the study, followed by weight loss, flatulence and abdominal pain. Headache and nausea were reported in up to 20% of subjects, and two subjects withdrew from the drug because of the development of an axonal neuropathy. Nonetheless, in exceptional circumstances, a licence for the use of miglustat (Zavesca) in adult patients with mild-to-moderate Gaucher's disease has been granted. A rigorous programme of intensive pharmacovigilance and clinical monitoring has been imposed on the company, Oxford GlycoSciences, which developed the drug, by the European Medicines Evaluation Agency (EMEA).

The licensing of miglustat for substrate reduction in Gaucher's disease offers the hope of further clinical development of other iminosugar analogues, such as NB-DGJ and the forthcoming late-phase analogues of the PDMP inhibitors, including GENZ 112638. Introduction of simple molecules that can be absorbed orally has the potential for much cheaper production than recombinant human glycoproteins that require further modification for effective delivery to the macrophage system. This observation offers the hope of increased availability of treatment for patients with Gaucher's disease who are unable to afford or obtain enzyme replacement therapy. Furthermore, the use of small-molecule inhibitors such as the iminosugars and morpholino compounds in severe neuronopathic lysosomal storage diseases can be considered where these two drugs may allow penetration into neural tissue and an improvement in the neurological injury resulting from pathological storage in this tissue. Further trials are in progress to determine whether or not substrate reduction therapy can synergise with enzyme replacement and whether the medication will indeed have any therapeutic value for patients suffering from otherwise intractable neuronopathic glycosphingolipidoses, including chronic neuronopathic Gaucher's disease. The data so far available, however, indicate that substrate reduction therapy remains a credible option for further therapeutic development and, if it should prove to be safe and effective in the long term, will be more attractive than enzyme infusions for many patients.

Development of pharmacological chaperone therapy

In many diseases due to mutations affecting a single polypeptide, the deficiency results from misfolding and aggregation of the protein before it reaches its intracellular site of action. In Gaucher's disease, there is evidence that some mutant glucocerebrosidase variants are misfolded and retained in the endoplasmic reticulum; thereafter they are transported via a quality-control pathway to the cytosol for proteolytic degradation, thus escaping delivery to the lysosome.

Pharmacological chaperones are molecules designed to bind to the nascent protein variant and alter its conformation, thus facilitating normal folding. They may serve as temporary inhibitors of the enzyme, often by binding at the active site; but in the case of lysosomal enzymes, binding at the neutral pH of the endoplasmic reticulum to accelerate folding may be only be temporary, since when the correctly folded protein reaches the acid environment of the lysosome, where further processing may occur, the affinity of the inhibitor is likely to be reduced.

Much research into pharmacological chaperones has been carried out in fibroblasts from patients with Fabry's disease and following the successful use of high-dose infusions of galactose given over the long term in one patient with the cardiac-restricted variant of this disease, clinical trials of the iminosugar, 1-deoxygalactonojirimycin, AT1001, a weak inhibitor of α-galactosidase A), are being conducted by the Amicus Company.

Numerous compounds have been evaluated as potential pharmacological chaperones for mutant glucocerebrosidases in Gaucher's disease; these also include iminosugar molecules. With encouraging studies of fibroblasts and other cells obtained from Gaucher's patients with different mutations, including the widespread N370S variant, multicentre phase I/II clinical trials are in progress using the agent AT2101 from Amicus. Although the belief that N370S represents a folding/aggregation mutant has been much disputed, isofagamine (AT2101) enhances its activity several-fold when studied in cultured cells obtained from patients by means of an in situ functional assay of lysosomal glucocerebrosidase using a novel fluorogenic substrate.

Although the clinical relevance of these studies has yet to be confirmed, the presence of the N370S variant protein in the cells of about 40% of the Gaucher's patients attending most clinics worldwide, renders this innovative option for oral therapy very attractive for rigorous clinical experimentation and testing.

Pathophysiology

The pathological macrophage of Gaucher's disease is a striking feature of the condition and provides a source of clues as the link between the storage of glycosphingolipid and the unexplained manifestations of the condition in many tissues. As set out above, Gaucher's disease is accompanied by weight loss, fatigue and increased metabolic rate, with a sustained inflammatory response accompanied by B-cell proliferation. Massive enlargement of the spleen and liver occur and there is pathological injury in the lung and brain as well as extensive destruction within bone. Recent studies have been reported in which the polymerase chain reaction has been used to identify genes whose transcriptional products are specifically increased in Gaucher's disease tissue. A recently described subtractive procedure was used to identify multiple genes, including a chemokine and others associated with the inflammatory response, whose expression was greatly increased. Northern and immunoblotting studies revealed increased mature forms of several cathepsin proteins identified in the gene expression profile and increased enzymatic activities of the proteinases, as well as cathepsins B, K and S, were identified in the tissue and in the serum of patients with Gaucher's disease. Increased cathepsin activities appear to be specific since they were not significantly elevated in the serum obtained from patients suffering from lysosomal disorders other than Gaucher's disease. Serum cathepsin activities correlated positively with objective clinical activity scores for Gaucher's disease. The relationship between the pulmonary activation-related chemokine (PARC) and a putative tumour-suppression gene is yet to be established in Gaucher's disease, but the study represented the first of many that will no doubt examine the secondary pathological gene expression in the condition. Further studies are likely to involve cDNA microarray analysis, which has already been used to identify upregulated genes in the spinal cords of mice suffering from Sandhoff disease, together with MHC class II–mediated responses in some way initiated by the GM_2 storage.

The Gaucher's cell is derived from a dedicated phagocytic lineage; but with the introduction of proteomics, using two-dimensional electrophoresis followed by mass spectroscopy of protein fragments, there is an obvious application to all the glycosphingolipid disorders. A glimpse of the extraordinary power of proteomics for investigating the molecular cell pathology of storage disorders has been provided by the characterization of mouse phagosome proteins after exposure of parent macrophages to solid particles of latex. More than 140 protein species including lysosomal cathepsins (and several already reported in the human Gaucher cDNA library) have been identified by this means. Clearly, the method has great potential for the systematic molecular investigation of cell activation and differentiation processes in the context of storage diseases.

In many respects Gaucher's disease, a rare disorder of the lysosome, carries with it a succession of productive achievements in translational research and, despite its rarity, is regarded as sufficiently important to attract substantial investment from at least five pharmaceutical companies eager to benefit from the introduction of innovative biological agents as well as small organic molecules for therapeutic use. The underlying pathophysiology of this unique macrophage disorder, with its ill-understood neurological manifestations, has many lessons for science and for the understanding of conditions apparently only remotely connected to the innate immune system.

Summary

Gaucher's disease is a model of an inborn error of metabolism and represents the most common disorder of a single organelle, the lysosome. Deficiency of a pathway for the breakdown of complex glycolipids in cell membranes leads to a multi-system disorder of varying severity that affects viscera, the nervous system and the skeleton. Recognition that lysosomal enzyme deficiencies can be complemented from the external fluid phase has led to spectacular therapeutic developments for an otherwise untreatable condition. Enzyme replacement therapy with targeted delivery to the pathological macrophages that serve as the cellular focus of this disease has been a singular success for the development of orphan drugs – and the biotechnology company Genzyme. Two additional recombinant protein molecules are in competitive late-phase development for enzyme replacement therapy. Other approaches, including marrow transplantation and a newly licensed orally active iminosugar designed to reduce the flow of new and incoming substrate, have been introduced for Gaucher's disease; the Genzyme Corporation also has an oral substrate-reducing agent in clinical trial based on unrelated chemistry. A further innovation has been the emergence of an experimental programme to develop pharmacological chaperones for Gaucher's disease and the glycosphingolipid lysosomal disorder Fabry disease.

Gaucher's disease has scientific ramifications in the fields of human genetics (it is over-represented in at least two population groups); cell biology; the pathobiology of the macrophage system; and glycosphingolipid metabolism in nervous tissue. The disease raises many questions of societal importance for the development of expensive agents to treat rare disorders and focuses awareness on the need for informative surrogate biomarkers that play a critical role in monitoring severity and the progress of treatment, – especially in cognate inherited diseases where recruitment for clinical trials is necessarily limited. About 4500 patients are receiving enzyme replacement therapy for Gaucher's disease: this is but a fraction of the global burden. Nonetheless, the signal success of the first definitive treatment for this fascinating lysosomal disease has stimulated continuing scientific development to address unmet and, at times, ill-understood medical needs.

Multiple-choice questions

1. Gaucher's disease is usually manifest in adults and children by:
   a. Splenomegaly and thrombocytopenia.
   b. Jaundice and abdominal pain.
   c. Blindness and neurodegeneration in childhood.
   d. Lytic lesions in bone.
   e. Ophthalmoplegia.
2. Gaucher's disease
   a. Is an inborn error of metabolism exclusively affecting Sephardic Jews.
   b. Is an inborn error of metabolism exclusively affecting Ashkenazi Jews.
   c. Is an inborn error affecting Menonite Jews.
   d. Is an inborn error of metabolism principally affecting boys and men.
   e. Is an inborn error of metabolism inherited as an autosomal recessive trait.
3. Gaucher's disease
   a. Is a lysosomal storage disorder.
   b. Is a protein aggregation disease.
   c. Is a peroxisomal membrane defect.
   d. Is a peroxisomal enzyme defect.
   e. Is not accessible to treatment.
4. Gaucher's disease
   a. Principally affects the cardiovascular system.
   b. Principally affects the mononuclear phagocyte system.

c. Principally affects the lymphatic drainage of the viscera.
   d. Principally affects the kidneys and disposal of unwanted proteins.
   e. Principally affects the liver and biliary system.
5. In Gaucher's disease, understanding the following processes has been important for therapeutic developments:
   a. The breakdown of carbohydrate stored in the body.
   b. The breakdown of membrane proteins.
   c. The metabolism of dietary lipids.
   d. The formation and breakdown of glycosphingolipids.
   e. The generation of intracellular signalling mechanisms in blood-forming organs.
6. The contemporary treatment of Gaucher's disease is
   a. An unlicensed orphan medication.
   b. A licensed drug.
   c. Two licensed drugs that can be purchased over the counter.
   d. Two licensed drugs available in many countries.
   e. Still at an experimental stage because of questionable efficacy in the long-term.

Answers

1 (a) is correct.
2 (e) is correct.
3 (a) is correct.
4 (b) is correct.
5 (d) is correct.
6 (d) is correct.

FURTHER READING

Abrahamov, A., Elstein, D., Gross-Tsur, V. *et al.* (1995). Gaucher disease variant characterized by progressive calcification of heart valves and unique genotype. *Lancet* **346,** 1000–3.

Aerts, J. M., Hollak, C., Boot, R., Groener, A. (2003). Biochemistry of glycosphingolipid storage disorders: implications for therapeutic intervention. *Philosophical Transactions of the Royal Society of London: Series B, Biological Sciences* **1433,** 905–14.

Barton, N. W., Brady, R. D., Drambrosia, J. M. *et al.* (1991). Replacement therapy for inherited enzyme deficiency – macrophage-targetted glucocerebrosidase for Gaucher's disease. *New England Journal of Medicine* **324,** 1464–70.

Beutler, E., Grabowski, G. A. (2001). Gaucher's disease. In Scriver, C. R., Valle, D., Beaudet, A. *et al.* (eds.). *The Metabolic and Molecular Bases of Inherited Disease.* Vol III. New York: McGraw-Hill, pp. 3635–68.

Boot, R. G., Verhoek, M., de Fost, M. *et al.* (2004). Marked elevation of the chemokine CCL18/PARC in Gaucher disease: a novel surrogate marker for assessing therapeutic intervention. *Blood* **103,** 33–9.

Brady, R. O., Kaufer, J. N., Bradley, R. M., Shapiro, D. (1966). Demonstration of a deficiency of glucocerebrosidase-cleaving enzyme in Gaucher's disease. *Journal of Clinical Investigation* **45,** 1112–15.

Butters, T. D., Dwek, R. A., Platt, F. M. (2003). New therapeutics for the treatment of glycosphingolipid lysosomal storage diseases. *Advances in Experimental Medicine and Biology* **535,** 219–26.

Cox, T., Lachmann, R., Hollak, C., Aerts, J. *et al.* (2000). A novel oral treatment of Gaucher's disease with N-butyldeoxynojirimycin (OGT 918) to decrease substrate biosynthesis. *Lancet* **355,** 1481–5.

Cox, T. M. (2002). Gaucher disease: understanding the molecular pathogenesis of sphingolipidoses. *Journal of Inherited Metabolic Disease* **24,** 106–21.

Dvir, H., Harel, M., McCarthy, A. A. *et al.* (2003). X-ray structure of human acid-β-glucosidase, the defective enzyme in Gaucher disease. *The EMBO Journal* **4,** 704–9.

Elstein, D., Hollak, C., Aerts, J. M. *et al.* (2004). Sustained therapeutic effects of oral miglustat (Zavesca, N-butyldeoxynojirimycin, OGT 918) in type 1 Gaucher disease. *Journal of Inherited Metabolic Disease* **41,** 4–14.

Fan, J. Q. (2003). A contradictory treatment for lysosomal storage disorders:inhibitors enhance mutant enzyme activity. *Trends in Pharmacological Sciences* **24,** 355–60.

Frustaci, A., Chimenti, C., Ricci, R. *et al.,* (2001). Improvement in cardiac function in the cardiac variant of Fabry's disease with galactose-infusion therapy. *New England Journal of Medicine* **345,** 25–32.

Hollak, C. E. M., van Weely, S., van Oers M. H. J., Aerts, J. M. F. G. (1994). Marked elevation of chitotriosidase activity. A novel hallmark of Gaucher disease. *Journal of Clinical Investigation* **93,** 1288–92.

Lachmann, R. H., Grant, I. R., Halsall, D., Cox, T. M. (2004). Twin pairs showing discordance of phenotype in adult Gaucher's disease. *Quarterly Journal of Medicine* **97,** 199–204.

Mistry, P. K., Davies, S., Corfield, A., Dixon, A. K., Cox, T. M. (1992). Successful treatment of bone marrow failure in Gaucher's disease with low-dose glucocerebrosidase. *Quarterly Journal of Medicine* **303,** 541–6.

Mistry, P. K., Wright, E. P., Cox, T. M. (1996). Delivery of proteins to macrophages: implications for treatment of Gaucher's disease. *Lancet* **348,** 1555–9.

Mizukami, H., Mi, Y., Wada, R. *et al.* (2002). Systemic inflammation in glucocerebrosidase-deficient mice with minimal glucosylceramide storage. *Journal of Clinical Investigation* **109,** 1215–21.

Moran, M. T., Schofield, J. P., Hayman, A. R. *et al.* (2000). Pathologic gene expression in Gaucher disease: up-regulation of cysteine proteinases including osteoclastic cathepsin K. *Blood* **96,** 1969–78.

Pastores, G. M., Weinreb, N. J., Aerts, H. *et al.* (2004). Therapeutic goals in the treatment of Gaucher disease. *Seminars in Hematology* **41**(4 Suppl 5), 4–14.

Street, R. A., Chung, S., Wustman, B. *et al.* (2006). The iminosugar isofagamine increases the activity of N370S β glucosidase in Gaucher fibroblasts by several mechanisms. *Proceedings of the National Academy of Sciences (USA)* **103,** 13813–18.

Von Figura, K., Hasilik, A. (1986). Lysosomal enzymes and their receptors. *Annual Review of Biochemistry* **55,** 167–93.

3

Obesity

J. Shakher, P. G. McTernan and Sudhesh Kumar

Obesity is a common metabolic disorder characterised by an excess of body fat to the extent that it leads to complications. In simple terms, obesity results from a chronic imbalance between energy intake and expenditure. Although this is the fundamental basis, the aetiology is multi-factorial, implicating genetic susceptibility, environmental and social influences and the dysfunction of the still incompletely understood physiological mechanisms regulating body weight through control of appetite and energy expenditure.

Epidemiology

The prevalence of obesity has been rising steadily in the past few decades. Where epidemiological data are available, based on body mass index (BMI), 64 million Americans are overweight and a further 44 million obese. A dramatic rise in the prevalence of obesity has been seen in England, where it has increased three-fold, from 6% to 17% in men and 8% to 20% in women between 1980 and 1998. Obesity, once thought to be mainly a problem of the affluent West, is now a major global problem, with increased prevalence in developing countries. Another worrying trend is the increasing numbers of children with obesity, resulting in an increase in the prevalence of childhood type 2 diabetes.

Definition and classification

Obesity is subjectively viewed as 'excess deposition of fat'. For health professionals there are various ways of measuring the degree of obesity; these include assessments of body weight in relation to height and also the distribution of body fat.

Body mass index (BMI)

BMI is calculated using the formula weight in kilograms/ height in metres^2. Based on BMI, the World Health Organization (WHO) has classified overweight and obesity in adults (Table 3.1). This measure of obesity has, however, some limitations:

1. The same BMI may reflect different degrees of fatness in different ethnic groups. For example, Black Americans have a higher BMI than Whites; by contrast, Chinese and other Asians have a lower BMI than Whites.
2. BMI would also be elevated in a more muscular person because excess of weight would be contributed by muscle, not fat.
3. There are problems with clearly defining BMI in growing children and adolescents.
4. Most importantly, BMI does not provide any information about the pattern of body fat distribution, such as central or abdominal obesity. Visceral fat, which is regarded as metabolically undesirable fat, is associated with increased risk of type 2 diabetes and other cardiovascular complications.

Topography of fat

Visceral or central fat is termed 'bad fat' as it is more metabolically active and, through lipolysis, releases large amounts of non-esterified fatty acids (NEFAs),

Table 3.1 WHO classification of overweight and obesity

BMI (kg/m^2)	Classification
< 18.5	Underweight
18.5–24.9	Normal range
25.0 or higher	Overweight
25.0–29.9	Pre-obese
30.0–34.9	Obese class I
35.0–39.9	Obese class II
40.0 or higher	Obese class III

which can drain directly into the portal circulation. Excessive flux of NEFAs into the liver and the peripheral circulation has been suggested to cause insulin resistance by interfering with the uptake and utilisation of glucose. A waist circumference of more than 102 cm in men and 88 cm in women results in increased risk of impaired glucose tolerance, diabetes mellitus, dyslipidaemia and hypertension, and these in turn compound the risk of coronary heart disease in these individuals.

Waist-to-hip ratio (WHR)

To measure central or abdominal obesity, the waist-to-hip ratio (WHR) is used. There are several ways of measuring waist circumference, and it is therefore important to clarify the method used to measure it. A common measurement used is the minimum circumference between the costal margin and iliac crest with the subject standing; the hip circumference is a maximum circumference over the buttocks. Both measurements are taken in the horizontal plane. Women with a WHR greater than 0.85 and men with WHR greater than 1.0 are said to have central obesity.

Waist circumference (WCR)

Waist circumference (WCR) alone may be used to classify a patient's level of risk of complications through obesity. Waist circumferences greater than 94 cm and 102 cm in men and greater than 80 cm and 88 cm in women approximate BMIs greater than 25 and 30 respectively and can add to the information gained through BMI alone.

Imaging

Computed tomography (CT) and magnetic resonance imaging (MRI) scans can give better direct measurements of fat distribution, but these methods are used only for research.

Skinfold thickness

Measurement of the subcutaneous layer using calibrated callipers has limitations, as it does not reflect central obesity; in severe obesity, moreover, the jaws of the callipers would not fit. However, this method may be useful in children. Four skinfold thickness measurements (biceps, triceps, subscapular and suprailiac) have been used to give a more accurate estimate of fatness.

Total body water (TBW)

Laboratory methods like estimation of total body water (TBW) or total body potassium are used mostly for research purposes. Body composition is assumed to be of two compartments, one consisting of fat mass (FM) and the other a mixture of non-fat components called fat-free mass (FFM). The FM can be derived from calculation of TBW by using isotope-labelled water. The fat is hydrophobic (anhydrous) and FFM contains approximately 73% water [FFM (kg) = TBW/0.73]. This principle is used in the measurement of body fat by 'fat monitoring scales' that use bioelectrical impedance to estimate TBW and derive a measure of body fat.

Aetiology of obesity

The cause of obesity is a multi-factorial and includes:
1. Genetic susceptibility
2. Environmental and social influences
3. Defective appetite regulation
4. Reduced energy expenditure
5. Obesity secondary to other causes (Table 3.2)
   a. Endocrine diseases (hypothyroidism, Cushing's syndrome)
   b. Drug-induced factors (neuroleptics, antidepressants)
   c. Psychological factors

Table 3.2 Secondary causes of obesity

Endocrine (determinants that play a minor role in the aetiology of obesity)
Cushing's Syndrome
Hypothyroidism
Polycystic ovarian syndrome
Drugs
Antidepressants (increase appetite)
Tricyclics (e.g. amitriptyline, imipramine, clomipramine)
Selective serotonin reuptake inhibitors (SSRIs; e.g. fluoxetine, paroxetine)
Benzodiazepines
Lithium
Antipsychotics (e.g. olanzapine)
Steroid hormones
Psychological
Binge-eating disorder (unlike bulimia, this does not involve induced vomiting)
Night eating syndrome (morning anorexia, evening hyperphagia, insomnia)

Genetic factors

The genetic influence on the regulation of body weight has been assessed by twin, adoption, population, and family studies. The inheritable risk of obesity is thought to be around 30%. Twin studies looking at twins reared apart and response to re-feeding experiments indicate genetic influence accounting for 70% of the difference in BMI. Overfeeding in identical pairs of male twins showed that two brothers from the same set of twins are more likely to respond similarly to overfeeding. Closer correlation in body weight is observed between monozygotic than dizygotic twins. The Danish adoption study involving 800 adoptees showed no relationship between the body weight of adoptees and their adopted parents but a close relationship with the body weight of their biological parents. Adoption studies indicate heritability of about 33%. Obesity also tends to run in families, and risk of obesity is higher if a person has obese parents. This could imply that both genetic and environmental factors are at work.

There are also rare genetic syndromes associated with obesity through unknown mechanisms, such as Prader-Willi, Alstrom and Laurence-Moon-Biedl syndromes.

Recently specific genetic mutations involved in appetite regulation in obesity have been described (Fig. 3.1).

1. Commonest is the mutation of MC4-R, which accounts for about 5% of childhood obesity. This condition is associated with morbid obesity with hyperphagia and continuous food-seeking behaviour.
2. Mutation of the leptin gene with deficiency of leptin has been identified in two children from consanguineous marriage. The children are born phenotypically normal and at the age of 3 to 4 months develop obesity, hyperphagia and failure to attain puberty (similar to gene mutation in the ob/ob mouse).
3. Mutation of the leptin receptor gene has also been described. In a French family, three sisters showed early onset of obesity, impaired linear growth and hypothalamic amenorrhoea.
4. POMC gene mutation results in the early onset of obesity, adrenal insufficiency and red hair pigmentation.
5. Mutation of the PPAR-γ gene results in marked obesity, and three out of four patients have type 2 diabetes.

Thrifty-genotype and thrifty-phenotype hypotheses

Obesity is increasing in developing countries, particularly in urban areas. Certain ethnic groups have a higher propensity to develop obesity (e.g. Pima Indians and Polynesians). It is thought that when these people move from a period of food deprivation to a period of plenty, the presence of the thrifty gene facilitates the expression of obesity. In contrast, the Barker hypothesis (thrifty-phenotype hypothesis) argues that it is poor intra-uterine nutrition that is important. Low-birth-weight babies appear to be at a higher risk of developing abdominal obesity, with complications such as hypertension, coronary heart disease and diabetes later in life, especially

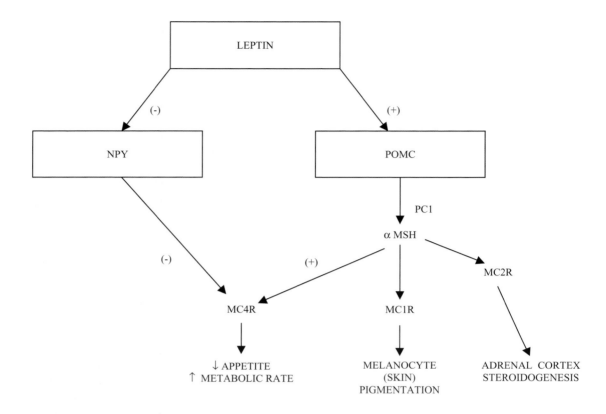

α MSH = melanocyte stimulating hormone
MCR   = melanocortin receptors
NPY   = neuropeptide Y
PCI   = proconvertase inhibitor
POMC   = pro-opiomelanocortin

Figure 3.1 Genetic mutations in appetite regulation in obesity.

when these children are exposed to high-fat foods and sedentary lifestyle.

Environmental factors

The rise in global epidemic of obesity has occurred over too short a period to implicate genetic factors as a major determinant; instead, environmental and social factors seem to play a major role. Modernisation has seen a parallel rise in obesity. A sedentary lifestyle and the availability of high-calorie diets in a genetically susceptible individual lead to obesity.

Automobiles and television are two obvious environmental culprits. There is a remarkably close association between indices of inactivity and the degree of obesity. The number of hours of television watching is directly associated with increases in body weight. In the USA, an increased in fat content in the diet over the years has mirrored the increase in obesity.

In developed societies, there is an inverse relationship between obesity and socio-economic status, particularly among women, lower economic status favouring the development of obesity. Adequate resources will allow someone to make a choice of healthy low-fat food and also enable him or her to indulge in recreational sporting activities.

Certain ethnic groups have different beliefs and perceptions about body weight. Exercise activity with a view to losing weight is still a relatively new concept and may not be readily acceptable in some ethnic groups. Obesity is more common among Black than White women, affecting 60% of middle-aged Black compared to 33% of White women.

Physiological mechanisms for the regulation of body weight

Regulation of appetite

Appetite is regulated at various levels, particularly at the hypothalamus (central regulator) and at the gastrointestinal tract and adipose tissue (peripheral regulators) through excitatory and inhibitory signals (Fig. 3.4).

Gastrointestinal signals

These include the following:

Cephalic signals: Appetite is stimulated even before the food is ingested. The thought, smell and sight of food results in the desire to eat; similarly, foods that are considered unpleasant can elicit a negative signal to the brain.

Taste signals: Once the food is in the mouth, appreciation of texture, particle size and temperature is achieved by the taste buds. Peptides such as substance P are released, which may play a role food preferences.

Gastric signals: Gastric factors such as hunger pangs or a sensation of fullness through gastric distention can influence appetite via the autonomic nervous system. The vagus nerve acts as a principal sensory relay to the hypothalamus via the medulla.

During the digestive process, peptides such as CCK, enterostatin and gastrin-releasing peptide (GRP) are released, which can decrease food intake. Some of these gastrointestinal or gut peptides are also found in the, brain and vice versa (brain–gut axis).

Cholecystokinin (CCK) is located in the duodenal and proximal jejunum and also in the central nervous system. Its principal action is to locally stimulate gall-bladder contraction and pancreatic enzyme secretion. It induces satiety by binding to CCK-A receptors via vagal afferent neurons. Although CCK-B receptors predominate in the brain, the action of CCK is peripheral, as it does not cross the blood-brain barrier and its effect is blocked by vagotomy.

Gastrin-releasing peptide, another gut peptide, is a 27–amino acid polypeptide sharing its biological activity with bombesin, which is found in the skin, brain and gut of frogs. Gastrin-releasing peptide releases gastrin from antral G cells and also acts as a neurotransmitter to enhance satiety.

Enterostatin can decrease food intake, particularly the intake of dietary fat. It is secreted from the pancreas in relation to fatty meals.

Incretin belongs to another family of gastrointestinal signals, of which glucagon-like peptide-1 (GLP-1) has been extensively studied. Glucagon-like peptide is 42–amino acid polypeptide found in mucosal cells in the duodenum, jejunum and ileum and is structurally similar to glucagon. It is released in response to foods like glucose, triglycerides and amino acids. It is also known as glucose-dependent insulinotrophic polypeptide, as it enhances insulin release in response to oral glucose loads.

The release of insulin facilitates glucose disposal, and a gradual dip of 7% to 10% of glucose triggers hunger signals (metabolic signal).

Nutrient signals, from nutrients such as glucose and fatty acids, can modulate food intake. Glucose, the major fuel of the brain, may act directly on the central nervous system to modulate appetite. Fatty acids and their metabolites can decrease food intake.

The sympathetic nervous system also has a role to play in generating satiety. Stimulation of the β-3 adrenal receptor on brown adipose tissue results in heat production, and this thermogenic effect may decrease food intake. Peripheral β-2 adrenal receptors may reduce food intake through a mechanism other than heat production.

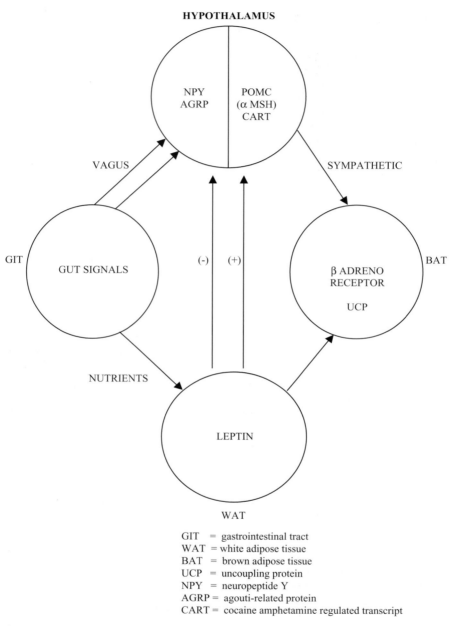

GIT   = gastrointestinal tract
WAT = white adipose tissue
BAT = brown adipose tissue
UCP = uncoupling protein
NPY = neuropeptide Y
AGRP = agouti-related protein
CART = cocaine amphetamine regulated transcript

Figure 3.2 The hypothalamus.

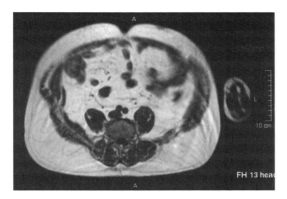

Figure 3.3 An MRI scan of the abdomen at level of L4, showing visceral fat in a patient with abdominal obesity. (Courtesy of Dr Arpan Bannerjee, Consultant Radiologist, Heartlands Hospital, Birmingham.)

Central regulation of appetite

The central appetite modulator is the hypothalamus and its connections to the pituitary gland. Broadly speaking, a lesion of ventral medial hypothalamus (VMH) results in hyperphagia, decreased energy expenditure and obesity. Whereas destruction of the lateral hypothalamus (LPH) has the opposite the effect, with a reduction of body fat. The paraventricular nucleus (PVN) acts as a centre for regulation of food intake by influencing composition of food, its size and the frequency of its consumption. These nuclei 'talk to each other' through neurotransmitters to maintain energy balance and body weight around a set point. These neurotransmitters may stimulate (orexigenic) or inhibit (anorexigenic) appetite (Table 3.3).

Neuropeptide Y (NPY) is the most powerful stimulatory peptide that promotes food intake and energy storage. A 36–amino acid peptide, it is structurally related to pancreatic polypeptides (PPs) and is distributed in the central and peripheral nervous system. Neuropeptide Y is synthesised in the neurons of the arcuate nucleus (ARC) of the hypothalamus. One pathway projects into the PVN, the centre of food regulation, and the other, into the reproductive axis. Neuropeptide Y has wide-ranging effects on food intake, reproduction, anxiety, memory reten-

Table 3.3 Endogenous factors regulating appetite

Stimulatory	Inhibitory
Neuropeptide Y	α melanocyte–stimulating hormone
Agouti-related protein	Corticotropin-releasing hormone (CRH)
Galanin	Glucagon-like peptide 1 (GLP-1)
Melanin-concentrating hormone (MCH)	Cocaine- and amphetamine-related transcript (CART)
Norepinephrine	Leptin
Orexins/hypocretin	Cholecystokinin

tion, thermal regulation and adrenal, cardiovascular and gastrointestinal regulation. It activates its receptors Y1 to Y6. Neuropeptides Y1 and Y5 modulate appetite and Y2 may acts as autoreceptor for NPY release.

Neuropeptide Y can also reduce energy expenditure by inhibiting the sympathetic stimulation of brown adipose tissues. It is negatively regulated by leptin and insulin.

Melanin-concentrating hormone (MCH) is another powerful stimulatory peptide identified in the hypothalamus. Mice with deletion of MCH develop hypophagia, an increased metabolic rate and lower body weight.

Others peptides, such as *galanin (GAL,)* preferentially stimulate fat intake, whereas *norepinephrine (NE)* stimulates carbohydrate ingestion.

Endogenous opiods can increase feeding behaviour; *dopamine* and the weaker orixegenic peptides *orexin A and, orexin B* (hypocretin 1 and 2) also modulate food intake.

Anorexigenic signals

Pro-opiomelanocortin (POMC)

The POMC gene is located on chromosome 2. It is synthesised in the pituitary, arcuate nucleus of the hypothalamus, solitary tract of the medulla, and several peripheral tissues such as the testes, ovary, placenta, duodenum, liver, kidneys, lungs, thymus, adrenal medulla and lymphocytes. It is most abundant in the corticotroph cells of the pituitary. Processing of POMC is tissue-specific; in the anterior pituitary, POMC is processed predominantly into adrenocorticotrophic hormone (ACTH); it is stimulated by corticotrophin-releasing hormone (CRH) and inhibited by glucocorticoids. In the hypothalamus, ACTH is further cleaved to form α melanocyte-stimulating hormone (MSH). The effect of POMC expression is probably mediated by α MSH through five melanocortin receptors (MC-1R to MC-5R). MC-3R and MC-4R are expressed in the hypothalamus and involved in energy homeostasis. Melanocortin receptor-4 is distributed through the brain but found in higher concentrations in the paraventricular nucleus (PVN) and lateral hypothalamus, important energy regulation sites. α-MSH acts on MC-4R and possibly MC-3R; it inhibits eating behaviour and increases energy expenditure. Melanocortin receptor-4 knockout mice show hyperphagia, hyperinsulinaemia and obesity. The human homologue is a relatively common single-gene defect associated with childhood-onset obesity.

Agouti-related protein (AGRP), an endogenous protein, is a potent antagonist to MC-3R and MC-4R. It acts as a stimulatory peptide and is co-expressed with the potent orexegenic NPY in the hypothalamus. Leptin negatively regulate these peptides as obese mice deficient in leptin (ob/ob mice) show increased levels of AGRP and NPY.

Corticotrophin-releasing hormone (CRH) is another food-inhibitory peptide, which probably acts on the PVN through its receptors CRH1 and CRH2. Urocortin, which is a member of the CRH family, is more potent in suppressing feeding behaviour.

Neuro-peptide CART (cocaine and amphetamine–regulated transcript), found in hypothalamic nuclei, probably inhibits feeding by instruction of NPY signalling.

Serotonin (5 HT) is derived from the amino acid tryptophan and is widely distributed in the brain and spinal cord. Sixteen 5 HT receptors are recognised, some of which are found in the anterior pituitary and hypothalamus. In the anterior pituitary, 5 HT receptors are involved in the secretion of LH, ACTH and prolactin; in the hypothalamus, they modulate food intake. Serotonin in general decreases food intake by acting through its receptors.

Leptin

The discovery of leptin in 1994 led to a paradigm shift in the view of adipose tissue from being primarily a depot of stored fat to a highly metabolically active specialised tissue participating in energy metabolism. Leptin is secreted by fat cells and feeds back to the hypothalamus where it activates POMC, the gene expression of which could also be affected by NPY, opiods, sex steroids, glucocorticoids, dopamine and CRH. Leptin circulates bound to plasma protein and affects appetite regulation centrally. Leptin can reach the brain through diffusion or through the cerebrospinal fluid, probably by binding to receptors in the choroid plexus. Leptin inhibits peptides like NPY, agouti-related peptide (AGrP) and MCH, and activates POMC, precursor of α MSH, to cause a decrease in food intake. Thus, leptin-deficient mice caused hyperphagia by rise in NPY and AGRP and a fall in α MSH and CART.

Leptin also has important peripheral actions that help to oxidise lipid, particularly in muscle, where it stimulates lipid oxidation by stimulating adenoside monophosphate-(AMP) related kinase. It is also possible that leptin may stimulate energy expenditure by increasing sympathetic outflow in brown adipose tissue in addition to its effects on lipid oxidation.

A leptin receptor (Ob-R) was first isolated by cloning from the murine choroid plexus. A receptor gene mRNA is processed differently in various tissue (choroid plexus, lungs, kidneys, hypothalamus) with at least five leptin receptors, ObR-a, Ob-Rb, Ob-Rc, Ob-Rd, Ob-Re and Ob-Rf. All of them share a common extra-cellular domain or leptin binding site and differ in intracellular sequence. Ob-Rb has an intercellular domain to initiate signalling of leptin effects. In the db/db mouse, a d/b mutation affects the intracellular signalling (similar to insulin resistance in type 2 diabetes, post-receptor defect).

Regulation of energy expenditure

This can be broadly considered under three headings:

1. Resting metabolic rate (RMR). This is energy produced while the subject is fasting or after the absorptive state to maintain the basic life-supporting process. This accounts for 50% to 70% of daily energy expenditure and is related to fat-free mass or lean body mass. Therefore RMR is high in males. Obese people are not shown to have impaired RMR.

2. Energy expenditure due to physical activity accounts for approximately one-third of energy expenditure. This is related to the duration and intensity of exercise. Obese persons spend more energy during physical activity, as an obese person has to move a greater mass. Most studies have shown that obese persons tend to be less active, and this is related to a reduced level of non-exercise energy expenditure.

3. Expenditure related to the metabolism of food results in an expenditure energy called the thermic effect of food (TEF). It is possible that obese person may have a depressed thermic effect.

Cellular mechanisms of thermogenesis

In mammals, brown adipose tissue (BAT) is a site of energy expenditure. Exposure to cold leads to sympathetic stimulation of brown adipocytes via norepinephrine (NE) binding to β-adrenergic receptors. The adrenergic receptors, especially β-3 receptors, are highly expressed in BAT. As in white fat, sympathetic stimulation promotes the hydrolysis of triglycerides (TGLs), with release of free fatty acids (FFAs) and glycerol. However, in BAT, most FFAs are immediately oxidised in mitochondria and, because of uncoupling proteins (UCPs), a large amount of heat is produced. [bypassing the adenosine triphosphate (ATP) synthesis pathway]. This process is part of what is called non-shivering thermogenesis. UCP1 is expressed mainly in the BAT in mice and is a vital mitochondrial protein. UCP expressions is upregulated by catecholamines, thyroid hormone and leptin and decreased by glucocorticoids. Two other uncoupling proteins UCP2 and UCP3, have been cloned. In human infants, BAT comprises up to 5% of body weight and then diminishes with age, virtually disappearing by adulthood. The human white fat does express β-3 receptors, albeit at very low levels. It is likely that there are alternative mechanisms for the control of energy expenditure in humans.

Consequences of obesity

The consequences of obesity are medical, psychological and economic.

Mortality

Obesity is related to increased risk of mortality. This begins to rise with a BMI greater than 25; BMI above 30 is associated with a 1.5 to 2.4 excess independent risk of mortality. In some ethinic groups (e.g. Indo-Asians), a higher risk is seen at a lower BMI of 25 kg/m^2.

Hypertension

The prevalence of hypertension is increased with greater BMI, especially with central obesity. Elevations in blood pressure above 140/90 are approximately three times more prevalent among obese persons than the non-obese. The exact mechanism of association of central obesity and hypertension is not fully defined. Insulin resistance is thought to be a metabolic link between hypertension and obesity. Hyperinsulinaemia as a consequence of insulin resistance is thought to increase blood pressure by enhancing sodium reabsorption directly through its effects on distal renal tubules and indirectly through central stimulation of the sympathetic nervous system as well as augmentation of angiotensin II–mediated aldosterone secretion.

Dyslipidaemia

Obesity is associated with an adverse lipid profile, increase in total cholesterol and, triglyceride, total and small dense low-density-lipoprotein (LDL) cholesterol, and in Apo-B. A low level of high-density-lipoprotein (HDL) cholesterol is an important contributor to the risk of CHD.

Coronary heart disease (CHD)/ cerebrovascular disease

Central obesity is associated with an increased risk of CHD. Along with this there is also an increased risk of a recurrent cardiac event after acute myocardial infarction. The increased CHD morbidity and mortality may be related to traditional risk factors such as hypertension and dyslipidaemia or the effect of obesity per se on the cardiovasculature. Obesity is associated with disturbances in cardiac function and structural changes in the absence of hypertension and underlying organic heart disease. There is an increase in total blood volume in proportion to body weight resulting in higher cardiac output. Volume overload of the left ventricle results in increased left ventricular stress, which stimulates eccentric hypertrophy of the ventricular wall with resultant diastolic dysfunction. Over time, excessive wall stress can cause ventricular dilatation, resulting in systolic dysfunction. This disorder is described as obesity cardiomyopathy. These factors also account for a two-fold increase in risk of stroke in obese persons compared to the non-obese.

Sleep apnoea/Pickwickian syndrome

Both obstructive and central sleep apnoea are more common in severely obese persons. Weight reduction is an effective therapy for sleep apnoea, possibly due to reduction of mechanical effects of excess fat in the neck, but other, as yet unclear, mechanisms may also apply. Morbid obesity can lead to hypoxaemia as well as carbon dioxide retention.

This combination is seen in obesity-hypoventilation syndrome.(Pickwian syndrome).

Other metabolic problems related to obesity include polycystic ovarian syndrome and increased risk of pregnancy related hypertension and gestational diabetes.

The risks of gallstones, osteoarthritis and cancer of the distal colon are reported to be increased with obesity.

Psychological

In western culture, obesity is perceived as unattractive. Poor self-image leads to a variety of psychological problems such as anxiety, depression, anger, guilt and somatic complaints. These, in turn, lead to a withdrawal syndrome with disruption of social relationships.

Economic

Besides medical complications, the financial cost directly attributed to obesity is much higher than the cost implicated in coronary heart disease or hypertension. Added to this is the indirect cost to the economy from loss of productivity due to sick leave or disability. The economic burden is doubled in developing countries, as the cost of health care is added on to the problem of fighting infection and undernutrition.

Insulin resistance (IR) and diabetes mellitus

Obesity is characterised by hyperinsulinaemia and IR. Despite this association, not all obese person develop diabetes. However, increase in weight is a major risk for the development of type 2 diabetes; this is especially true of central obesity. Indeed, the majority of type 2 diabetic patients are obese. It is postulated that non-esterified fatty acids (NEFAs) from a central fat depot cause IR by stimulating gluconeogenesis in liver and inhibiting glucose uptake and utilisation. The precise mechanisms for the obesity-associated IR are not fully understood. Recent advancements in adipocyte cell biology have improved our understanding of the adipose tissue as an 'endocrine organ' secreting various mediators and may help to explain the link between obesity and type 2 diabetes.

Resistin

In the early part of 2001, a protein encoded by a new adipocyte-specific gene called resistin was identified in murine adipose tissue. In addition to this, experiments determined that the protein was predominately expressed in adipose tissue, while thiazolidinediones (TZDs), specifically rosiglitazone, appeared to reduce its secretion from fat. The protein has been named resistin, for resistance to insulin. Studies with mice have shown that resistin is increased markedly by both genetic and diet-induced obesity. In contrast, administration of resistin to these models demonstrated impairment of both glucose tolerance and insulin action in normal mice. Therefore resistin appears to be a possible candidate to explain the anti-diabetic effects of TZDs as well as suggesting a mechanism by which excess adiposity leads to insulin resistance. However, the physiological role of resistin in human subjects is still not well understood.

Adiponectin

Thiazolidinediones also appears to regulate the secretion of a substance called adiponectin by raising the levels of adiponectin following adminstration of TZD. In obese humans and people with type 2 diabetes, plasma levels of adiponectin are reduced. It is proposed that the reduced level of adiponectin in these diseases could cause hyperinsulinaemia, hyperglycaemia, perhaps insulin resistance, and increased NEFA. In animals, these metabolic changes are reversed by the administration of adiponectin.

Tumour necrosis factor α (TNF-α)

Tumour necrosis factor α is an inflammatory cytokine produced by macrophages; it is also secreted by adipose tissue. Levels of TNF-α are elevated in obese animals and during insulin resistance. It may cause insulin resistance by decreasing glucose transport (GLUT 4 transport), interfering with insulin receptor and with the post-receptor signalling pathway. It reduces the activity of lipoprotein lipase and increases hormone-sensitive lipase (two key enzymes involved in regulating of lipolysis and lipogenesis respectively), resulting in increases in NEFAs.

Interleukins

Interleukins 6 and 8 are also cytokines, which are secreted by adipocytes. Interleukin 6 increases lipolysis similar to TNF-α, resulting in elevated NEFA levels.

Treatment of obesity

Treatment of obesity requires a multi-disciplinary team approach involving dieticians, psychologists, physicians and surgeons, where appropriate. The cornerstone of obesity management is lifestyle modification, leading to small but permanent changes in food choices and increased levels of physical activity.

Assessment of the obese patient

Clinical assessment of obesity includes measuring BMI, waist circumference and pattern of obesity. Age of onset and factors contributing to obesity are recorded. The food diary is a useful way of ascertaining the caloric intake, food preferences and any abnormal eating pattern or behaviour that would require an additional psychological input. The presence of osteoarthritis or heart disease would influence the exercise-management programme. Treatment of associated risk factors such as diabetes, hypertension and lipid profile would need to be addressed. Secondary causes of obesity, such as hypothyroidism, must also be considered where appropriate. Drugs including antidepressants may need to be reviewed. Motivation is the key factor that will determine the success of the treatment plan.

The support of family members is equally important if long-term weight loss is to be achieved. Subsequently, realistic goals are set with an aim of losing about 5% to 10% of total body weight. Once all these considerations have been reviewed, the lifestyle programme is drawn up, tailored to each individual's needs and expectations.

Dietary therapy

Diet must be nutritionally adequate and suitable for the individual patient. Too rigid a diet, very low in calories, is likely to succeed in the short term, but ultimate failure is likely and the patient will resume over-eating. Long-term dieting is necessary to lose fat through regular follow-up and feedback. Changes in eating habits are necessary to maintain the initial weight loss. Dietary therapy alone has limited success, as no more than 10% of obese persons achieve a successful outcome. Very low calorie diets (VLCDs) restricted to less than 800 calories per day with delivery of high-protein supplements can be tried. These diets must be followed under careful medical supervision and can induce weight loss of up to 1.5 to 2.5 kg a week. A VLCD is associated with partial regaining of weight in the long term; it also has side effects such as orthostatic hypotension, fatigue, dry skin, hair loss, menstrual irregularities and an increased incidence of gallstones. In view of this, it is better to adopt a diet that is moderately restricted in calories, amounting to a deficit of 500 to 1000 calories per day, which the patients are likely to follow in the long term.

Behaviour modification

Both psychoanalysis and psychotherapy are useful adjunctive process. Behavioural therapy helps to change the eating behaviour of a person in the long term. It can be done in groups, often headed by a psychologist. Cognitive behavioural therapy is useful in some obese people with abnormal eating patterns.

Exercise

Obese persons tend to be inactive, and physical exercise is essential to maintain weight loss. The aim is to build up the duration of physical activity over days and months. If patients are unable to pursue more vigorous exercise, the most commonly recommended alternative is walking for about 10 to 15 min per day twice weekly initially and gradually increasing to 30 to 45 min every other day.

Drug therapy

Several drugs have been used over many years and some have been withdrawn because of side effects. For example, amphetamines decreases appetite but causes elevated mood, sleep disturbance, agitation, and psychosis; they also have addictive properties. Fenfluramine is a centrally acting agent that was withdrawn because of associated cardiac valvulopathy.

The two drugs most commonly used today are orlistat (Xenical) and sibutramine (Meridia).

Orlistat is an inhibitor of gastric and pancreatic lipase, enzymes necessary for breakdown of fat. Inhibition of lipases reduces absorption of dietary fat by about 25% to 35%, which results in an increased fat load in the colon. Side effects include fatty and oily stools, faecal urgency, incontinence and flatulence. Side effects are more common if the patient has increased his or her fat intake to more than 30%. The drug is licensed for obese persons or persons with a BMI of 28 kg/m$^($ with associated risk factors. Orlistat is given as 120 mg three times daily with meals. Orlistat is now commonly prescribed on a long-term basis and has been shown to help maintain weight loss. Theoretically, long-term administration can cause malabsorption of the fat-soluble vitamins (A, D, E and K); a vitamin supplement is therefore recommended.

Centrally active drugs

Sibutramine acts centrally to inhibit reuptake of serotonin and noradrenaline, thus enhancing satiety. The dosage is 10 mg per day, which may be increased to 15 mg per day if the initial weight loss is less than 2 kg after 4 weeks of treatment. If there is less than 5% weight loss in 3 months or if the patient regains as much as 3 kg, treatment may have to be discontinued. Sibutramine's side effects are dryness of mouth, insomnia and an increase in blood pressure. Blood pressure must be monitored every fortnight for the first 2 months and thereafter on a monthly basis. Sibutramine can be given for a year to patients 18 to 65 years old with a BMI above 30 or a BMI of 27 with 'co-morbidities'. It is contraindicated in people with organic causes of obesity, neuropsychiatric disorders, coronary artery disease, heart failure, blood pressure above 145/95, and those on antidepressants,.

Newer agents under evaluation include lipase inhibitors, β-3 receptor agonists, the anticonvulsant topiramate and cannabinoid receptor antagonists. Rimonabant is a selective antagonist of the central cannabinoid CB1 receptor, which suppresses appetite and also facilitates smoking cessation.

Surgery

Surgery is for people with grade 3 obesity and severe co-morbid conditions. Patients should be well informed and motivated and selected by a multidisciplinary team comprised of medical, surgical and dietary expertise, as well as a psychiatrist. There are two types of obesity surgery: (1) restrictive and (2) combined restrictive and malabsorptive.

Restrictive surgery uses bands or staples to restrict food intake. The bands or staples are surgically placed near the top of the stomach to section off a small portion often called a stomach pouch. A small outlet is left at the bottom of the pouch, allowing the food to remain in the pouch longer and thus create a sensation of fullness.

- Vertical banded gastroplasty (VBG) is a restrictive surgery, since it involves surgically creating a stomach pouch. It required the use of bands and staples and was the most frequently performed procedure in the early 1990s.
- Gastric banding involves the use of a band to create the stomach pouch.
- Laparoscopic gastric banding (Lap-Band) is a 'keyhole' procedure whereby an inflatable silicone cuff or band is placed around the upper part of the stomach. The band can be inflated with a small volume of fluid through an injection port under the skin in order to achieve a stomach pouch of the desired capacity.

Both VBG and laparoscopic banding produce about 50% to 60% loss of excess weight over the first 2 years postoperatively. Side effects are due to the small capacity of the stomach pouch (approximately 1 cup of food). Eating too much at once or not chewing enough to break down the food can cause nausea, stomach discomfort and vomiting. Other side effects are heartburn and abdominal pain.

Possible complications include the leakage of stomach juices into the abdomen, injury to the spleen, band slippage, erosion of the band, breakdown of the staple line, and stretching of the stomach pouch from overeating. Infection or death has been reported in less than 1% of patients. Patients must learn to eat smaller amounts of food at any one time, chew their food well and eat slowly. Failure to adjust eating habits may inhibit weight loss.

Combined restrictive and malabsorptive surgery is a combination of restrictive surgery (stomach pouch) with bypass (malabsorptive surgery), in which the stomach is connected to the jejunum or ileum of the small intestine, bypassing the duodenum.

- Roux-en-Y gastric bypass (RGB) is the most commonly performed gastric bypass procedure, RGB involves the creation of a stomach pouch to restrict food intake. A direct connection, which is Y-shaped, is made from the ileum or jejunum to the stomach pouch to ensure malabsorption. The longer the segment of small intestine bypassed, the greater the malabsorption component and the greater the weight loss.
- Biliopancreatic diversion (BPD) is the most extensive and complicated obesity surgery. A portion of the stomach is removed and the remaining section is connected to the ileum. This procedure successfully promotes weight loss, but it is typically used only for persons with severe obesity who have a BMI of 50 or more.

There is a greater weight loss in gastric bypass compared to gastroplasty after 1 year. Over 2 years, gastric bypass surgery patients have been shown to lose two-thirds of their excess weight. The success rate for weight loss for RGB is 68% to 72% over a 3-year period; the analogous success rate for BPD is 75%.

Side effects are due to the rapid transit of food, whereby food moves too quickly through the small intestine, causing nausea, weakness, sweating, faintness, and sometimes diarrhoea after eating ('dumping syndrome'). There can also be an inability to eat sweets without severe, debilitating weakness and sweating. Dairy intolerance, constipation, headache, hair loss and depression are other possible side effects.

There is a risk of nutritional deficiency due to bypass of the duodenum and part of the jejunum, where many nutrients are absorbed. Nutritional deficiencies include malabsorption of vitamin B12, leading to anaemia and iron deficiency. The reduction in vitamin D and calcium absorption can cause osteoporosis and other bone disease. Lifelong use of nutritional supplements such as multivitamins, vitamin B12, vitamin D and calcium is necessary.

Weight loss usually occurs soon after obesity surgery and continues for 18 months to 2 years. Most patients regain some weight after this time; after five years, however, patients have reported maintaining a weight loss of 60%.

Medical benefits include an enhanced quality of life, improved mobility and stamina, as well as better mood and self-esteem. There is also improvement diabetes mellitus, glucose intolerance, high cholesterol/triglycerides, hypertension and sleep apnoea. In general, 60% of patients with obesity-related medical conditions are no longer on medication for these conditions 3 years after surgery.

Clinical scenarios

1. A 40-year-old woman with a history of fatigue, lethargy and weight gain over the preceding 6 months presented to the medical clinic. She also noticed excessive loss of her scalp hair.
   What is the likely diagnosis?

What test would you do to confirm the diagnosis?
What is the treatment?
   Answer: Her symptoms are suggestive of hypothyroidism. A thyroid function test would confirm the diagnosis. Replacement with thyroxin may help to control weight gain.

2. A 30-year-old weight lifter became depressed after his wife left him. He stopped going to the gym and subsequently was started on an antidepressant by his general practitioner. He gained about 10 kg in weight.
   What factors contributed to his weight gain?
   What would be the best management of his condition?
   The two likely factors in causing his weight gain are lack of exercise and the antidepressant drug. Management would involve gradual withdrawal of the medication, assessment by psychologist, and resumption of exercise.

3. A 32-year-old obese woman with BMI of 40 was referred to obesity clinic. She had a poor self-image, remained confined to her home and was socially isolated. She had a history of sexual abuse as a child.
   What is the underlying cause of her obesity?
   What treatment apart from diet and exercise would be beneficial?
   Her depressive illness with comfort eating and lack of activity could have contributed to her obesity. Psychological assessment and treatment would help her to gain self-confidence.

4. A 19-year-old Asian girl with BMI of 42 is seen at the obesity clinic. She is unable to control her food intake and admits to binge eating. All her family members are obese, and her 7-year-old brother weighs 80 kg. Her brother and she would regularly buy food from a nearby Indian 'take away' at night, even though they had had their dinner. Their mother would give them money for food and sweets.
   What is the reason for her weight gain and what treatment would be helpful?
   The reason for her weight gain is an excess intake of calories. Her eating behaviour has been

influenced by her home environment. The treatment would have to be directed towards the entire family, especially the mother, in order to have a successful outcome.

Multiple-choice questions (true or false)

1. Obesity is
   a. confined to western society
   b. commoner in the lower socio-economic class
   c. a condition in which endocrine factors play a major role
   d. a condition to which genetic factors contribute about 30%
2. Central obesity is associated with
   a. an increase in type 2 diabetes
   b. decreased insulin resistance
   c. hyperlipidaemia
   d. hypertension
3. Appetite stimulatory peptides are
   a. neuropeptide Y
   b. AGRP
   c. MCH
   d. α MSH
4. Leptin
   a. is secreted by the hypothalamus
   b. inhibits appetite
   c. acts through its receptors
   d. can stimulate energy expenditure
5. Body mass index (BMI)
   a. accurately reflects central obesity
   b. is useful to define childhood obesity
   c. is higher in muscular person
   d. is helpful in grading obesity

Answers

1 a, F; b, T; c, F; d, T
2 a, T; b, F; c, T; d, T
3 a, T; b, T; c, T; d, F
4 a, F; b, T; c, T; d, T
5 a, F; b, F; c, T; d, T

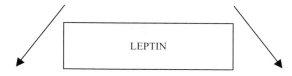

Figure 3.4

FURTHER READING

Alpert, M. A. (1993). Obesity and the heart. *American Journal of Medical Science* **306,** 117.

Barnett, A. H., Kumar S. (2004). *Obesity and Diabetes.* New York: John Wiley & Sons.

Barsh, G. S., Farooqi, I. S., O'Rahilly, S. (2000). Genetics of body-weight regulation. *Nature* **404,** 644–51.

Bhopal, R. (2002). Epidemic of cardiovascular disease in South Asians. *British Medical Journal* **324,** 625–6.

Bray, G. A., Tartaglia, L. A. (2000). Medicinal strategies in the treatment of obesity. *Nature* **404,** 672–7.

Bray, G. A. (1996). Health hazards of obesity. *Endocrinology and Metabolism Clinics of North America* **25,** 907–19.

Bray, G. A. (1999). Clinical evaluation of the obese patient. *Baillieres Best Practices Research Clinical Endocrinology and Metabolism* **13,** 71–92.

Campfield, L. A., Smith, F. J. (1999). The pathogenesis of obesity. *Baillieres Best Practices Research Clinical Endocrinology and Metabolism* **13,** 13–30.

DeFronzo, R. A. (1991). Insulin resistance syndrome. *Diabetes Care* **14,** 173.

De Fronzo, R. A. (1975). The effect of insulin on renal handling of sodium, potassium, calcium, and phosphate in man. *Journal of Clinical Investigation* **55,** 845–55.

DeGroot, L. J., Jameson, J. L. (2001). *Endocrinology* 4th edn. Philadelphia: W. B. Saunders Company.

Despres, J. P. (1996). Hyperinsulinaemia as an independent risk factor for ischemic heart disease. *New England Journal of Medicine* **334,** 952–7.

Despres, J. P. (1998). The insulin resistance syndrome of visceral obesity: effect on patients' risk. *Obesity Research* **6(Suppl 1**), 8S–17S.

Faloia, E., Giacchetti, G., Mantero, F. (2000). Obesity and hypertension. *Journal of Endocrinological Investigation* **23,** 54–62.

Flier, J. S. (2001). Diabetes: The missing link with obesity? *Nature* **409,** 292–3.

Forouhi, N. G. (2001). Relation of CRP to cardiovascular risks in European and South Asians. *International Journal of Obesity* **25,** 1327–31.

Ford, E. S. (2002). Prevalence of the metabolic syndrome among US adults: findings from the Third National Health and Nutrition Examination Survey. *Journal of the American Medical Association* **287,** 356.

Greenspan, F. S. (2003). *Basic and Clinical Endocrinology*, 7th edn. Stamford, CT: Appleton & Lange.

Heck, A. M., Yanovski, J. A., Calis, K. A. (2000). Orlistat, a new lipase inhibitor for the management of obesity. *Pharmacotherapy* **20,** 270–9.

Hotamisligil, G. S. (1993). Adipose expression of TNF-α: direct role in obesity linked insulin resistance. *Science* **259,** 87–91.

Hubert H. B. (1983). Obesity as an independent risk factor for cardiovascular disease: a 26 year follow-up of participants in the Framingham Heart Study. *Circulation* **67,** 968–77.

James, W. P. T., Astrup, A., Finer, N. *et al.*, for the STORM Study Group (2002). Effect of sibutramine on weight maintenance after weight loss: randomised trial. *Lancet* **356,** 119–25.

Kahn, B. B., Flier, J. S. (2000). Obesity and insulin resistance. *Journal of Clinical Investigation* **106,** 473–81.

Kopelman, P. G. (1998). Obesity as a medical problem. *Nature* **404,** 635–43.

Leptin: Review article. *Nature* **395,** 763–70.

Montague, C. T., Farooqi, I. S., Whitehead, J. P. *et al.* (1997). Congenital leptin deficiency is associated with severe early-onset obesity in humans. *Nature* **387,** 903–8.

Montague, C. T., O'Rahilly, S. (2000). The perils of portliness: causes and consequences of visceral adiposity. *Diabetes* **49,** 883–8.

Neel, J. V. (1962). Diabetes mellitus: a thrifty genotype rendered detrimental by process. *American Journal of Human Genetics* **14,** 353–62.

National Obesity Forum: Guideline on Management of Adult Obesity. www.nationalobesityforum.org.uk.

Niewoehner, C. B. (2004). *Endocrine Pathophysiology*, 2nd edn. Raleigh, NC: Hayes Barton Press.

NICE Guidelines on obesity. www.nice.org.uk.

NIH Consensus Statement (1991). *Gastrointestinal surgery for severe obesity*. **9,** 1–20.

Per Bjorntorp (2001). *International Textbook of Obesity*. West Sussex, UK: John Wiley & Sons.

Rea, T. D. (2001). Body mass index and the risk of recurrent coronary events following acute myocardial infarction. *American Journal of Cardiology* **88,** 467–72.

Reaven, G. M. (1996). The role of insulin resistance and the sympathoadrenal system. *New England Journal of Medicine* **334,** 374.

Ross, R. (1999). Atherosclerosis – an inflammatory disease. *New England Journal of Medicine* **340,** 115–26.

Schwartz, M. W., Woods, S. C., Porte, D. Jr. (2000). Central nervous system control of food intake. *Nature* **404,** 661–71.

Seidell, J. C. (1998). Epidemiology: definition and classification of obesity. In Kopelman P. G., Stock, M. (eds.). *Clinical Obesity*. Oxford, UK: Blackwell Science, pp. 1–17.

Seidell, J, C. (2000). Obesity, insulin resistance and diabetes – a worldwide epidemic. *British Journal of Nutrition* **83(Suppl 1),** S5–8.

Sjostrom, L. V. (1992). Mortality of severely obese subjects. *American Journal of Clinical Nutrition* **55,** 516S.

Sjostrom, L. V. (1992). Morbidity of severely obese subjects. *American Journal of Clinical Nutrition* **55(Suppl 2),** 508S–515S.

Steppan, C. M. (2001). The hormone resistin links obesity to diabetes. *Nature* **409,** 307.

Stunkard, A. J., Wadden, T. A. (1992). Psychological aspects of severe obesity. *American Journal of Clinical Nutrition* **55,** 524S–32S.

Stunkard, A. J., Sorensen, T. I., Hanis, C. *et al.*(1986). Adoption study of human obesity. *New England Journal of Medicine* **314,** 193–8.

Stunkard, A. J., Foch, T. T., Hrubec, Z. (1986). A twin study of human obesity. *Journal of the American Medical Association* **256,** 51–4.

Tartaglia, L. A. (1997). The leptin receptor. *Journal of Biological Chemistry* **272,** 6093–6.

Wardlaw, S. L. (2000). Clinical review 127: obesity as neuroendocrine disease: lessons to be learned from proopiomelanocortin and melanocortin receptor mutations in mice and men, *Journal of Clinical Endocrinology and Metabolism* **86,** 1442–6.

Weyer, C. Hypoadiponectinemia in obesity and type 2 diabetes: close association with insulin resistance and hyperinsulinemia. *Journal of Clinical Endocrinology and Metabolism* 2001; 86:1930.

Weatherall, D. J., Ledingham, J. G. G., Wareell, D. A. (1996). *Oxford Textbook of Medicine*, 3rd edn. Oxford, UK: Oxford University Press.

Wilding, J. P. H. (1997). Obesity treatment – science, medicine and the future. *British Medical Journal* **315,** 997–1000.

World Health Organisation (1998). *Obesity: Preventing and Managing Global Epidemic*. Geneva: World Health Organisation.

4

Autoimmune mechanisms

Anthony P. Weetman

Key points

- Most autoreactive T and B cells are removed or inactivated during foetal development; several mechanisms normally control the remainder. Disorders in these mechanisms cause autoimmune disease.
- Susceptibility to most autoimmune disease is dependent on both genetic and environmental factors. Genes in the major histocompatibility complex, called HLA in humans, have an important role in determining whether an immune response (including autoimmunity) occurs.
- Autoimmune disease is produced by humoral (antibody) or cell–mediated (T cell–dependent) mechanisms.
- There is a spectrum of autoimmune diseases ranging from organ-specific disease, such as those conditions affecting the endocrine system (see also Chapter 7), to non-organ-specific diseases, such as rheumatological disorders.
- Autoimmune thyroid disease may result in hyperthyroidism (Graves' disease), caused by TSH receptor–stimulating antibodies, or hypothyroidism (Hashimoto's thyroiditis or primary myxoedema), caused mainly by antibodies against thyroid peroxidase and by T cell–mediated injury to thyroid follicular cells.

The immune system evolved to protect the organism against infection and, probably later, against malignancy. The devastating effects of congenital or acquired immunological deficiency states, result-ing in infection and neoplasia, are proof of this central role. Protection must be effective against the vast array of infectious agents likely to be encountered, and it operates via two flexible recognition systems: the T cells and B cells. These recognise foreign antigens by specific cell surface receptors: the T-cell receptor (TCR) and surface-bound immunoglobulin or antibody. By recombination events, dealt with below, a vast array of antigens can be recognised by these receptors, but such huge diversity brings the penalty that, occasionally, self- or autoantigens will be targets for the immune response.

At the beginning of the twentieth century, it was generally believed that the body was incapable of reacting against itself, a postulate termed *horror autotoxicus* by Paul Ehrlich. The reasons for this were not understood, and much of the study of immunology for the next 50 years was devoted to the immunochemistry of antigens and antibodies. Then, however, the investigation of transplantation and rejection by Medawar, Owen, and others, and the demonstration of autoimmune disease in animals and humans by Witebsky, Rose, Doniach and Roitt marked a new era in which immunobiology and its application to clinical problems became dominant. Thanks to the ideas of Jerne and Burnet, attention focused on the selection of antibodies by antigen as a means of ensuring a restricted and yet appropriate response by particular clones of B cells. By comparison, 'clonal abortion' was postulated as a mechanism whereby autoreactive cells were destroyed by their contact with self antigens at a critical stage of fetal development: failure of clonal abortion would cause autoimmune disease.

Since the early 1960s, these initial precepts have been expanded to include T cells, which lie at the heart of the immune response. The recent application of molecular techniques has led to spectacular developments in our understanding of how the T and B cells most likely to be beneficial are selected, and how tolerance to self antigens is imposed on potentially dangerous cells recognising these autoantigens. The same methods have greatly increased our knowledge of how cells of the immune system communicate with each other, through an enormous array of receptor–ligand pairs and soluble mediators called cytokines.

The normal immune response

Autoimmune mechanisms of disease can be understood only by reference to the normal immunological response to an exogenous antigen. A brief outline follows, taking in sequence the steps of antigen presentation, activation of T cells and B-cell stimulation (Fig. 4.1).

Antigen presentation

Extracellular bacteria, viruses, and proteins are taken up by endocytosis (via binding to receptors on the cell surface) or phagocytosis and processed by the antigen-presenting cell (APC) before presentation to the T cell. This processing occurs in acidic endosomes or lysosomes, resulting in short peptide fragments of around 20 amino acid residues. These peptides then associate with one of a particular group of polymorphic molecules encoded by the class II region of the major histocompatibility complex (MHC) genes. This complex is termed human leucocyte antigen (HLA) in humans, and three types of class II gene product are expressed: HLA-DR, HLA-DQ and HLA-DP (Fig. 4.2). The intracellular association between antigenic peptide and class II

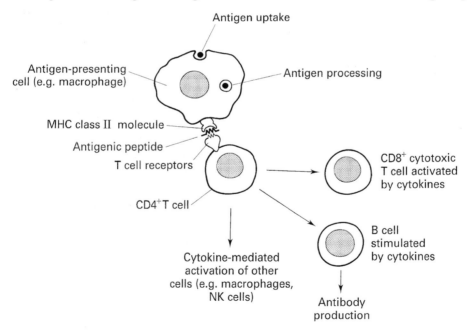

Figure 4.1 Antigen presentation to a CD4$^+$ T cell induces helper activity for CD8$^+$ T cells or antibody production and is mediated by cytokines. Such cytokines can also activate other cells, for example, natural killer (NK) cells.

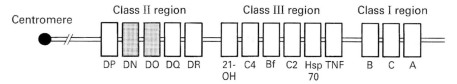

Figure 4.2 Sequence of the major loci in the HLA complex on chromosome 6. The entire complex covers over 300 kb and is not drawn to scale. Shaded gane loci are not expressed. TNF, tumour necrosis factor; hsp, heat shock protein; 21-OH, A, B loci encoding 21-hydroxylase; C4, Bf and C2 are complement components.

molecule stabilises the latter; this association occurs predominantly in distinct vesicles following the synthesis of class II molecules in the Golgi apparatus. Antigen binding to class II molecules on the antigen-presenting cell (APC) surface is not a major pathway, because class II molecules bind processed peptides with high affinity and are, therefore, already complexed when expressed.

The peptide sequence of an antigen recognised by a T cell is termed the *epitope*. Each epitope constitutes around 10 amino acid residues that lie in an antigen-binding groove of the class II molecule during presentation; the ends of peptide that are not part of the epitope protrude from either side of the groove (Fig. 4.3). The polymorphic structure of class II molecules ensures that only certain peptides fit each particular groove, accounting for the influence of class II genes in determining immune responses. Selection is also imposed during the next step in the immune response, because the peptide–class II molecule complex is recognised by a specific T-cell receptor (TCR). If a suitable TCR is not available, no response to this particular epitope is possible. Most foreign antigens contain several T-cell epitopes; therefore a response can be mounted by genetically diverse individuals.

T-cell stimulation

The major class of TCR is a heterodimer composed of an α- and a ß-chain (Fig. 4.4), each with a constant (C) and variable (V) region, joined by junctional (J) and diversity-generating (D) sequences. Epitope recognition is primarily determined by the V region and,

to a lesser extent, the D and J sequences. A minor population of T cells expresses a TCR comprising a γ- and a σ-chain; the exact function of these cells is not clear. The structure of the TCR is similar to that of the immunoglobulin molecule. There are around 100 different $V\alpha$ and $V\beta$ gene segments in humans and these can pair with over 50 $J\alpha$ and 13 $J\beta$ segments, as well as two D regions in the case of the β-chain. In addition, nucleotides can be added between the V–J, V–D, and D–J regions during gene rearrangement, a process not encoded in the germ line. The result is a vast repertoire of different TCRs, only a

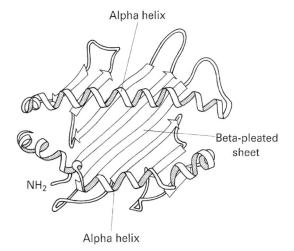

Figure 4.3 Model of the antigen-binding groove on the HLA-A2 molecule (after Bjorkman *et al.*, 1987. *Nature*, 329, 506). Class II molecules have a similar structure. The most polymorphic residues line the groove, either on the α-helices or the β-pleated sheet floor.

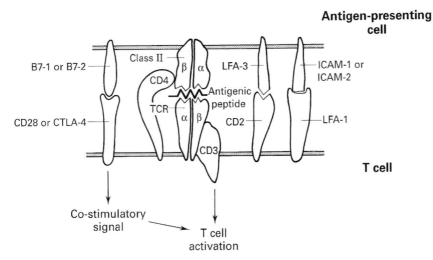

Figure 4.4 Major molecules involved in antigen presentation to a CD4+ T cell. Soluble cytokines (e.g. IL-1) are also involved. LFA, lymphocyte function-associated antigen; ICAM, intercellular adhesion molecule.

small fraction of which is ever used. Many TCRs formed during development will, by chance, recognise self antigens, and such T cells will (hopefully) be deleted.

The trimolecular interaction between an $\alpha\beta$ TCR and the MHC class II–peptide complex results in T-cell activation through signal transduction mediated by CD3, a complex of proteins non-covalently associated with the TCR (Fig. 4.4). This leads to the production of interleukin-2 (IL-2) and the IL-2 receptor by the T cell, which in turn promote proliferation and further activation. However, several other accessory molecules are required for the interaction of the TCR and the APC to occur efficiently: T cells at different stages of development require varying combinations of accessory molecules (Fig. 4.4). Foremost among these are:

1. Adhesion molecules; these allow binding between the cells: some of these interactions partially activate the T cell. Some adhesion molecules contribute to the binding of T cells to any APC; others are restricted to interactions with certain types of cell.

2. The CD4 and CD8 glycoproteins; these recognise cells carrying MHC class I and II molecules, respectively. The T-cell CD4 molecule stabilises the interaction between the class II molecule–peptide complex and the TCR by binding to a non-polymorphic region on the MHC molecule. As CD4 is expressed only on a subset of T cells, these alone can interact with class II molecule–peptide complexes. The reciprocal T-cell subset expresses CD8, which binds to class I MHC molecules. These present endogenous antigens (such as viral proteins synthesised within a target cell) rather than antigens of exogenous origin. Therefore a major role for the CD8+ subset is recognition (and destruction) of virally infected cells.

3. Co-stimulatory molecules, particularly B7–1 and B7–2 (CD80 and CD86); these are present on APCs and provide an essential second signal to CD4+ cells by binding to CD28 and CTLA-4 on these T cells. In the absence of this co-stimulatory signal, CD4 T cells are not stimulated by the class II molecule–peptide complex and, in many cases, instead become inactivated. This process is called *anergy*. Anergic T cells are paralysed, failing to respond to antigen subsequently even if this is presented with the correct second signals.

Table 4.1 Profile of cytokines produced by the two main CD4$^+$ T Cell subsets, T_H1 and T_H2, in humans. Naive T cells may only secrete IL-2 after initial stimulation and some activated cells have cytokine profiles that do not fall into these two categories

	T_H1	T_H2
γ-IFN	++	0
TNF	++	+
Lymphotoxin	++	−
IL-2	++	+
IL-4	−	++
IL-6	−	++
IL-10	+	+
Function	Macrophage activation, producing delayed-type hypersensitivity responses	B cell stimulation leading to antibody formation, eosinophil and mast cell production

Note:

IL, interleukin; γ-IFN, γ-interferon; TNF, tumour necrosis factor.

CD4$^+$ T cells are often called T-helper (TH) cells. Once a CD4$^+$ T cell has been activated, it can proliferate and express a number of different cytokines. Two broad patterns of cytokine production can be identified (Table 4.1), which correspond to the main effector functions of CD4$^+$ T cells – namely, producing an inflammatory or *delayed-type hypersensitivity* response (TH1 cells) and providing help for antibody production by B cells (TH2 cells). The cytokines produced by each CD4$^+$ subset reciprocally inhibit the other, resulting in either a predominantly delayed-type hypersensitivity or a humoral response, mediated by whichever subset is initially activated. Cytokines released by stimulated CD4$^+$ T cells are also essential to the activation of CD8$^+$ T cells, which can then mediate cytotoxicity against antigen-specific targets.

B cells and antibody production

Antibodies are the second type of molecule involved in specific antigen recognition. Each comprises two heavy and two light chains. The amino-terminus in both sets of chains contains a V-region domain, analogous to the TCR and also responsible for antigen binding. The V region determines the antibody specificity – that is, what antigen the antibody will recognise. Unlike the TCR, antibodies usually recognise conformational determinants on an antigen that depend on its tertiary structure.

Antibody diversity is generated by recombination events similar to those responsible for TCR diversity, with the important addition of somatic mutation (see also Chapter). An enormous number of different immunoglobulin molecules can be generated by (1) the large number of genomic immunoglobulin *V* gene segments whose mRNA can be spliced with different *D* and *J* segments; (2) nucleotide addition at the regions coding for the heavy chain VDJ and light chain VJ junctions; (3) pairing between the different types of heavy and light chain; and (4) somatic mutation, which changes nucleotides coding for the key parts of the immunoglobulin V region involved in antigen recognition, resulting in slightly different V regions derived from a primordial *V* gene segment. The last mechanism is particularly important in determining fine specificity, and most B cells express V regions that have undergone somatic mutation.

Antibodies are synthesised by B cells after antigen-specific triggering of the TCR induces T-cell activation and the provision of cytokines that cause B-cell

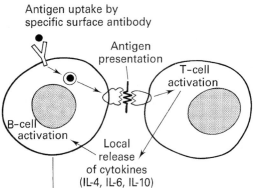

Figure 4.5 Role of B cells in antigen presentation. Surface immunoglobulin allows presentation of specific antigen: close contact with the T cell permits local delivery of non-specific cytokines to the appropriate B cell.

activation (Fig. 4.2). However, B cells can also serve as APCs to amplify the immune response. The presence of specific antibodies on the B-cell surface allows them to focus on a particular antigen, which can be taken up and processed. This leads to a close collaboration between the T and B cell, resulting in amplification of the immune response (Fig. 4.5).

Discrimination between self and non-self

The best way to prevent autoimmune disease is not to generate T cells and B cells that recognise self. However, the random events of recombination for both TCRs and antibodies, which are necessary to generate diversity, ensure that autoreactive cells *will* be produced. A hierarchy of defences has evolved to deal with this threat (Table 4.2); different autoantigens evoke different control mechanisms.

Clonal deletion of T cells

Two kinds of experiment have supported Burnet's hypothesis of clonal abortion or deletion. The first utilised the knowledge that a particular kind of TCR, encoded by the *V* gene segment termed $V\beta17a$, recognises the MHC class II molecule I-E, which occurs in some strains of mice. Strains of animals not expressing I-E have $V\beta17a^+$ T cells, but crossing these mice with a strain expressing I-E results in the near absence of $V\beta17a^+$ T cells in the offspring. Sequential study of these animals revealed that $V\beta17a^+$ T cells were present in the thymus early in T-cell development, at a stage when CD4 and CD8 are both expressed. However, these cells were deleted as they matured into the distinct $CD4^+$ and $CD8^+$ populations, following recognition of I-E at a critical stage in their development. The second kind of experiment

Table 4.2 Hierarchy of defence mechanisms normally preventing autoimmune disease: clonal deletion of autoreactive T cells is the most secure; sequestered autoantigen, the least

Mechanism	Comment
1. Clonal deletion	Some T cells inevitably escape
2. Clonal anergy	Can be bypassed, e.g. if excessive IL-2 is provided
3. Functional ignorance	Certain self antigens may not be susceptible to processing by APCs; exact importance unknown
4. Active suppression	Requires active and continuing suppression of autoreactive T cells and, therefore, is likely to become defective with time
5. Lack of T cell help	Autoreactive $CD8^+$ T cells and B cells are only harmful if specific $CD4^+$ T cells are stimulated
6. Sequestered autoantigen	Accidental exposure to antigen will rapidly induce an autoimmune response

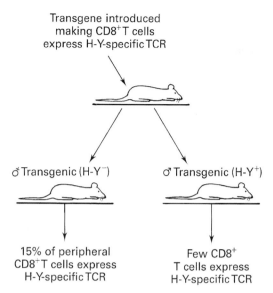

Transgene introduced
making CD8$^+$ T cells
express H-Y-specific TCR

♂ Transgenic (H-Y$^-$)

♂ Transgenic (H-Y$^+$)

15% of peripheral
CD8$^+$ T cells express
H-Y-specific TCR

Few CD8$^+$
T cells express
H-Y-specific TCR

Figure 4.6 Demonstration of intrathymic clonal deletion in transgenic mice. Male mice constitutively expressing the male transplantation antigen H-Y delete the majority of CD8$^+$ T cells bearing the transgenic H-Y-specific TCR during intrathymic development. Those that escape deletion have low levels of CD8, which may limit their pathogenicity.

used transgenic mice to demonstrate clonal deletion (Fig. 4.6) with similar results.

The thymus can also positively select T cells, again shown most elegantly in transgenic experiments. Such selection occurs at an earlier stage of T-cell development than negative selection and ensures that the T-cell repertoire contains T cells that react appropriately with self MHC molecules. T cells with an absent or very high affinity for MHC molecules (the latter, therefore, likely to be dangerous) die. Although the molecular events causing positive and negative selection are only now becoming clarified, it seems certain that the developing T cell must encounter appropriate adhesion molecules, cytokines and co-stimulators as well as self MHC to mature: inappropriate or inadequate recognition of self MHC leads to deletion by programmed cell death (apoptosis).

It has recently become clear that many self antigens are expressed within the thyroid during development on specialised APCs and that a single defect in a gene called *AIRE* (standing for 'autoimmune regulator') can interfere with this process. Individuals with a mutation in *AIRE* develop autoimmune polyglandular syndrome type 1 in childhood. Typically in this autoimmune recessive condition, there is a combination of autoimmune disease of the parathyroid glands, causing hypoparathyroidism, and adrenal cortex, causing Addison's disease, together with a susceptibility to chronic mucocutaneous *Candida* infections. Several other autoimmune disorders, including thyroid disease, also occur in these patients.

These observations clearly show the importance of clonal deletion in eliminating the bulk of autoreactive T cells, but they also show that deletion is not complete, even for self antigens that are in abundance. The huge number of potential autoantigens, which may not be expressed at the appropriate time for deletion to occur, poses one limitation on this mechanism. It is also difficult to envisage the intrathymic expression of all self antigens, such as tightly regulated cell surface receptors and intracellular enzymes. This is because only soluble or cell-bound antigens in the blood are likely to enter the thymic medulla, where they can be presented to T cells by dendritic cells and epithelial cells.

The failure to delete T cells capable of reacting with tissue-specific autoantigens may not be a problem provided that the antigen remains sequestered. Autoreactive CD8$^+$ T cells can also be permitted provided that CD4$^+$ T cells with the same specificity are firmly controlled or *tolerised*, as the CD8$^+$ subset will not respond unless appropriate help is provided for their activation. Both of these are rather dangerous strategies to prevent autoimmune disease, because infections and local inflammation in an organ may lead to the release of hitherto hidden self antigens or provide indiscriminate cytokine-mediated help, resulting in an autoimmune response. Therefore additional mechanisms have evolved to control autoreactive T cells that have escaped intrathymic deletion.

Anergy and T cells

Anergy is an incompletely understood process by which autoreactive T cells are not deleted but are somehow disabled so that they no longer respond to autoantigen. As long as an anergic T cell continues to ignore an autoantigen, no danger of autoimmune disease exists, but there is always a potential risk that anergy may be reversed. Anergy may occur in the thymus or in the periphery. As an example, *intrathymic tolerance* imposed during development can be demonstrated in mice for T cells reactive with endogenous Mls (minor lymphocyte-stimulating) antigens. The Mls-1ᵃ autoantigen is recognised by T cells expressing a TCR that includes the Vβ6 element. If a strain of mouse that possesses the Mls-1ᵇ rather than the Mls-1ᵃ autoantigen is immunised with Mls-1ᵃ cells, the animal does not mount a response against Mls-1ᵃ, but also it does not delete the Vβ6⁺ T cells, which can still be detected in the recipient. By using a chimaeric animal in which the bone marrow and thymus are derived from different strains, it can be shown that anergy is induced in the thymus.

Peripheral tolerance has been most clearly demonstrated in transgenic animals. For example, if I-E⁻ murine β cells (in the islets of Langerhans of the pancreas) express an I-E transgene, they become I-E⁺, and it might be predicted that Vβ17a⁺ T cells (discussed above) present in these otherwise I-E⁻ mice would recognise and attack the β cell. However, this is not the case, nor are the Vβ17a⁺ T cells absent, showing that insufficient I-E finds its way into the developing thymus of the transgenic mice to delete those 'self-reactive' T cells (Fig. 4.7). Instead, the T cells become anergic, ignoring the β cells (although it must be said that this anomalous expression of I-E class II molecules by the β cell alters intracellular processes, which ultimately leads to β-cell death and diabetes).

Intrathymic and peripheral anergy both occur because an antigen-specific TCR encounters a class II molecule–antigen complex in the absence of a co-stimulatory signal, particularly B7–1 and B7–2. This results in a fundamental change in intracellular tyrosine kinase activation by the TCR, together with an

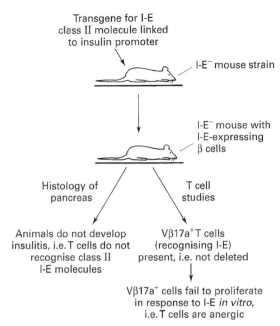

Figure 4.7 Demonstration of peripheral tolerance in transgenic mice. Mice expressing the MHC class II molecule I-E normally delete T cells with the Vβ17a TCR; these cells are only found in I-E⁻ animals. If the I-E molecule is expressed by pancreatic β cells in I-E⁻ mice, Vβ17a⁺ T cells are not deleted but become anergic becaused the β cells fail to express the necessary co-stimulatory signal.

alteration in inositol phosphates and intracellular free calcium. These changes prevent the T cell from producing IL-2. In the thymus, it is likely that thymic epithelial cells that do not express co-stimulators are responsible for anergy, particularly for those T cells specific for epithelial cell peptides not expressed by thymic dendritic cells.

However, under normal circumstances, pancreatic β cells (and most other cells in the body) do not express class II, which is largely a property of 'professional' APCs such as macrophages, dendritic cells and B cells. At first sight, therefore, peripheral tolerance hardly seems important, but class II expression can be induced by cytokines, particularly γ-interferon (γ-IFN). As these cytokines are released locally in inflammation, the resulting capacity to induce anergy could prevent autoimmune attack at the exact time and place when it is likely to occur. It is also now known that T-cell deletion can occur in the periphery as well as in the thymus. This could be an extreme outcome of the same mechanisms that result in anergy. The affinity of interaction between the TCR and MHC class II molecule–peptide complex may determine the ultimate fate of the T cell both within the thymus and in the post-thymic environment.

T-cell suppression

Anergy only operates on certain T cells, depending mainly on their maturational state. There are also theoretical problems with anergy as an explanation for control of all autoreactive T cells. First, it is hard to imagine how thymic epithelial cells can both positively select and anergise T cells, but this may depend on different properties of medullary and cortical epithelial cells and on the stage of T-cell development. Second, anergy could be bypassed, for instance by conditions that supply sufficient IL-2 to overcome the anergic state. Finally, 'professional' APCs are present in most tissues, and these might be expected to deliver appropriate co-stimulatory signals if self antigens are processed, thus overcoming peripheral tolerance.

The concept of suppressor T cells has been controversial, but there are now many examples suggesting that self-reactive T cells that have escaped deletion or anergy are prevented from causing autoimmune disease. The best example currently of this mechanism is that mediated by a population of T cells characterised in mice through their expression of CD4 and high levels of the IL-2 receptor CD25. Such cells have been termed T-regulatory cells (Tregs for short). Animal experiments using models of autoimmune endocrine disease produce by neonatal thymectomy have shown that such Tregs can prevent autoimmunity if transferred from animals without disease. There is accumulating evidence that such Tregs also mediate similar functions in humans, and ways to upregulate their activity could be a novel way to suppress autoimmune disease in the future.

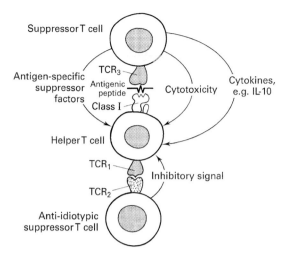

Figure 4.8 Possible mechanisms to explain T cell-mediated suppression of autoreactive T cells. The importance of these remains to be determined, although it is now clear that T_H1 and T_H2 cells can inhibit each other by cytokines. Anti-idiotypic T cells may react with fragments of the TCR on the helper cell (TCR_1) presented by MHC class I or II molecules.

In more refined experiments in which an autoantigen is recognised by a specific TCR, vaccination with fragments of this TCR can prevent disease, probably through the activation of T cells whose TCRs recognise these peptides (Fig. 4.8). This is an example of a network between idiotypes (the disease-associated TCR) and anti-idiotypes (the induced TCR), terms originally applied by Jerne to a control network of antibodies. Stimulation of one part of the network (e.g. an increase in idiotype) results in compensation in another part (increase in anti-idiotype), and the balance is restored. Other possibilities also exist to account for immunoregulation (Fig. 4.8), including the release of cytokines that either reduce the immune response generally or cause inhibition of an ongoing TH1 or TH2 response by the reciprocal inhibition mentioned previously.

B-cell tolerance

In the absence of T-cell help, autoreactive B cells will not produce high-affinity IgG-class autoantibodies.

Therefore the need for T-cell tolerance is of key importance, but B-cell tolerance is also necessary to prevent the emergence of self-reactive B cells as a result of somatic mutation. In addition, the accidental supply of B-cell help arising, for instance, from a T cell responding to a microbial antigen that cross-reacts with a self antigen, could be disastrous. As with T-cell tolerance, transgenic mice have been used to show that autoreactive B cells are subject to both deletion and anergy.

In the first such experiment, the offspring from two transgenic mice were studied, the parents expressing either hen egg lysozyme (HEL) or antibodies against HEL (anti-HEL). In this situation, the mice treat the transgenic HEL as a self antigen. The doubly transgenic progeny did not delete anti-HEL-expressing B cells, which could readily be detected using a specific marker on this particular antibody. However, the B cells did not produce anti-HEL even after stimulation *in vitro*, indicating that they were anergic. Such cells had reduced levels of IgM but still expressed IgD on their surface. Clonal deletion has also been demonstrated in doubly transgenic mice expressing both a novel MHC class I gene in their liver and antibodies against the class I product. These animals delete almost all of the B cells synthesising class I antibody in the spleen and lymph nodes and neither make such antibodies nor have detectable transgene-expressing B cells.

Multivalent antigens on cell surfaces seem particularly good at inducing deletion, whereas soluble, univalent antigens induce anergy. This presumably reflects an important role for the affinity of the antigen binding to the surface immunoglobulin on the immature B cell in determining outcome. The maturational state of the B cell is also important, with antibody-producing plasma cells being very resistant to deletion and anergy.

Initiation of autoimmune disease

Given these complexities and the realisation that even more levels of control probably operate in the intact animal, it hardly seems surprising that autoimmune diseases arise through a breakdown in tolerance. The following are the most likely points at which the control of autoreactive lymphocytes may be disturbed.

1. Autoreactive lymphocytes are not deleted. This may arise in particular strains of animal where particular MHC molecules cannot present self antigen. Failure of deletion could occur in all members of a species if an organ-specific autoantigen does not appear in the thymus at the requisite time; autoimmune disease then arises in those individuals who fail to control such T cells subsequently.

2. Failure of intrathymic anergy. For T cells, this may result in autoimmune disease if sufficient IL-2 or other signals are supplied to overcome the anergic state. Anergic B cells may also be activated by sufficient help in the form of T cell–derived cytokines.

3. Failure of peripheral tolerance and suppression. Drugs and thymectomy may alter an animal's capacity to provide active T-cell suppression, or local APCs may provide co-stimulatory signals to overwhelm peripheral tolerance.

4. Cross-reactivity. If an immune response is mounted against a foreign antigen that is by chance sufficiently similar to self (i.e. *cross-reactive*), then autoimmunity may result. The participating T cells are not tolerised, perhaps because they have a relatively low affinity for the self antigen, but their activation by foreign antigen leads to a strong response that is then sufficient to cause problems.

5. Exposure of sequestered autoantigens. Certain antigens, such as lens protein, may never gain access to the immune system under normal conditions and therefore do not induce tolerance of any kind. This is usually trouble-free, but leakage and exposure of the antigen in adult life results in a severe autoimmune response. With lens protein, this causes sympathetic ophthalmitis, which damages the intact eye when the other eye is injured.

Whether autoimmune disease appears in an individual depends on one or more of these malfunctions occurring. The chances of this happening are related to exogenous and endogenous factors:

the simplest example is the eye trauma just mentioned. However, most autoimmune diseases are the result of a complex interplay between genetic susceptibility and non-genetic influences, which operate on the (imperfect) state of self-tolerance, making it more or less likely that such conditions will arise.

Immunogenetics and autoimmunity

Genetic susceptibility is demonstrated in many of the more common autoimmune diseases by the increased frequency of these disorders in family members. Inheritance does not follow a clear pattern and, even in genetically identical monozygotic twins, there is only 30% to 50% concordance (i.e. disease occurring in both individuals) for disorders such as type I diabetes mellitus, rheumatoid arthritis, and Graves' disease. There are two explanations for this. First, the random nature of immunoglobulin and TCR gene rearrangements means that each family member, including twins, generates a unique T- and B-cell repertoire, which can modify disease expression. Second, and of greater importance, nongenetic factors also contribute to susceptibility. As a result, autoimmune diseases show incomplete

penetrance, and a susceptible individual without the disease is at continued risk of developing it, depending on exposure to appropriate environmental factors. It is also now clear that several genes are involved in determining whether an individual develops an autoimmune disease, and some of these are (apparently) protective, making analysis of the complex roles of different genes very difficult.

The role of MHC class I and II genes

Autoimmune responses are not uniquely influenced by genetic factors; the production and strength of all immune responses are in part determined by the genetic background of the individual. This can be studied far more readily in inbred laboratory animals than in humans, and the results have provided vital information about the genes contributing to autoimmunity. In the seminal experiments performed by Rosenthal and Shevach in 1973, immune responsiveness to synthetic antigens in guinea pigs was shown to be linked to MHC loci encoding products expressed by macrophages, now known as class II molecules (Table 4.3). At about the same, Zinkernagel and Doherty demonstrated the role of MHC class I molecules in the genetic restriction

Table 4.3 Effect of MHC-encoded immune response genes in guinea pigs immunised with synthetic peptide antigens. Strain 2 (but not strain 13) guinea pigs were known to respond to the antigens DNP-PLL and glutamyl alanine co-polymer; strain 13 (but not strain 2) animals respond to glutamyl tyrosine co-polymer. Macrophages from two strains and one hybrid were used to present antigen to T cells from immunised animals. The T cell proliferative response determines whether the antigen has been presented. The results show that strain governs the ability of macrophages to present antigen. Because the responses were blocked in separate experiments by antibodies against strain-specific MHC class II molecules, these molecules must determine whether antigen presentation occurs.

Peptide antigen	Response of strain 2 T cells with macrophages from strain			Response of strain 13 T cells with macrophages from strain		
	2	13	$(2 \times 13)F_1$	2	13	$(2 \times 13)F_1$
DNP-PLL	+	0	+	0	0	0
Glutamyl alanine co-polymer	+	0	+	0	0	0
Glutamyl tyrosine co-polymer	0	0	0	0	+	+

Note:

$(2 \times 13)F_1$ is the first generation hybrids from strain 2 and strain 13 matings. +, T cell response; O, no T cell response.

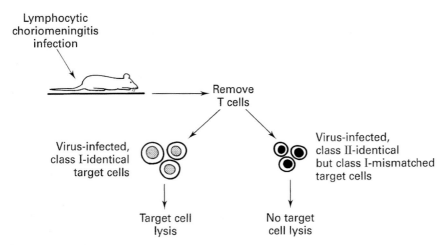

Figure 4.9 Demonstration of MHC class I restriction of CD8$^+$ cytotoxic T cells in mice infected with a virus. A variety of class I molecules exist that present different viral antigens.

of cytotoxic T cells (Fig. 4.9). These results focused attention on the critical role of the MHC in immunogenetics, although there is still incomplete understanding of the organisation and function of this huge complex (Fig. 4.2).

The basic structure of MHC class I and II molecules is similar. For class I molecules, a large polymorphic α-chain is non-covalently linked to the invariant β2-microglobulin, whereas two polymorphic chains, α and β, associate for a class II molecule. In both cases, this structure results in an antigen-binding groove composed of two α-helices with a β-pleated sheet floor (Fig. 4.3). The groove is surrounded by the most polymorphic residues in the MHC molecule, encoded by the different class I or II alleles and creating a series of different grooves. Whether a peptide epitope can bind to a particular groove and be presented to a T cell, therefore, depends on the fit, which in turn is determined by the MHC alleles the individual has inherited.

The class I and II MHC genes may control immune responsiveness by a combination of the following mechanisms.
1. Determinant selection. The various MHC alleles inherited by an individual determine which antigenic peptides can be presented to T cells. If a particular peptide cannot bind to the range of grooves in an APC, the individual will not mount an immune response against that antigenic determinant.
2. Clonal selection. By a similar process but operating during T-cell development, certain MHC molecules may tolerise particular T cells by deletion or anergy and positively select others. The MHC alleles, therefore, shape to the individual's T-cell repertoire.

Other MHC genes

There are several other MHC genes that can influence immune responsiveness. One product, tumour necrosis factor (TNF), is a cytokine that is encoded in the MHC and has many important immunological effects; cytotoxicity against tumour cells is actually not its major property. Genetic variation in TNF levels could contribute to the strength of an immune response. Certain components of complement are also encoded in the class III region (Fig. 4.2), including C4. In individuals with deficiency of C4, caused by the presence of one or two null alleles of the gene for C4A, there is impaired complement activation that prevents the normal clearance of immune complexes. These may be deposited in various tissues, giving rise to the autoimmune disorder systemic lupus erythematosus (SLE).

This example is also important as it illustrates an important feature of MHC loci, *linkage disequilibrium*, by which certain alleles are found together more frequently than would be expected by chance. Linkage disequilibrium arises because recombination within the MHC is not random, being particularly restricted to sites called 'hot spots'. The loci between such hot spots are, therefore, inherited in a block, and selection has allowed certain combinations of alleles (termed a *haplotype*) to become frequent in the population. In Caucasians, the *HLA-A1*, *HLA-B8*, *HLA-DR3* haplotype is common, and this haplotype also includes a C4A null allele. Systemic lupus erythematosus is apparently associated with these particular class I and II alleles, but the likely mechanism is through the C4 class III allele in linkage disequilibrium.

Non-MHC genes

The role of these is at present unclear, but there is no doubt that several non-MHC loci determine immune and autoimmune responses. For example, a gene on murine chromosome 19 has been discovered that encodes the Fas antigen, which plays a fundamental role in negative selection in the thymus. Mice with a defective *fas* gene fail to delete autoreactive T cells and develop a condition resembling SLE. Another example is the gene *NOD2*, which was discovered by genome screening to be involved in the susceptibility to inflammatory bowel disease. Although the reasons for this are still not clear, this gene encodes an intracellular protein that is activated by peptidoglycan (a bacterial wall component). *NOD2* polymorphisms may encode forms of the protein that result in defective production of anti-inflammatory cytokines in response to bacteria encountered in the gut. Polymorphisms in the gene encoding the key immunoregulatory molecule CTLA-4 have been associated with increased susceptibility to organ-specific autoimmune diseases, presumably because the variant form of the pro-

tein permits a more prolonged immune response (and hence increased chance of an autoimmune response). This hypothesis is borne out by experiments in mice in which *CTLA-4* has been knocked out: these animals develop a generalised lymphoproliferative disorder with autoimmunity. The role of *AIRE* in autoimmune polyglandular syndrome type 1 has been mentioned previously. Evidence so far suggests that polymorphisms in *AIRE* do not contribute to the susceptibility to more common and sporadic autoimmune disorders. A second example of a single gene defect causing autoimmunity is the lethal syndrome of immune dysfunction, polyendocrinopathy and enteropathy, X-linked (IPEX), which may be treatable with bone marrow transplantation. This condition results from a defect in a gene (*FOXP3*) that controls the development of T-regulatory cells.

Non-genetic factors in autoimmunity

Females are more prone to autoimmune disease; this is in part due to female sex steroids, because the sex difference generally becomes apparent after puberty, and oestrogens confer enhanced susceptibility in animal models of autoimmunity. Oestrogens generally enhance any immune response. In contrast, testosterone given to female animals reduces their risk of developing autoimmunity. Stress may precipitate autoimmunity via neuroendocrine effects on the immune response. Glucocorticoids are particularly important, having suppressive effects that may impair the regulation of autoreactive T cells. However, lymphocytes possess receptors for many hormones and for other regulatory molecules whose levels are altered by stress, and the sympathetic innervation of lymphoid organs can mediate effects of central nervous system stimulation.

Infections have been proposed as precipitating agents in many autoimmune diseases, but good evidence exists for only a few conditions. Possible mechanisms are as follows:

1. Direct infection of a cell by a virus leads to release of relatively hidden autoantigens or modifies cell surface molecules, making them immunogenic.

2. Infection affects the cells of the immune system, enhancing incipient autoimmune responses indirectly.
3. Amino acid sequences within endogenous proteins of the infecting organism sufficiently resemble self antigen that an immune response against the infection leads to recognition of the cross-reactive autoantigen. This is termed *molecular mimicry*. It accounts for the myocardial damage (rheumatic heart disease) resulting from streptococcal infections in some individuals, as there is cross-reactivity between antigens in this organism and the heart.

Infections do not always precipitate autoimmunity. In some experimental models, autoimmune diseases occur more frequently if the animal is raised in a germ-free environment. Presumably non-specific immune stimulation from commensal organisms is required to maintain immunoregulation of autoreactive lymphocytes. Drugs can also induce autoimmune diseases by molecular mimicry or by combining with a self antigen to create novel antigens to which tolerance does not exist. Environmental toxins may likewise be involved.

Effector mechanisms

It is usual to consider the effector mechanisms in autoimmune disease as cell-mediated and humoral (i.e. antibody-mediated); the various possibilities are shown in Table 4.4. However, both types of response occur in most autoimmune diseases, and deciding which is the most important in initiation can be difficult (Table 4.5). In some cases, autoantibodies arise after the tissue is injured, but even in this secondary phase, they may be important determinants of disease outcome. The presence of circulating autoantibodies can be assessed by a number of immunoassays, and the results of these are extremely valuable in diagnosis. Several tests are available to determine cell-mediated autoimmune responses, but these tend to be used for research purposes only, as their clinical relevance is not established. The results are often difficult to interpret, in part because the lymphocytes that can be most easily tested come from the circulation, but it is usually inaccessible T cells infiltrating the target organ that contain the major autoreactive population. The target organ also contains B cells making autoantibodies, but these also secrete antibodies into the circulation, making serological testing feasible.

Treatment of autoimmune disease

Many autoimmune diseases require no immunological treatment, as the condition is mild or simple treatment is sufficient (for instance, hormone replacement in some autoimmune endocrine disorders). Other conditions are more serious, and

Table 4.4 Effector mechanisms in autoimmune disease

Antibody-mediated mechanisms
Complement fixation
Antibody-dependent cell-mediated cytotoxicity (ADCC): NK cells bind to antibodies on the target cell via Fc receptors and kill it
Direct effects, e.g. enzyme inhibition
Receptor stimulation or blockade

Cell-mediated mechanisms
CD8+ T cell-mediated cytotoxicity
Release of cytokines with direct effects on the target cell
Indirect effects of cytokines, stimulating bystander lymphocytes and macrophages, which then exacerbate tissue injury

Table 4.5 Features distinguishing between humoral and cell-mediated autoimmune disease

	Humoral	Cell mediated
Antibodies against a specific autoantigen in all patients	Yes	No
T cells reacting against a specific autoantigen in all patients	Yes[a]	Yes
Autoantibody detectable in target organ	Yes	No
T cells present on target organ	Possibly	Yes
Disease in neonates of mothers with disease	Yes	No
Disease transferred to animals by T cells	No	Yes
Disease transferred to animals by serum	Yes	No
T cell removal improves disease	Yes[a]	Yes
Antibody removal (e.g. plasma exchange) improves disease	Yes	No

Note:

[a]Autoantibody production requires T cell help.

an immunotherapeutic solution would be optimal, yet at present the risks outweigh the benefits. For example, type 1 (insulin-dependent) diabetes mellitus causes considerable late morbidity, yet intensive insulin replacement provides the best current option (Chapter 7). Finally, some disorders are so pressing that immunological treatment is justified, although current regimens are relatively crude and non-specific (Table 4.6).

Glucocorticoids have a number of non-specific immunosuppressive actions and are used in several autoimmune disorders; however, they cause severe side effects when given at high dosage for a prolonged period. Other agents, like penicillamine and gold, have been found empirically to modify the immune response in rheumatoid arthritis, while newer immunosuppressive agents, such as cyclosporine and tacrolimus, have been developed

Table 4.6 Current treatments commonly used for autoimmune disease

Treatment	Comment
Glucocorticoids	Anti-inflammatory and, at high dosage, immunosuppressive
Cytotoxic drugs (e.g. azathioprine, cyclophosphamide, methotrexate)	Non-specifically inhibit cell proliferation, particularly rapidly dividing lymphocytes
Disease-modifiying treatment (gold, penicillamine, chloroquine, sulphasalazine)	Diverse agents found to influence the course of rheumatoid arthritis and other non-organ-specific disorders; they have a variety of immunological effects
Cyclosporin A; tacrolimus	Non-specifically inhibit T cell function; also used in transplantation
Plasma exchange	Useful for severe antibody-mediated disease (e.g. myasthenia gravis) but only temporary effects if used alone
Intravenous immunoglobulin	Pooled normal immunoglobulin may contain naturally occurring anti-idiotypic antibodies that restore immunoregulatory networks

Table 4.7 Major examples in the spectrum of autoimmune disease

Spectrum	Disease	System affected
Organ-specific disease		
	Hashimoto's thyroiditis	Thyroid
	Type 1 diabetes mellitus	Pancreatic β cells
	Pernicious anaemia	Gastric parietal cells
	Addison's disease	Adrenal (sometimes ovary)
	Graves' disease	Thyroid, orbit (sometimes skin)
	Myasthenia gravis	Skeletal muscles
	Pemphigus vulgaris	Skin, mucous membranes
	Primary biliary cirrhosis	Intrahepatic bile ducts[a]
	Chronic active hepatitis	Liver[a]
	Sjögren's syndrome	Salivary and lacrimal glands[a]
	Rheumatoid arthritis	Jointsa
	Scleroderma	Skin, joints, kidney, gut, lungs
Non-organic specific disease	Systemic lupus erythematosus	Widespread

Note:

[a]Associated with other features in some patients.

as successful treatment for transplantation rejection; their non-specific effects also make them useful in severe autoimmune disorders. Plasma exchange aims to remove circulating antibodies and immune complexes, but these recur unless immunosuppressive therapy is also started. All these treatments can suppress beneficial as well as harmful immune responses, so the complications of infection and certain malignancies are not surprising with prolonged usage.

Exciting preliminary results in non-organ-specific autoimmune disorders (Table 4.7) have been obtained using monoclonal antibodies to delete or block certain T-cell populations. This is becoming more acceptable as mouse or rat monoclonal antibodies can be engineered to contain human C region sequences, thereby preventing an immune response to these animal proteins. Monoclonal antibodies against key cytokines like TNF may also suppress autoimmune responses. Long-term results are not yet available, but lasting remission has occurred in some cases. This suggests that correcting only a single component in the complex sequence of

events causing autoimmune disease is sufficient for innate immunoregulatory mechanisms to restore and maintain control over autoreactive lymphocytes.

More specific immunotherapy is possible, based on the results from animal models of autoimmunity (Fig. 4.10). These treatments require further advances in our understanding for their application to humans. In particular, it will be important to identify individuals at risk of developing autoimmune disease so as to enable early treatment, as autoimmune responses diversify with disease duration. By the time a disease becomes clinically apparent, the number of autoantigens and TCRs involved is usually too great to make specific therapy feasible. Furthermore, target organ destruction may be irreversible. Immunogenetic markers could be of key importance in predicting those at risk, particularly if combined with markers of an early phase in the autoimmune response. Of course, if some of these approaches to restoring tolerance turn out to be innocuous (e.g. orally induced tolerance), they could be universally applied, but considerable effort will be needed to

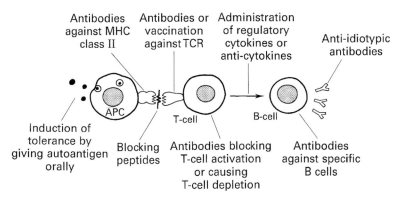

Figure 4.10 Sites of action for novel forms of immunotherapy in autoimmune disease. These have been explored generally in animal models so far.

ensure that such strategies do not actually cause disease in certain individuals.

The spectrum of autoimmune disease

The range of autoimmune disease is often considered as a spectrum, with organ-specific conditions at one end and non-organ-specific conditions at the other (Table 4.7). The various organ systems involved depend on the tissue distribution of the autoantigen, an ubiquitous autoantigen inducing non-organ-specific disorders. The organ-specific conditions tend to be associated with each other and there is quite extensive overlap in the autoimmune responses seen in the non-organ-specific disorders, to the point that a definite diagnostic label cannot be attached to certain patients. Shared immunogenetic susceptibility may be partly responsible for these associations, and the consequences of tissue injury in non-organ-specific disease can also result in a diverse autoimmune response.

Autoimmune thyroid disease

The exemplar condition in this chapter is autoimmune thyroid disease, which includes both destruction of the thyroid (autoimmune hypothyroidism)

and hyperthyroidism (Graves' disease). Some patients show a transition from one extreme to the other, and immune responses against the same thyroid autoantigens can be detected in both conditions. Autoimmune hypothyroidism is usually divided into two forms: Hashimoto's thyroiditis, in which there is a goitre (enlargement of the thyroid gland), and atrophic thyroiditis, in which the gland is smaller than normal. The goitre results from pronounced lymphocytic infiltration, whereas there is predominantly fibrosis in atrophic thyroiditis. Some patients with Hashimoto's thyroiditis can develop atrophy and fibrosis, so that these two forms of autoimmune thyroiditis may be a continuum.

Autoimmune hypothyroidism

Autoimmune hypothyroidism is common, affecting about 1% of women and 0.1% of men; it is an example of a predominantly cell-mediated autoimmune disease. However, in keeping with many autoimmune conditions, autoantibodies against thyroid antigens can easily be detected in these patients: antibodies against thyroglobulin (TG) were the first clear example of an autoimmune response to be described in humans. Thyroglobulin is a large protein that stores thyroid hormone in the colloid filling thyroid follicles. Antibodies to TG and other thyroid autoantigens are diagnostically useful, but their role in causing tissue injury is uncertain (see below). The major clinical features of autoimmune hypothyroidism are shown in Fig. 4.11.

The condition is caused by destruction of thyroid cells, so that few thyroid follicles remain. The remaining thyroid epithelial cells may show hyperplasia because they are stimulated by excessive thyroid-stimulating hormone (TSH) (Fig. 4.12). Some also show a vacuolated, eosinophilic cytoplasm because of an increase in mitrochondria and are termed Hurthle or Askanazy cells. Fibrosis predominates in atrophic thyroiditis, whereas lymphocytic infiltration, with the formation of germinal centres (as in lymph node cortex), is prominent in Hashimoto's thyroiditis. Both elements are present to varying degrees in most affected thyroids.

Lessons from experimental autoimmune thyroiditis

Experimental autoimmune thyroiditis (EAT) is the archetypal animal model of autoimmune disease. In 1956, the same year that TG antibodies were described in Hashimoto's thyroiditis, Rose and Witebsky showed that immunisation of rabbits with rabbit TG induced thyroid lymphocytic infiltration (i.e. thyroiditis) and TG antibody formation. To do this, TG had to be given with an adjuvant, a mixture of substances empirically found to enhance the immune response to an antigen. In this case, the adjuvant was a mixture of mineral oil and killed mycobacteria (called complete Freund's adjuvant), which probably enhances immunogenicity because the oil allows persistence of the antigen and the mycobacteria produce non-specific stimulation of a wide variety of immune responses, increasing the likelihood of specific antigen recognition.

These experiments showed that self-reactive T and B cells exist in healthy normal animals and, under extreme circumstances, can be provoked into responses against tissue-specific autoantigens. Subsequently, EAT was induced in a variety of species by the same technique, with most work being performed using mice. As a result of the availability of

inbred mouse strains, it was soon appreciated that the autoimmune response to TG was influenced by MHC class II genes, which determined whether an animal was a good responder or a poor responder. This distinction presumably reflects the ability of certain class II molecules to bind TG epitopes and to influence the T-cell repertoire. Other genes may also contribute to susceptibility. In particular, MHC class I genes may operate by determining whether or not a particular TG epitope, recognised by CD8$^+$ cytotoxic T cells, is expressed with class I molecules on the thyroid cell surface.

Using monoclonal antibodies to deplete T-cell subsets, it can be shown that both CD4$^+$ and CD8$^+$ T cells are essential for the development of EAT after immunisation. TG-specific CD4$^+$ T cells can be cloned from diseased animals and grown in tissue culture: small numbers of these cells will produce EAT when transferred to a healthy recipient. Thyroglobulin- and MHC class I–specific CD8$^+$ T cells are responsible for thyroid cell killing, whereas TG antibodies have little effect on thyroid cells *in vitro* or *in vivo*. Therefore, this is clearly a T cell–mediated disease, with CD4$^+$ T cells being involved in initiation and CD8$^+$ T cells in tissue injury.

The central role T cells play in EAT is further demonstrated by manipulating the T-cell repertoire without TG immunisation. In certain strains of mice and rats, removal of the thymus at a critical stage in T-cell development can induce severe EAT, with TG antibody formation and lymphocytic thyroiditis. Two mechanisms contribute to this. Thymectomy may result in the persistence of autoreactive T cells due to be deleted later in development and may also deplete the animals of critical immunoregulatory (CD4$^+$, CD25$^+$) T cells that keep non-tolerised TG-specific T cells in check. The latter possibility is supported by transfer experiments: EAT gets better in animals receiving T cells from healthy donors, whose immunoregulatory network is intact. Thymectomy and other forms of T-cell depletion will induce other autoimmune diseases, such as pernicious anaemia, oophoritis and type 1 diabetes mellitus, depending on the strain of the animal as well as on environmental factors. Given the influence of MHC genes

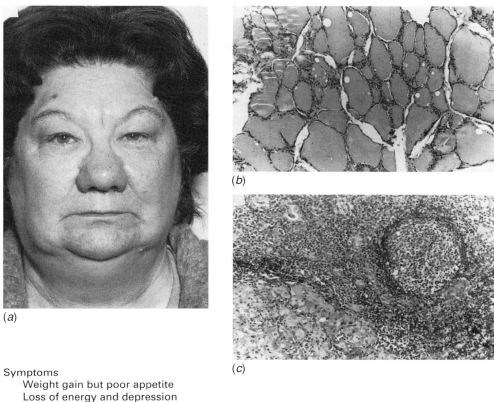

(a)

(b)

(c)

Symptoms
    Weight gain but poor appetite
    Loss of energy and depression
    Dry skin and hair
    Feeling cold
    Constipation
    Altered period (menorrhagia, oligomenorrhoea)

Signs
    Cool dry skin
    Slow pulse (bradycardia)
    Slow relaxing tendon reflexes
    Obesity
    Diffuse hair loss
    Goitre (in Hashimoto's thyroiditis)

Diagnosis
    Elevated TSH, low free T_4
    Thyroglobulin and thyroid peroxidase antibodies
    (detected by immunofluorescence,
    haemagglutination or ELISA methods)

Figure 4.11 Major clinical features of autoimmune hypothyroidism. (*a*) Facial appearance of a patient with Hashimoto's thyroiditis. (*b*) Thyroid section from a normal thyroid. (*c*) Thyroid section from a patient with Hashimoto's thyroiditis. Note destruction of thyroid follicles and the lymphocytic infiltration. (Original magnification ×200; photomicrographs courtesy of Dr T. J. Stephenson, Sheffield.)

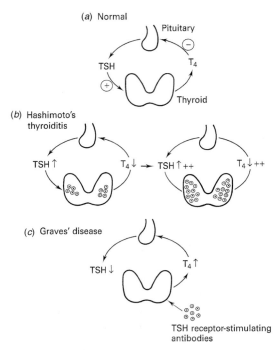

Figure 4.12 Effect of autoimmune thyroid disease on the pituitary–thyroid axis. (*a*) The normal feedback loop. (*b*) In the early stage of Hashimoto's thyroiditis (left), a decline in thyroxine (T_4) production leads to an increase in TSH. This can stimulate the remaining thyroid cells to make sufficient T_4 to maintain values within the normal reference range. After months of years of continuing destruction (right), the TSH can no longer compensate and the T_4 levels become sub-normal. (*c*) In Graves' disease, there is production of TSH receptor-stimulating antibodies by B cells within and outside the thyroid. The antibodies induce hyperthyroidism and pituitary TSH secretion declines.

in shaping the T-cell repertoire, this genetic component is not surprising.

A third type of EAT arises spontaneously in certain animal strains and therefore most closely resembles autoimmune hypothyroidism in humans (Table 4.8). In one such example, the obese strain (OS) chicken, three separate genetic elements determine susceptibility. One lies within the MHC, another controls T-cell regulation, and the third determines the

thyroid response to autoimmunity. The exact loci involved have not been delineated, but the idea of genetic susceptibility being in part target organ–specific is appealing as an explanation for the striking specificity of many autoimmune disorders.

The development of thyroiditis in OS chickens is critically dependent on T cells, although thyroid antibodies may also be important effectors of tissue damage by complement fixation and by antibody-dependent cell-mediated cytotoxicity (ADCC). Thyroglobulin is a heavily iodinated molecule because of the need for iodine in thyroid hormone synthesis. Thyroglobulin antibody formation in OS chickens depends on how much iodine is present in the diet: TG with a low iodine content does not induce antibody formation, presumably because the iodine is crucial to epitopes recognised by both T cells and B cells. Furthermore, murine EAT induced by TG immunisation results in T-cell recognition of an epitope containing iodine at a critical site in the TG molecule where thyroid hormones are formed. Therefore dietary iodine is an example of an environmental factor operating with genetic susceptibility to determine whether autoimmune thyroid disease is induced.

Immunogenetics of autoimmune hypothyroidism

In Whites, autoimmune hypothyroidism is associated with the class II specificity HLA-DR3, which can now be divided by molecular techniques into two alleles, DRB1*0301 and DRB1*0302. So far it is not clear whether one or both of these alleles is responsible for the association, and in certain White populations there are additional HLA-DR associations. The simplest way of determining whether an allele contributes to genetic susceptibility is to measure the frequency in patients and healthy subjects and determine the relative risk (Table 4.9), which gives some idea of how important a factor is for the individual. An alternative figure, the aetiological fraction, indicates how much of a disease may be attributed to the genetic factor. By both measures, the contribution of HLA-DR3 to the development

Table 4.8 Animal models of spontaneous autoimmune thyroiditis

	Obese strain (OS) chicken	Buffalo strain rat	BB strain rat	Non-obese diabetic mouse
Thyroiditis (incidence,%)	>90	<25	Variable: up to 60	Variable: up to 90
TG antibodies	Yes	Yes	Yes	Yes
T cell dependent	Yes	Yes	Yes	Probably
Female preponderance	No	Yes	Yes	No
Dietary iodine exacerbates disease	Yes	Yes	Yes	Not tested
Hypothyroid	Yes	No	No	Not tested
Autoimmune diabetes also present	No	No	Yes	Yes

of autoimmune hypothyroidism is quite small and does not explain the entire genetic contribution to susceptibility.

Furthermore, different class II alleles are associated with autoimmune hypothyroidism in non-White populations; in Whites, only a small proportion of individuals with the HLA-DR3 specificity develop the disease. These facts show that HLA-DR3 itself cannot be responsible for autoimmune hypothyroidism, acting instead as a risk factor whose impact will be determined by other, unknown genes influencing the autoimmune response and by environmental factors. It is therefore not surprising that autoimmune hypothyroidism in juveniles shows a much stronger tendency to be inherited than the same condition in adults. If a potent combination of genes is inherited, autoimmune disease will result early in life without much need for an environmental

Table 4.9 Measuring the strength of an association between an allele (HLA-X) and a disease. Data are obtained on N_1 plus N_2 patients and N_3 plus N_4 healthy controls, divided according to the presence or absence of HLA-X.

	HLA-X$^+$	HLA-X$^-$
Patients	N_1	N_3
Control subjects	N_2	N_4

Note:
The relative risk is $(N_1 \times N_4)/(N_2 \times N_3)$.

contribution, whereas a mild immunogenetic susceptibility will cause disease only in combination with the appropriate non-genetic factors, which requires time for the exposure to occur.

The mechanism by which HLA-DR3 increases susceptibility is not known, but a number of other autoimmune diseases are also associated with HLA-DR3, particularly the DRB1*0302 allele. This is in linkage disequilibrium with HLA-A1, HLA-B8 (and other MHC alleles) and forms a common haplotype in Whites. A number of non-specific immunological functions are altered in healthy HLA-A1, HLA-B8, HLA-DR3–positive individuals, including enhanced TNF production (as a result of a TNF allele also in linkage disequilibrium), and some survival advantage is probably conferred by this haplotype. Although heightened immune responsiveness against foreign microbial antigens may have been a beneficial result, the same non-specific enhancement exacerbates any autoimmune response, explaining the frequent association of this haplotype and autoimmune diseases.

An alternative way to assess genetic contribution is to measure linkage. If a marker is associated with a disease, then it should segregate with the disease in a family with multiple affected members. The presence of disease in a family member without the marker is compelling evidence against its importance. Recently, linkage analysis has shown little evidence for HLA markers determining susceptibility to autoimmune thyroid disease. This is still in keeping with a role for *HLA-DR3* in the autoimmune response but suggests that other genes outside the MHC are also important. So far, the only genes known to contribute to thyroid autoimmunity are two, both involved in T-cell regulation, namely, *CTLA-4* (mentioned above) and *PTPN22*, which encodes lymphoid-specific phosphatase, an enzyme that has a major role In terminating T-cell responses.

Non-genetic factors

The clearest non-genetic factor is the influence of hormones on the autoimmune response (although of course an individual's hormone profile is in part genetically determined). Autoimmune hypothyroidism is 4 to 10 times more common in women, this sex difference beginning after puberty. Experiments in EAT show that disease can be prevented by giving testosterone to female animals and is exacerbated by oestrogens or castration in males, indicating that sex hormones are the important factors in this. Pregnancy also alters the autoimmune response, with a decline in disease activity during pregnancy and a post-partum rebound in the year after delivery (Fig. 4.13). Although it is not as yet entirely clear why these changes occur, they seem likely to be related to the variations in sex and other hormones with pregnancy. In the majority of women, immunoregulatory mechanisms lead to recovery from the disease with few effects, but in some patients the post-partum exacerbation of pre-existing mild autoimmune thyroiditis may be severe enough to result in permanent clinical hypothyroidism. Therefore pregnancy is a risk factor for the development of autoimmune hypothyroidism, further increasing the proportion of women with this disorder.

As in EAT, iodine intake is another factor determining susceptibility. An increase in dietary iodide in the West has been blamed for an apparent rise in Hashimoto's thyroiditis, but exact figures are not available to confirm this. There is no clear evidence that infection is important. Viral (or subacute) thyroiditis is not usually followed by autoimmune hypothyroidism and viruses have not been detected in affected thyroid tissue. However, it is possible that

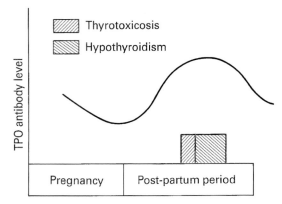

Figure 4.13 Post-partum thyroiditis in a woman with thyroid peroxidase (TPO) antibodies before conception. TPO antibody levels, reflecting the severity of autoimmune thyroiditis, decline during pregnancy but rise in the post-partum period. At the peak of this rise, there may be sufficient thyroid injury to release stored thyroid hormones, causing transient thyrotoxicosis. If the injury continues, the stores are depleted and the patient becomes hypothyroid. When the antibody levels fall, the normal thyroid function is restored but the patient is at risk of autoimmune thyroid disease in the future.

a viral (or bacterial) infection may trigger autoimmunity months or years before the condition becomes apparent clinically. At this stage, the absence of an infecting organism would be expected. Finally treatment with immunomodulatory drugs, in particular α-IFN, can precipitate autoimmune thyroid disease in some patients.

Autoimmune responses to thyroid autoantigens

There are three major thyroid autoantigens: TG; thyroid peroxidase (TPO), the key enzyme involved in thyroid hormone synthesis; and the TSH receptor, which transmits the stimulatory signal from pituitary-derived TSH to the thyroid cell (Fig. 4.12). The immune response to the TSH receptor was discussed previously. T cells recognising and reacting to TG and TPO can be detected in patients with autoimmune hypothyroidism and occasionally, in much lower frequency, in healthy controls. This suggests that some thyroid-specific T cells escape thymic tolerance but are normally kept under control by immunoregulatory networks. Whether a primary defect in control contributes to the initiation of thyroid autoimmunity is unknown, as it is difficult to examine patients at the initiation of the autoimmune response.

By the time of clinical presentation, a number of different TG and TPO epitopes are recognised by polyclonal T cells expressing heterogeneous TCRs. This may represent *determinant spreading*, following the response to only a single dominant epitope in the initial phase of the illness. Once an autoimmune response starts, it spreads to involve other (cryptic) epitopes because the localised inflammation brings together activated APCs and T cells releasing cytokines, which overcome any tolerance to these cryptic determinants. As a consequence, attempts to limit immune damage by using modified epitopes or influencing specific TCRs are unlikely to succeed by the time disease becomes apparent. Fortunately, this is not necessary in autoimmune hypothyroidism, as thyroxine replacement is sufficient treatment, but similar diversification occurs in some serious autoimmune disorders where such treatment would be beneficial.

The B-cell response to TG and TPO is also polyclonal. Antibodies to TG in particular are frequent in healthy subjects, but these are generally IgM class and of low affinity and specificity, so-called *natural* autoantibodies. During the autoimmune process, the B-cell response matures because specific B cells are stimulated by thyroid-reactive T cells. These autoantibodies are IgG and have high affinity and specificity. They are also present at high concentrations, and their presence is useful in determining that autoimmunity is the cause of hypothyroidism in a newly diagnosed patient (Fig. 4.12). Thyroglobulin antibodies do not fix complement because the B cell epitopes are too widely spread to allow complement fixation, which requires two or more immunoglobulin Fc regions in proximity. Thyroid peroxidase antibodies do fix complement and can also mediate antibody-dependent cell-mediated cytotoxicity (ADCC) and inhibit the enzymatic activity of TPO *in vitro*.

These antibodies, therefore, contribute to the development of autoimmune hypothyroidism, but it also seems likely that cytotoxic T cells play an important role in thyroid cell damage (Fig. 4.14). In addition, the cytokines released by the infiltrating T cells and macrophages (especially (γ-IFN and TNF)

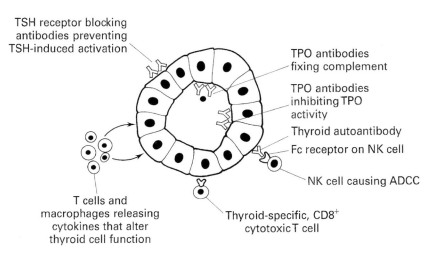

Figure 4.14 Mechanisms causing thyroid cell injury and hypothyroidism in autoimmune hypothyroidism.

have a number of adverse effects on thyroid cells, directly inhibiting function and inducing expression of MHC class II molecules and adhesion molecules such as intercellular adhesion molecule-1 (ICAM-1). The role of this 'aberrant' class II expression in thyroid autoimmunity is not yet clear. Although it was originally suggested that class II–positive thyroid cells would present autoantigens to T cells, exacerbating the autoimmune response, there is no evidence that these cells can provide a second, costimulatory signal. Therefore, thyroid cell class II expression may result in peripheral tolerance. The appearance of ICAM-1 on thyroid cells stimulates the adherence of lymphocytes expressing LFA-1 (lymphocyte function–associated antigen 1) (Fig. 4.4), and *in vitro* experiments show that this increases the killing of thyroid cells by cytotoxic T cells.

Graves' disease

In contrast to most cases of hypothyroidism, this is an example of a predominantly antibody-mediated autoimmune disease; TSH receptor autoantibodies bind to and stimulate the receptor, leading to hyperthyroidism (Fig. 4.12). The excessive production of thyroid hormones results in the main clinical features of the disease (Fig. 4.15). Graves' disease is frequently associated with a number of eye signs and symptoms, called ophthalmopathy; this complication is discussed below. There is no animal model yet of Graves' disease.

The Graves' thyroid is enlarged as a result of hypertrophy and hyperplasia of the thyroid follicles, which have tall columnar epithelium with little colloid. There is also widespread lymphocytic infiltration and occasional germinal centre formation. Antibodies to TG and TPO are found in most patients with Graves' disease. In view of the shared autoimmune response against these two autoantigens, it is not surprising that some patients may have autoimmune hypothyroidism and then develop Graves' disease, and vice versa. Indeed, spontaneous hypothyroidism may occur in up to 25% of Graves' patients followed for 20 years.

Precipitating factors

Graves' disease occurs in around 1% of women and 0.1% of men. There is a 30% to 50% concordance for Graves' disease in monozygotic twins, compared with around 7% concordance in HLA-identical siblings. These facts indicate the importance of both genetic and non-genetic factors in susceptibility and tell us that non-HLA genes make an important contribution. As in autoimmune hypothyroidism, *HLA-DR3* is associated with Graves' disease, but the location of other susceptibility genes is unknown except for *PTPN22*, which has been associated with Graves' disease, and *CTLA-4*, which has an equal role in Graves' disease and autoimmune hypothyroidism. It is possible that polymorphisms in genes such as that encoding the TSH receptor could account for the development of Graves' disease, specifically in a patient predisposed to thyroid autoimmunity.

Pregnancy and sex hormones, as well as dietary iodide, are important non-genetic factors in precipitating Graves' disease. Stress – as measured by the frequency of adverse events such as divorce, bereavement and difficulties at work – can also initiate the condition. The effects of stress probably depend on altered neuroendocrine input into the immune system, altering regulation of the autoimmune response. There have been suggestions that infection may induce Graves' disease, although the evidence so far is fragmentary. Certainly *Yersinia* and other microorganisms contain proteins that cross-react with the TSH receptor, making molecular mimicry a possibility. If this does occur, it can be a factor in only a small proportion of patients, as most have no evidence of such infections. Nonetheless, it is important to appreciate that several different combinations of susceptibility factors, genetic and non-genetic, may induce the same clinical disorder.

TSH receptor antibodies

Several lines of evidence show that TSH receptor antibodies cause Graves' disease. First, they are

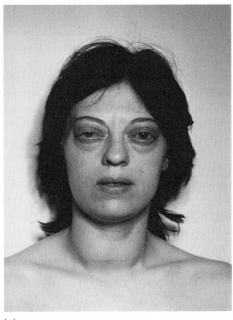

(a)

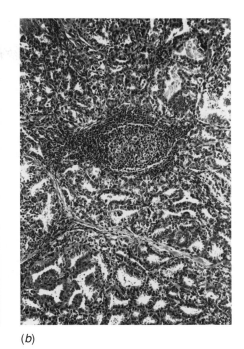

(b)

Symptoms
    Weight loss and increased appetite
    Irritability
    Feeling the heat; excessive sweating
    Tremor
    Palpitations
    Altered periods (oligomenorrhoea)

Signs
    Hot, sweaty palms
    Fine tremor of hands
    Fast pulse (sinus tachycarcia, sometimes atrial fibrillation)
    Thin
    Diffuse firm goitre
    Eye signs (ophthalmopathy) in 60%

Diagnosis
    Suppressed TSH, elevated free T_4 and T_3 (triiodothyronine)
    TG and TPO antibodies in 75%
    TSH receptor antibodies in >95% (research assays;
    not in general clinical use)

Figure 4.15 Major clinical features of Graves' disease. (*a*) Facial appearance of a patient with Graves' disease. Note the prominent eyes (proptosis) and swelling around the eyes (periorbital oedema), which are features of thyroic-associated opthalmopathy. (*b*) Thyroid section from a patient with Graves' disease (normal thyroid section in shown in Fig. 4.11*b*). Note the lymphocytic infiltration (centre). (Original magnification ×200; photomicrograph courtesy of Dr T. J. Stephenson, Sheffield.)

detected in almost all Graves' patients, and when TSH receptor antibody levels fall, there is remission of the disease. Those without such antibodies have mild disease; therefore the antibody level may be below the current level of detectability or the antibodies may be being made in the thyroid itself but do not appear in the serum. Second, thyroid stimulation can be produced by administration of the antibodies. Adams and colleagues demonstrated in 1956 that radioiodine could be released from the thyroid gland of animals by administration of Graves' serum. Purified Graves' IgG stimulates thyroid cells *in vitro* and, using recombinant TSH receptors transfected into mammalian cells, can be shown to operate exclusively via this receptor. Finally, the babies born to mothers with high levels of TSH receptor–stimulating antibodies have transient thyrotoxicosis, produced by the placental transfer of maternal IgG. The severity of this neonatal thyrotoxicosis correlates well with the activity of TSH receptor antibodies in the mother's serum.

The production of TSH receptor antibodies is T cell–dependent. Like the response against TPO and TG, this T-cell response is polyclonal. The TSH receptor antibodies that cause Graves' disease bind to the extracellular domain of the TSH receptor and activate it, leading to an increase in intracellular cyclic AMP. This is the same pathway used by TSH, but the effects of TSH receptor antibodies may be longer lasting because of the high affinity of antibody binding to the receptor. Not all TSH receptor antibodies cause thyroid cell stimulation, however. Some bind to a different epitope on the receptor, which does not activate it but instead prevents TSH from doing so. These blocking antibodies, therefore, have the opposite effect to the stimulating antibodies, yet both may occur in the same patient, so that thyroid function is determined by the balance between the two. TSH receptor–blocking antibodies also occur in patients with goitrous and atrophic autoimmune hypothyroidism, in whom they may contribute to the impaired thyroid activity. Transient hypothyroidism can occur in babies born to such mothers, again because the antibodies cross the placenta.

Thyroid-associated ophthalmopathy

Eye signs can be found in around two-thirds of Graves' patients (Fig. 4.15) and occasionally appear in Hashimoto's thyroiditis. These changes are caused by enlargement of the extraocular muscles, which are infiltrated by activated lymphocytes. As a result of cytokine production, fibroblasts in the muscles are stimulated, leading to increased production of glycosaminoglycans and collagen (Fig. 4.16). From studies using imaging techniques such as computed tomography, it is apparent that almost all Graves' patients have some extraocular muscle enlargement and hence thyroid-associated ophthalmopathy. This suggests that the tissue-infiltrating lymphocytes in the thyroid and extraocular muscles may be recognising a similar (but unidentified) cross-reactive antigen present in the two sites. One obvious candidate is the TSH receptor, and recent preliminary experiments have shown the presence of a truncated form of the receptor in extraocular muscle. Smoking is a risk factor for the development of severe ophthalmopathy in Graves' disease, but the mechanism responsible is not known.

Summary

The first evidence that the body could mount an immune response against itself came from experiments showing that rabbits immunized with thyroid extract produced antibodies against thyroglobulin, and in these same animals there was development of a lymphocytic infiltrate of the thyroid gland. In the six decades since that discovery, it has become clear that many previously obscure diseases are caused by autoimmunity, and indeed reaction against self components can be interpreted as part of the normal immune response that results in disease only when control goes awry. As well as being the archetype of this type of disease mechanism, autoimmune thyroid diseases comprise the commonest examples of these disorders, and the various types of thyroid autoimmunity demonstrate the different ways that autoimmune mechanisms can cause tissue dysfunction. These can typically be categorised as those

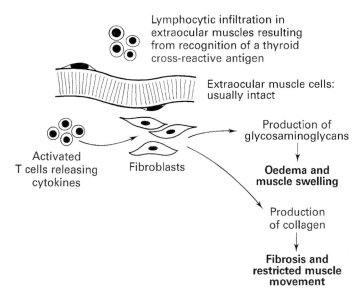

Lymphocytic infiltration in extraocular muscles resulting from recognition of a thyroid cross-reactive antigen

Extraocular muscle cells: usually intact

Activated T cells releasing cytokines

Fibroblasts

Production of glycosaminoglycans

Oedema and muscle swelling

Production of collagen

Fibrosis and restricted muscle movement

Figure 4.16 Possible mechanisms involved in thyroid-associated ophthalmopathy. The nature of the shared autoantigen in thyroid and extraocular muscle in not known.

resulting from antibody-mediated mechanisms (e.g. Graves' disease caused by antibodies that stimulate the TSH receptor) and cell-mediated mechanisms (such as autoimmune hypothyroidism caused by T cell–mediated destruction of thyroid cells).

Clinical scenarios

Thyroid-associated ophthalmopathy

A 26-year-old woman presented with discomfort behind the right eye and over 6 weeks developed diplopia in all directions of gaze, particularly noticeable when looking up and out. She had also noticed that the soft tissues around the eyes were swollen, particularly on waking. Although there were no symptoms or signs of thyroid disease on examination, biochemical testing revealed positive thyroid peroxidase antibodies and a TSH of 0.1 (reference range 0.5 – 4.5 mU/l). The patient was advised to stop smoking, sleep with the head of the bed propped up and given temporary prisms to correct the diplopia.

Over the course of the next 2 months, the TSH fell further and thyrotoxicosis was diagnosed clinically and biochemically. The patient was treated with carbimazole, which controlled the thyroid disease, but despite achieving euthyroidism after stopping antithyroid drugs, she required corrective surgery to the extra-ocular muscles to finally resolve the diplopia.

This case demonstrates that ophthalmopathy can sometimes present before thyroid disease becomes established. However, in the 5% or so of cases in which this is the pattern, there is usually subtle evidence of thyroid autoimmunity, such as positive thyroid peroxidase antibodies or an abnormal TSH. Close follow-up is required, as these patients are clearly at risk of developing thyroid disease. Biochemical control of abnormal thyroid function is important in helping to stabilise ophthalmopathy, as is smoking cessation.

Around 75% of patients obtain benefit from high-dose corticosteroid treatment for severe forms of eye disease, but this patient refused such treatment.

Finally the disease entered a quiescent phase, which allowed surgery to be undertaken to realign the extraocular muscles. The underlying process is believed to be a cross reaction, with an unknown antigen shared between the thyroid and orbit causing T-cell activation and release of cytokines, which in the orbit results in fibroblast activation. The most likely current candidate for the shared antigen is the TSH receptor.

Postpartum thyroiditis

A 22-year-old woman with a family history of thyroid autoimmunity noticed shaking of her hands and mild sweating 4 months after the birth of her first child. By the time she attended the endocrine clinic 4 weeks later, these symptoms had been replaced with a feeling of tiredness. Blood tests taken at the time of the onset of symptoms showed a suppressed TSH and raised free T4, whereas 4 weeks later the TSH was elevated and the free T4 was suppressed. In view of the symptoms, the patient was given thyroxine and monitored closely. She improved over the following 2 months, and the TSH returned to normal. Treatment was stopped 1 year after delivery and she remained well. Strongly positive levels of thyroid peroxidase antibodies were found at original presentation to the clinic, and although these declined in level, they were still present 1 year after delivery.

This patient has had postpartum thyroiditis, a common condition occurring in 5% of women in the year after pregnancy. In over 90% of cases, this is a transient disturbance of thyroid function, typically comprising an episode of thyrotoxicosis followed by a slightly longer phase of hypothyroidism. Treatment is usually not necessary, although a β blocker can be given during the thyrotoxic phase to ameliorate symptoms, and some patients with severe hypothyroid symptoms benefit from a short course of thyroxine.

Women with postpartum thyroiditis often have a family history of thyroid autoimmunity and prior to pregnancy have low levels of thyroid antibodies, marking a low-grade focal thyroiditis. During pregnancy, immune responses tend to be suppressed, but in the postpartum period (for unknown reasons) immune responses can be exacerbated; it is during this time that the autoimmune thyroid process may declare itself clinically. Although most such patients recover, long-term follow-up is essential, as the autoimmune process can progress to overt hypothyroidism in around 20% of cases over 5 to 10 years.

Graves' disease and other autoimmune disorders

A 53-year-old woman presented with shaking, weight loss, palpitations and itchy skin. She had a long history of vitiligo. Thyrotoxicosis was confirmed biochemically, and further examination showed evidence of ophthalmopathy, with slight proptosis and bilateral lid retraction. There was a small, firm, diffuse mobile goitre on examination, and thyroid peroxidase antibodies were positive. The patient was treated initially with antithyroid drugs but relapsed 2 years after the antithyroid drugs were stopped; thereafter she received radioactive iodine as definitive treatment for her Graves' disease. At the time of that treatment there was no active evidence of ophthalmopathy and the patient did not smoke. This meant that she was at low risk of developing the exacerbation of ophthalmopathy which can sometimes occur after radioiodine treatment. therefore she was not considered as a candidate for short-term corticosteroids to prevent such an exacerbation.

Six months after the radioactive iodine treatment, the patient complained of feeling tired, a symptom that had been present for a few months. In addition, she had recently noticed that her tongue had become sore. Although it was initially suspected that this woman had hypothyroidism following her radioactive iodine, further investigations revealed a low haemoglobin with a raised mean cell volume (MCV), suggesting the diagnosis of pernicious anaemia. This was confirmed by finding a low vitamin B12 level and positive antibodies to gastric parietal cells and intrinsic factor. She responded to treatment with vitamin B12 injections.

This case illustrates the common association of autoimmune diseases: up to 50% of patients with pernicious anaemia will have positive thyroid autoantibodies, and the frequency of pernicious anaemia in Graves' disease is around 2%, compared to a population prevalence of 0.15%. Patients with vitiligo have an eight-fold increased risk of developing autoimmune thyroid disease compared to the healthy population. Other associated autoimmune diseases include type 1 diabetes mellitus, Addisons's disease, coeliac disease, alopecia areata, rheumatoid arthritis and systemic lupus erythematosus. The most likely explanation for these associations of autoimmune diseases is sharing of common genetic susceptibility factors.

Multiple-choice questions (true or false)

1. Concerning the immune system:
   a. C8 T cells are cytotoxic.
   b. C4 cells recognise antigen presented by class I MHC molecules.
   c. C4 cells synthesise IL-4.
   d. C4 cells synthesise γ-interferon.
   e. CD8 cells provide help for B cells to make antibodies.
2. The following are mechanisms by which autoimmunity can be precipitated:
   a. Molecular mimicry by infectious agents
   b. Exposure of sequestered autoantigens
   c. Failure of peripheral tolerance
   d. Neonatal thymectomy in certain animal strains.
   e. As a result of a single gene defect
3. With regard to autoimmune hypothyroidism,
   a. The frequency is 5% in women.
   b. Men have twice the frequency of women.
   c. Antibodies occur against thyroglobulin and thyroid peroxidase.
   d. Fibrosis predominates in Hashimoto's thyroiditis.
   e. Germinal centres can be found in the thyroid.
4. With regard to Graves' disease,
   a. The diseases is caused by blocking antibodies against the TSH receptor.
   b. Babies born to mothers with Graves' disease may develop neonatal thyrotoxicosis.
   c. Dietary iodide may be a precipitating factor.
   d. The frequency of Graves' disease is around 1% in women.
   e. There is typically no lymphocytic infiltration in the thyroid in Graves' disease.

Answers

1 a, T; b, F; c, T; d, T; e, F
2 a, T; b, T; c, T; d, T; e, T
3 a, F; b, F; c, T; d, F; e, T
4 a, F; b, T; c, T; d, T; e, F

FURTHER READING

General

Feldmann, M., Steinman, L. (2005). Design of effective immunotherapy for human autoimmunity. *Nature* **435,** 612–19.

Goodnow, C. C. (2001). Pathways for self-tolerance and the treatment of autoimmune diseases. *Lancet* **357,** 2115–21.

Mackay, I. R. (2000). Tolerance and autoimmunity. *British Medical Journal* **321,** 93–6.

Pugliese, A. (2003). Central and peripheral autoantigen presentation in immune tolerance. *Immunology* **111,** 138–46.

Ramsdell, F., Fowlkes, B. J. (1990). Clonal deletion versus clonal anergy; the role of the thymus in inducing self tolerance. *Science* **248,** 1332–40.

Rioux, J. D., Abbas, A. K. (2005). Paths to understanding the genetic basis of autoimmune disease. *Nature* **435,** 584–89.

Schwartz, R. S. (2003). Diversity of the immune repertoire and immunoregulation. *New England Journal of Medicine* **348,** 1017–26.

Sprent, J, Surh C. D. (2003). Knowing one's self: central tolerance revisited. *Nature Immunology* **4,** 303–4.

Venanzi, E. S., Benoist, C. Mathis, D. (2004). Good riddance: thymocyte clonal deletion prevents autoimmunity. *Current Opinion in Immunology* **16,** 197–202.

Weetman, A. P. (1991). *Autoimmune Endocrine Disease.* Cambridge, UK: Cambridge University Press.

Weetman, A. P., McGregor, A M. (1994). Autoimmune thyroid disease: further developments in our understanding. *Endocrine Reviews* **15,** 788–830.

Specific topics

Bahn, R. S. (2003) Pathophysiology of Graves' ophthalmopathy: the cycle of disease. *Journal of Clinical Endocrinology and Metabolism* **88,** 1939–46.

Eisenbarth, G. S., Gottlieb, P. A. (2004). Autoimmune polyendocrine syndromes. *New England Journal of Medicine* **350,** 2068–79.

Pearce, E. N., Farwell, A. P., Braverman, L. E. (2003). Thyroiditis. *New England Journal of Medicine* **348,** 2646–55.

Rapoport, B. McLachlan, S. M. (2001) Thyroid autoimmunity. *Journal of Clinical Investigation* **108,** 1253–9.

Roberts, C. G. P., Ladenson, P. W. (2004) Hypothyroidism. *Lancet*. **363,** 793–803.

Schwartz, K. M., Fatourechi, V., Ahmed, D. D. F., Pond, G. R. (2002) Dermopathy of Graves' disease (pretibial myxedema): long-term outcome. *Journal of Clinical Endocrinology and Metabolism* **87,** 438–46.

Vaidya, B., Kendall-Taylor, P., Pearce, S. H. S. (2002). The genetics of autoimmune thyroid disease. *Journal of Clinical Endocrinology and Metabolism* **87,** 5385–97.

Weetman, A. P. (2000). Graves' disease. *New England Journal of Medicine* **343,** 1236–48.

Wiersinga, W. M. (ed.) (2005). Autoimmune endocrine disorders. *Best Practice and Research. Clinical Endocrinology and Metabolism*. Volume 19, Number 1, Amsterdam: Elsevier.

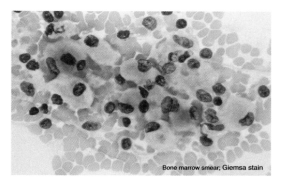

Bone marrow smear; Giemsa stain

Figure 2.2 Gaucher Cells – note the large abnormal Macrophages in marrow aspirate stained by the Giemsa method.

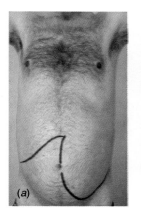

(a)

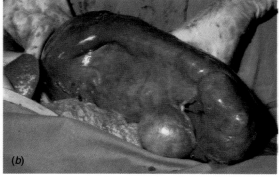

(b)

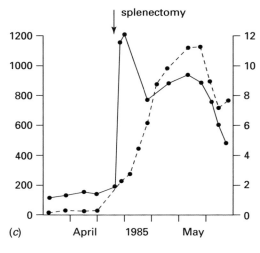

splenectomy

1200 — 12

1000 — 10

800 — 8

600 — 6

400 — 4

200 — 2

0 — 0

(c)

April   1985   May

Figure 2.3 (a) Massive hepatosplenomegaly in a young man with Gaucher's disease and haemorrhage. Treatment before 1991: (b) splenectomy specimen; (c) effect of splenectomy on leucocyte and platelet counts.

mast cells and basophils

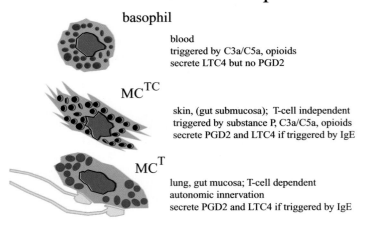

basophil

blood
triggered by C3a/C5a, opioids
secrete LTC4 but no PGD2

MC^{TC}

skin, (gut submucosa); T-cell independent
triggered by substance P, C3a/C5a, opioids
secrete PGD2 and LTC4 if triggered by IgE

MC^{T}

lung, gut mucosa; T-cell dependent
autonomic innervation
secrete PGD2 and LTC4 if triggered by IgE

Figure 5.2 Mast cells and basophils. MC^{T} indicates mast cell with granules containing tryptase; MC^{TC} indicates mast cells with granules containing tryptase and chymase. The granules of all three types contain histamine and proteoglycans, including heparin and chondroitin sulphate. All three are triggered by IgE as indicated in Fig. 5.4 to release their granule contents and secrete mediators, such as arachidonic acid derivatives.

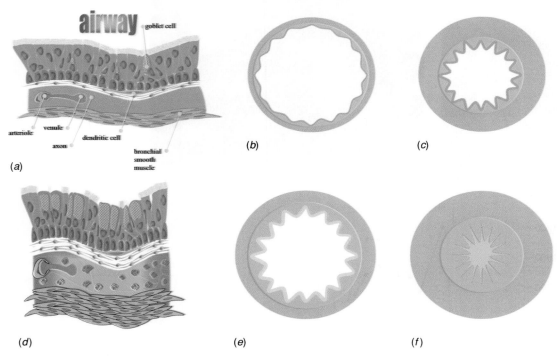

Figure 5.3 Allergic response in the lungs. A and B represent high-magnification and low-magnification views of a cross-section of a normal bronchiole, whereas D and E represent the corresponding views of a bronchiole from an asthmatic. Repeated or persistent allergic responses lead to remodelling of the airways. The main changes are mucous metaplasia/hyperplasia in the epithelium, thickening and stiffening of the lamina reticularis, thickening of the bronchial smooth muscle, infiltration of the airway walls with inflammatory cells (eosinophils, lymphocytes, plasma cells, mast cells) and an increase in small blood vessels and nerve fibres. The consequence of these changes is that an allergic response can lead to more severe obstruction in those with airways remodelling (C and F).

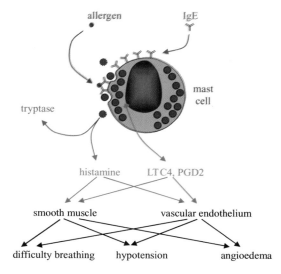

Figure 5.4 Mast cell activation during an allergic reaction. Adjacent IgE molecules, attached to the surface membrane of the mast cell *via* the high affinity IgE receptor (FcεRI), are bridged by binding to allergen. This leads to externalisation of the mast cell granules near the bridged receptors; thus, major activation in anaphylaxis will cause degranulation of the whole cell. Arachidonic acid is then released from the nuclear membrane by phospholipase A2 and converted to prostaglandin and leukotrienes (LTC4, PGD2), which are then secreted. These mediators then act on their respective receptors on smooth muscle, endothelial cells, secretory cells and so on to cause the clinical features of anaphylaxis.

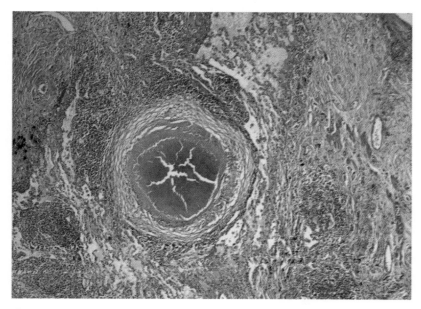

Figure 6.4 Histological section showing a typical TB granuloma with central caseous necrosis, mononuclear cell infiltrate and fibrosis. (Kindly supplied by the Department of Anatomical Pathology, Faculty of Health Sciences, University of Cape Town.)

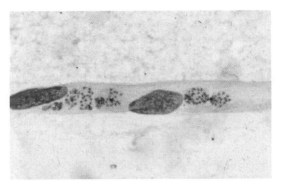

Figure 7.1 *Plasmodium falciparum* schizonts in cerebral venule, from post-mortem brain smear in child with cerebral malaria.

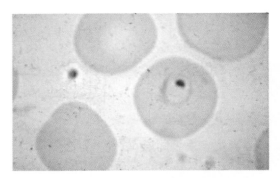

Figure 7.2 Thin blood film (Field's stain) with ring-stage asexual *P. falciparum* trophozoite in apparently normal erythrocyte (× 4000).

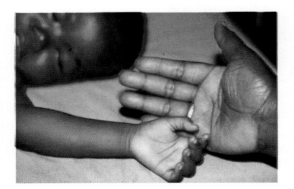

Figure 7.3 Pallor of palm of an infant with severe malarial anaemia.

Cardiac Output↓

renal	neurohumoral	myocardial
kidney perfusion ↓ ⇨Na⁺/ H₂O retention	periph. resistance ↑ by AII, NA, ET, etc.	changes in gene programme

further Cardiac Output↓

Figure 9.3 The three pathophysiological pathways leading to the development of heart failure. All three contribute to the progressive weakening of the heart muscle. They also correspond to the three major theories about heart failure developed over the last 100 years (in temporal order, from left to right). Upward and downward pointing arrows indicate increase or decrease, respectively. The pathways obviously interact, e.g. an increase in catecholamines will contribute to downregulation of myocardial adrenoceptors, etc. Abbreviations: AII: angiotensin II; NA: noradrenaline; ET: endothelin.

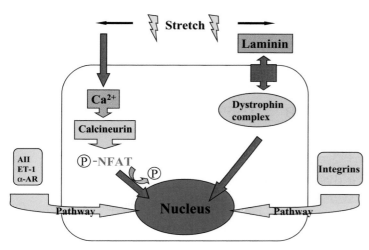

Figure 9.4 Simplified schematic of the molecular mechanisms leading to cardiac hypertrophy and failure. Stretch-dependent and independent pathways have been identified. Stretch usually results from mechanical overload (e.g. aortic stenosis, arterial hypertension), but may also stem from abnormal contractility of the myocardial cell itself, e.g. in hypertrophic cardiomyopathy. This latter condition mostly arises from a mutation in a contractile protein. Stretch may trigger one of two events: either an increase in intracellular calcium levels at each heart beat (through as yet unknown mechanisms). This will activate the calcium/calmodulin-dependent phosphatase calcineurin in the cytosol. A protein of the transcription factor family NFAT, which reside in the cytoplasm in their phosphorylated form, will be dephosphorylated and translocate to the nucleus where they induce the expression of genes typical of hypertrophy. In the other stretch-related pathway, stretch is thought to act on the extracellular matrix. This signal will be transmitted through the membrane via laminin (extracellular) and dystroglycan (dark square) or the integrin family of proteins.

There are also molecular mechanisms which are conducive to hypertrophy independent of stretch. These are mostly thought to be mediated by receptors which are coupled to G-proteins (largely Gq). Stimulation of the receptors for angiotensin II, endothelin, and the alpha adrenergic receptor by their cognate ligands is well documented to be sufficient for the induction of hypertrophy (and failure). The unresolved question is, which pathway(s) are relevant in human cardiac hypertrophy. It appears likely that a distinctive set of mechanisms variably combine in different clinical situations.

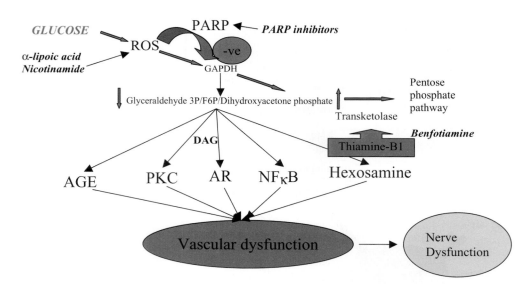

Figure 11.1 Possible mechanisms involved in the diversion of substrate (glucose) flux leading to diabetic neuropathy. Abbreviations: ROS: reactive oxygen species; PARP: poly(ADP-ribose) polymerase; DAG: diacylglycerol; AGE: advanced glycation end-product; PKC: protein kinase C; AR: aldose reductase, NF$\kappa\beta$; GADPH: glyceraldehyde–phosphate dehydrogenase.

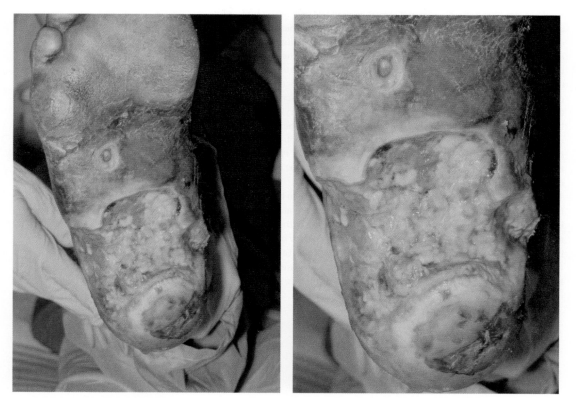

Figure 11.2 Plantar ulceration with necrosis.

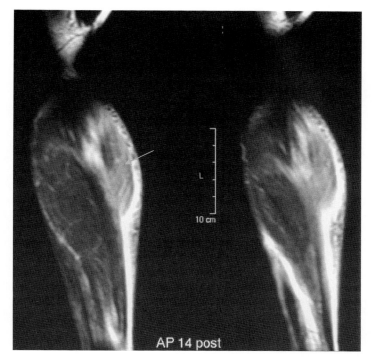

Figure 11.3 MR axial fat suppressed T2 weighted turbo spin-echo sagittal sequences were performed through the right calf demonstrating an extensive high signal abnormality throughout the medial head of the gastrocnemius muscle (→) and adjacent tissue with normal lateral head.

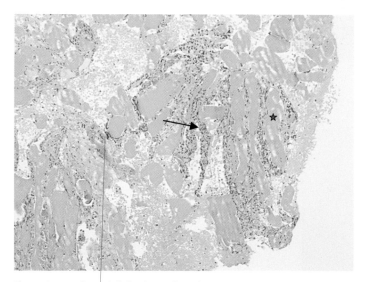

Figure 11.4 Inflamed skeletal muscle with a severe active chronic inflammatory cell infiltrate (→) between individual myocytes showing varying degrees of necrosis (*) characterized by loss of cross striations and nuclei together with fragmentation (H&E, ×100).

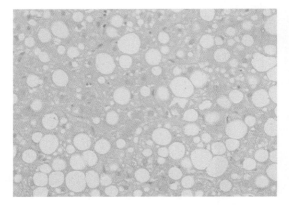

Figure 13.4 Alcoholic liver disease, fatty liver.

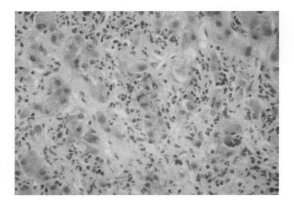

Figure 13.5 Alcoholic hepatitis (severe).

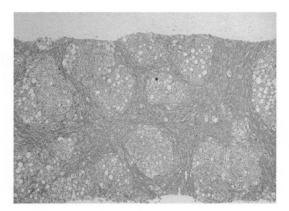

Figure 13.6 Alcoholic liver disease, micronodular cirrhosis.

5

Mechanisms of disease – allergy and anaphylaxis

Richard S. H. Pumphrey

Mechanisms of acute hypersensitivity reactions

Introduction

Allergy causes a vast range of illness. As might be expected for a process caused by inappropriate activation of the immune system, allergy mostly affects the body's interface with the environment – skin, conjunctivae, airways and gut – but any organ can be affected when the reaction involves the microvasculature. Although allergic reactions can cause behavioural changes, it is just as common for learned illness behaviour to mimic allergy; this is seldom mentioned in basic medical textbooks and commonly causes diagnostic confusion, so this chapter starts with an account of the behavioural aspects and works downward through the layers of complexity to the molecular processes that underlie allergy.

The most severe manifestation of acute allergic reaction is anaphylaxis. Its variability makes it difficult to diagnose in time to give treatment that could prevent its progression and consequently it may be fatal, either because of shock or asphyxia. The shock may be due to volume redistribution or direct effects of mediators on the heart, and the asphyxia may be due to upper or lower airways obstruction by the effects of the allergic reaction. This chapter ends with guidance for its recognition and management.

The nomenclature of allergy, hypersensitivity, and intolerance reactions causes confusion and remains controversial. Different terms are used in the USA and Europe. The European/WHO terminology (EAACI, 2001; Johansson *et al.*, 2004) is used in this chapter: for each manifestation of hypersensitivity, the primary division is into *non-immunological hypersensitivity* and *allergy* – the general synonym for immunological hypersensitivity of all types. Allergy is then divided into *IgE-mediated* and *non–IgE-mediated*. An older classification is still widely used, with IgE-mediated reactions called "type I hypersensitivity" and non–IgE-mediated allergy divided into types II through IV (Gell and Coombs, eds., 1962).

Behaviour mimicking hypersensitivity

Some patients claim allergy to hair sprays, disinfectants, household cleaning agents, paint, diesel exhaust and similar smells. Attacks may come on within seconds of exposure – too fast for an immunological process – leading to the conclusion that a neurological mechanism is more likely. Symptoms are variable but may include difficulty breathing, faintness, dizziness, palpitations, aches and pains, fatigue, impaired concentration and so on. Other triggers may cause this type of illness: an unusual patient claimed to be 'allergic to electricity'. She first suffered symptoms after a frightening lightning strike on her home, but later these recurred whenever lights or kitchen equipment were switched on near her. This group of conditions has been called 'idiopathic environmental intolerance' and may be a manifestation of panic disorder (Staudenmayer *et al.*, 2003; Tarlo *et al.*, 2002).

Intermittent or paroxysmal attacks of upper airway obstruction due to tight apposition of the vocal chords have commonly been misdiagnosed as allergic reactions (Matorell *et al.*, 1999). Symptoms may be very similar to laryngeal oedema, and such patients may have an attack following eating or in circumstances that lead to a diagnosis of allergy. Allergy is so common that allergy tests may be positive, adding to the confusion. Attacks commonly come on too quickly for genuine allergy, which usually takes at least 10 min before breathing becomes difficult and may recover more quickly; genuine angioedema takes many minutes to resolve, even following treatment. Diagnosis is confirmed by seeing the inappropriate chord movement using fibre-optic laryngoscopy; management ranges from proton pump inhibitors for symptoms associated with gastro-oesophageal reflux (Halstead, 2005) to speech therapy if the condition is psychogenic (Vertigan *et al.*, 2005).

Patients commonly attribute their ailments to what they have eaten. It can be difficult to sort out imagined associations from those that are real (Sampson, 1999). Each symptom may have a functional or an organic cause – for example, the abdominal bloating could be due to either to aerophagy or to non-allergic lactose hypersensitivity (Houghton and Whorwell, 2005) (Fig. 5.1). Dizziness and fatigue a few hours after eating may be due to hypoglycaemia; this has been reported in patients on self-imposed low-carbohydrate diets because of suspicion of carbohydrate intolerance (Bethune, Gompels and Spickett, 1999); the symptoms were caused by the diet they followed in the hope of avoiding the symptoms. Reactions triggered by sight, taste, or smell of the food can be distinguished from hypersensitivity by challenging under double-blind conditions: for example, a population study in an English town showed a perceived prevalence of food intolerance of almost 20%, but double-blind food challenge provided objective evidence of symptoms related to food in fewer than 2% of subjects (Young *et al.*, 1996). Without proper management, the list of avoided foods may grow inexorably, leading to malnutrition.

Behavioural aspects of allergic reactions

Sneezing and coughing are reflex responses to airways irritation, which may commonly occur during acute allergic reactions. Similarly, allergic reactions affecting the stomach trigger vomiting. Panic is so common in severe generalised reactions as to raise the suspicion that it is a reflex response. It may be recognised by a sense of 'impending doom' – the feeling that one is about to die – a common sensation during anaphylactic reactions.

It has been claimed (Russell *et al.*, 1984; MacQueen *et al.*, 1989) that after Pavlovian conditioning in experimental animals, the conditioning stimulus can replace allergen for mast cell activation and cause release of the same chemical mediators as did the allergen. Similar conditioned responses could account for reactions in allergic patients who, following genuine severe allergic reactions, have symptoms in similar or stressful circumstances in the absence of the allergic trigger.

Patients' appreciation of their allergic symptoms is variable and susceptible to the placebo effect. Because of this, 'alternative' treatment has a good chance of success, and it is hard to prove the effectiveness of new treatments for allergic disease.

Target organs

Although allergic responses are commonly restricted to the area of contact in skin or mucosa, spread of the allergen by blood or lymph can lead to generalised reactions. Each organ responds in a way determined by its structure: in the skin there may be urticaria or angioedema; reactions in the gut cause vomiting, colic, or diarrhoea; in the lungs there may be bronchoconstriction and mucus secretion; in the nose, blockage, secretion and sneezing; in the eyes, conjunctival oedema and redness, pain and lachrymation. Although the microvasculature is involved in all allergic reactions, the rest of the cardiovascular system is only affected by severe generalised reactions, when there may be shock.

IgE-mediated allergic reactions were previously called 'immediate-type hypersensitivity' because of

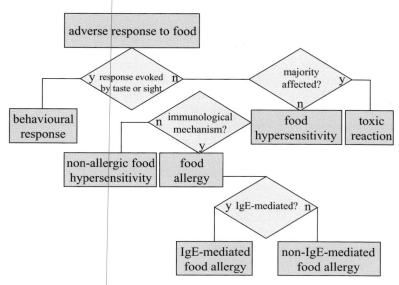

Figure 5.1 Classification of adverse reactions to foods. Not all adverse reactions to foods are due to allergy. Those with pseudo-allergy commonly attribute their symptoms to foods. They do not suffer the symptoms consistently when challenged with the suspected food under double-blind conditions. Non-allergic lactose hypersensitivity is a common condition in the natural human adult state, with the majority of the world's population hypersensitive to dietary lactose as adults. In infants, lactase digests lactose; but with increasing age, the levels of this enzyme in the gut fall and dietary lactose is left for the gut bacteria to convert into methane and hydrogen (which cause bloating and flatulence) and a variety of irritant acidic metabolites. In Europe, where the majority of adults retain enough lactase to cope with moderate quantities of milk, this is classified as non-allergic food hypersensitivity (formerly 'food intolerance'). In the rest of the world, where the majority of adults lack lactase, this could be classified as a toxic reaction. Non-allergic food hypersensitivity may be (rather arbitrarily) divided into reactions due to enzyme deficiency (e.g. lactase deficiency), direct pharmacological activity (such as high doses of monosodium glutamate causing Kwok's disease or tyramine causing migraine), and reactions that do not fall into these two categories.

their rapid onset, commonly peaking at 15 min after exposure and resolving within the hour if the amount of the agent is close to the least that will trigger a reaction. If there is exposure to much larger quantities, the reaction may spread beyond the initial point of contact, and it may be prolonged. In cases of extreme sensitivity, even the minute quantities introduced in a skin-prick test may lead to a generalised reaction. Delay in onset of a reaction may be due to delay in absorption of the allergen

(Inomata *et al.*, 2005) or the need for some chemical change in the structure of the allergen following (or in the case of dietary allergens, preceding) absorption. Delay in resolution of a reaction may be due to slow, continuing release of allergen from the gut or some other reservoir or to some secondary process triggered by the initial reaction. Thus, it is not unusual for persistent urticaria to follow an initial acute allergic reaction. When this happens, consideration should be given to the possibility that the initial 'reaction' was part of the continuing idiopathic (non-IgE–mediated) urticaria/angioedema, and the attribution to an allergic cause may have been mistaken.

All the symptoms of an IgE-mediated allergic reaction can be caused in other ways, but the time course will usually differ. Thus, non-IgE–mediated urticaria (which has many causes) commonly has a slower onset and lasts longer – sometimes months or years. Another example is asthma, rhinitis and nasal polyposis associated with aspirin sensitivity; this is not an allergy but instead may be due to interference with arachidonic acid metabolism in susceptible people. It may be difficult to tell when symptoms are genuinely due to allergy, when they are due to a non-allergic process causing similar symptoms, or when both allergic and non-allergic processes are acting synergistically.

Tissues affected by IgE-mediated allergic responses

Most tissues can be affected in one way or another by allergic responses. The microvasculature is a main target for the mediators of allergic reactions. Leakage of fluid from the venules in the upper dermis causes urticaria, in deeper tissues, angioedema. When angioedema affects the upper airway, it may cause difficulty breathing and sometimes death.

As tissues have a limited number of ways they can respond, their response during an allergic reaction is often similar to responses triggered by other stimuli. For example, bradykinin has similar actions to histamine on the microvasculature (Kaplan and Silverberg, 2002). In clinical practice, bradykinin tends to cause angioedema rather than urticaria, and the time course of these swellings is slower. An example is hereditary angioedema, where patients suffer attacks of swelling (often visible in deep subcutaneous tissues, when the swelling commonly follows minor trauma, but more commonly round the gut, causing abdominal pain or even obstruction) taking a few hours to reach their worst and persisting for a day or two; attacks of swelling commonly recur at 2- to 4-week intervals. Hereditary angioedema is due to deficiency of C1 esterase inhibitor, which allows

more rapid generation of bradykinin by the contact system (factor XIIa's action on kallikreinogen and kallikrein's on high-molecular-weight kininogen-releasing bradykinin are inhibited by C1 esterase inhibitor). Similar bradykinin-mediated swelling may follow treatment with angiotensin converting enzyme (ACE) inhibitors (Nikpoor, Duan and Rouleau, 2005): This is one pathway for the destruction of bradykinin. Both hereditary angioedema and adverse reactions to ACE inhibitors have been fatal when the angioedema blocked the upper airway, and reactions have been confused with allergy.

Other mediators released in allergic reactions also affect the microvasculature. Prostaglandins, leucotrienes, and cytokines act on endothelial cells and vascular smooth muscle, contributing to the acute allergic response (Lilly, 2005; Christie and Henderson, 2002). Their action on bronchial smooth muscle is probably more important than that of histamine. Detailed study of the tissues of the lower respiratory tract during asthmatic reactions has revealed the great complexity of primary and secondary mediators and their varied acute and chronic actions on the tissues and structure of the lung (Davies *et al.*, 2003).

Histamine causes relaxation of arteriolar smooth muscle but contraction of smooth muscle in the uterus, bronchioles and gut. The first experiments by Henry Dale into mechanisms of immediate-type allergic responses (Dale, 1953) used the contraction of uterine smooth muscle as the indicator. This demonstrated the need for sensitisation by a serum factor (IgE antibodies) before challenge by the allergen, and although histamine was known to have a similar action, it was 14 years before histamine was identified as the mediator for this type of reaction.

The nervous system plays an important part in acute allergic responses. The typical IgE-mediated allergic response to a skin-prick test (where a minute quantity of an allergen extract is pricked in through the epidermis) is a 'wheal and flare' response. The wheal is due to leakage of fluid from the venules caused by histamine, and the flare is due to reflex vasodilatation caused by substance P released from sensory fibres following the retrograde transmission of the pain signal from histamine (Okabe, 2001).

Similar sensory fibre responses trigger sneezing and coughing. Many mast cells (particularly those in the mucosa) are associated with autonomic nerve fibres, and these cells can be activated to secrete mediators neurologically (Suzuki, 2003). For this to explain how Pavlovian conditioning might cause mediator release (MacQueen et al., 1989), there would have to be an afferent sensory and efferent autonomic pathway with central processing: proof of such a mechanism has yet to be published.

Secondary effects of allergic reactions on tissues

Mucosal epithelial cells are affected by acute allergic reactions. The interactions are complex and involve autonomic nerves as well as mediators produced by the underlying tissues in response to allergen (Shimizu et al., 2004). Goblet cells in the epithelium and mucous glands are induced to secrete mucus, and the mucus genes are induced in ciliated epithelial cells and their precursors, leading to mucous metaplasia and hyperplasia (Hoshino et al., 2005). Thus repeated allergic stimulation leads to structural changes with enhanced mucus production.

This is just one change among many induced in the lungs in asthma. Detailed analysis leads to a picture of tissues awash with cytokines and other inflammatory mediators, produced by many different cell types and acting on many other cell types, with secondary, tertiary and higher-order effects (Holgate et al., 2000).

Treatment of asthma with β-2 agonists alone may relieve bronchoconstriction but does nothing to prevent the inflammatory response that goes with remodelling. Adequate doses of steroids have a limited effect on remodeling (Ward and Walters, 2005), but do protect against life-threatening attacks of asthma (Alvarez et al., 2005); they are an essential component of asthma management.

Release of mediators

The primary mediators of an acute allergic reaction come from a variety of specialised cells with histamine-containing granules (Fig. 5.2). These comprise two main types of mast cell, distinguishable by their granule content and structure, and basophils. These specialised cells are all triggered in a similar way by allergen bridging between two IgE molecules that are bound to the high-affinity IgE receptor (FcRεI) (Oliver et al., 2004). A cascade of events in these cells leads to the release of their granules, which then release pre-formed stored mediators (Fig. 5.3).

Each type of cell has a variety of other receptors that can activate the cell by non-IgE–mediated pathways and can increase or decrease the sensitivity of the cell to activation by IgE (Valent et al., 2002).

Immune responses leading to IgE antibodies

The first antibodies made in an immune response are IgM (the primary antibody response). The genes for immunoglobulin heavy chains are strung along the heavy chain locus on chromosome 14, with the library of V genes at the 5' (upstream) end, then D and J segments, then IgM and the other classes of heavy chain. During the maturation of antibody responses, the intervening heavy chain genes are looped out, bringing the VDJ rearranged gene next to the active heavy chain. The signals increasing the probability of the active heavy chain gene being the epsilon (ε) include the effects of IL-4 and IL-13 (produced by Th2 cells) on the B cell, but many other factors are involved (Bacharier, Jabara and Geha, 2005); principal among these are the effects of the dendritic cells in regulating immunoglobulin class switching. Many immune responses induce a brief, low burst of IgE production: the difference in allergic responses is the higher level and persistence of the IgE response. What causes this persistence is poorly understood: some factors are associated with the host (manifest as "atopy"), some with the timing and route of exposure and some with the immunising substance (the allergen together with other factors – adjuvants – that modify the immune response to the allergen).

Atopy and the timing of exposure

People are not all equally susceptible to allergy. Studies of inheritance suggest a multigenic pattern, and

mast cells and basophils

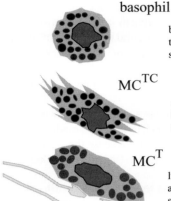

basophil

blood
triggered by C3a/C5a, opioids
secrete LTC4 but no PGD2

MC^{TC}

skin, (gut submucosa); T-cell independent
triggered by substance P, C3a/C5a, opioids
secrete PGD2 and LTC4 if triggered by IgE

MC^{T}

lung, gut mucosa; T-cell dependent
autonomic innervation
secrete PGD2 and LTC4 if triggered by IgE

Figure 5.2 Mast cells and basophils. MC^T indicates mast cell with granules containing tryptase; MC^{TC} indicates mast cells with granules containing tryptase and chymase. The granules of all three types contain histamine and proteoglycans, including heparin and chondroitin sulphate. All three are triggered by IgE as indicated in Fig. 5.4 to release their granule contents and secrete mediators, such as arachidonic acid derivatives. (See colour plate section.)

recently some genes have been identified whose allotypes seem able to modify the probability or severity of asthma or atopy; however, many of these genes cause their effects in concert with environmental factors (Arruda *et al.*, 2005) (Table 5.1). The consequence of so many genetic variants determining the atopic tendency is that the population must contain a wide spread of susceptibility, from those who are unlikely ever to mount an allergic response to those who react to very many environmental allergens with an IgE-dominated response. The recent trend for increasing prevalence of atopy suggests that environmental factors are facilitating the appearance of this state in those with lower genetic potential.

What are the new factors in the environment that are causing those with a lower innate tendency to become atopic? As atopy is manifest so early in life, attention has been focussed on gestation and infancy. A leading contender is the hygiene hypoth-

esis. In various studies associations have been found between infant immunisation (increases), infant use of antibiotics (increases), minor infant infections (decreases), exposure to endotoxin (decreases) (Waser *et al.*, 2004), and the later prevalence of atopy and asthma. The idea is emerging that certain infections such as hepatitis A may in certain patients be particularly effective at permanently switching off allergic responses (Umetsu, McIntire and DeKruff, 2005). Dendritic cells control the balance between Th1 and Th2 responses and may, in those destined to be atopic, alter this in favour of Th2 at the crucial time when the infant is exposed to potential allergens. Th2 lymphocytes include those secreting IL-4 and IL-13 – the key cytokines that not only support IgE antibody production in susceptible people but also increase mast cell reactivity and induce mucous metaplasia in the airways. There are, of course, many other potential environmental factors that will influence the appearance of atopy – level of

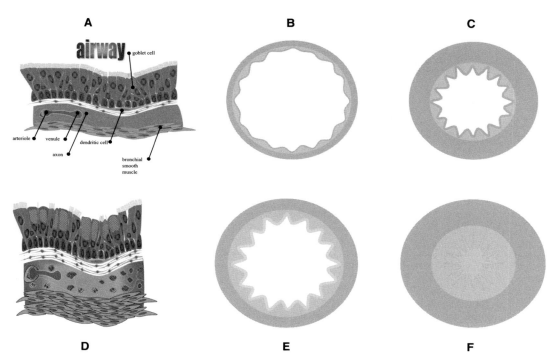

Figure 5.3 Allergic response in the lungs. A and B represent high-magnification and low-magnification views of a cross-section of a normal bronchiole, whereas D and E represent the corresponding views of a bronchiole from an asthmatic. Repeated or persistent allergic responses lead to remodelling of the airways. The main changes are mucous metaplasia/hyperplasia in the epithelium, thickening and stiffening of the lamina reticularis, thickening of the bronchial smooth muscle, infiltration of the airway walls with inflammatory cells (eosinophils, lymphocytes, plasma cells, mast cells) and an increase in small blood vessels and nerve fibres. The consequence of these changes is that an allergic response can lead to more severe obstruction in those with airways remodelling (C and F). (See colour plate section.)

allergen exposure in infancy, parental smoking and so on.

The nature of allergens

Some substances are more likely to cause an allergic response than others. It seems that the number of proteins associated with strong IgE antibody responses is limited. For example, of all the myriad plant proteins eaten in a normal diet, common allergens fall into a few structural families and a restricted range of functions – many being related to the plants defence against pathogens (pathogenesis related proteins) (Mills *et al.*, 2004). Curiously,

other key allergens are related to defence or attack – venom in wasp or jellyfish stings, antibiotics. and so on. What is it about these that make them allergens? It has not proved possible to identify any protein structure that is specifically associated with a tendency to cause an IgE response other than perhaps resistance to degradation before processing by antigen-presenting cell. On the other hand, there is evidence that other factors associated with the initial exposure to the protein do influence the type of response. These factors include the route, the timing and accompanying agents that act as adjuvants.

An adjuvant is a factor accompanying the antigen that alters the immune response. For example, many

Table 5.1 Disease-modifying genes for atopy and asthma*

Gene for	Location	Actions of disease modifying allotypes
CD14	5q 31	High-affinity receptor for LPS: favours Th1 over Th2 responses
IL-10		In presence of LPS, favours Th1 over Th2
		Promotes bronchial hyper-reactivity after RSV infection
IL-4	5q	
IL-13	5q	IgE promotion (favours Th2 responses)
IL-4R	16p12	Increases sensitivity of mast cells
		Promotes mucous metaplasia/hyperplasia in the airways
IgE	12q	IgE antibody characteristics
FcεRIβ	11q13	Mast cell responsiveness
		Modifies mast cell responsiveness to IgE-mediated signalling
β2-AR	5q 31–32	Disease modifier for bronchospasm
		Nocturnal asthma, bronchial hyper-responsiveness, increased IgE levels, asthma severity

*Many genes on at least 20 chromosomes affect the manifestation of atopy and/or asthma. Other genes are associated with eczema and other atopic conditions such as rhinitis. The examples here are a few which have been the subject of recent research.

immunising agents are adsorbed onto aluminium hydroxide. This insoluble matrix increases the uptake of the antigen into antigen-presenting cells, promoting a good antibody response. In some mouse models, aluminium hydroxide increases anaphylactic antibody production to the adsorbed protein (Yamanishi *et al.*, 2004); but in humans, repeated increasing doses of alum-conjugated allergen extracts are used to suppress IgE-mediated allergy (Corrigan *et al.*, 2005). Some foods seem much more potent than others in causing allergic responses, perhaps because there is some factor in the food that acts as an IgE-promoting adjuvant. Stings commonly lead to IgE responses in atopics and non-atopics alike: the venom contains toxins that will injure or destroy lymphocytes and antigen-presenting cells, opening up the possibility that the immune response may be diverted towards IgE production by these effects.

Evolution of allergic responses

IgE is a mammalian class of immunoglobulin. Why did it evolve? The cascade of events following activation of an allergic response described in this chapter is wholly disadvantageous, so there must

be some benefit conferred under different circumstances. Part of the answer lies with the defensive immune response against parasitic infestation (Hagel *et al.*, 2004). Parasitic helminths in particular cause immune responses with dominant IgE and eosinophils components, but proof that this IgE response is protective is limited to a few experimental models involving nematodes. Additionally, parasitic infestation can switch off the ability to produce allergic responses to proteins that otherwise act as allergens. As infestation by parasites was almost certainly endemic throughout most of human history; this seems yet another line of evidence that we today live under too hygienic conditions for a balanced immune system.

Anaphylaxis

Charles Richet wrote, '*ANAPHYLAXIS is the opposite condition to protection (phylaxis). I coined the word in 1902 to describe the peculiar attribute which certain poisons possess of increasing instead of diminishing the sensitivity of an organism to their action*' (Richet, 1913). It took many years before the processes causing such reactions were understood, and during that time, the meaning of the word

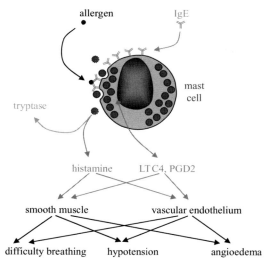

Figure 5.4 Mast cell activation during an allergic reaction. Adjacent IgE molecules, attached to the surface membrane of the mast cell *via* the high affinity IgE receptor (FcεRI), are bridged by binding to allergen. This leads to externalisation of the mast cell granules near the bridged receptors; thus, major activation in anaphylaxis will cause degranulation of the whole cell. Arachidonic acid is then released from the nuclear membrane by phospholipase A2 and converted to prostaglandin and leukotrienes (LTC4, PGD2), which are then secreted. These mediators then act on their respective receptors on smooth muscle, endothelial cells, secretory cells and so on to cause the clinical features of anaphylaxis. (See colour plate section.)

'anaphylaxis' drifted. It was clear that not all sudden, severe hypersensitivity reactions had the same mechanism, and the term 'anaphylactoid' was introduced to distinguish non-IgE–mediated reactions (Hanzlik and Karsner, 1920).

Anaphylaxis has recently been redefined. The new definition is: '*Anaphylaxis is a severe, life-threatening, generalised or systemic hypersensitivity reaction*'. Anaphylaxis is divided into allergic anaphylaxis and non-allergic anaphylaxis, and allergic anaphylaxis is divided into IgE-mediated anaphylaxis and non-IgE–mediated anaphylaxis. It is suggested that the term 'anaphylactoid' should no longer be used. This proposal has not been universally accepted.

An authoritative recent American practice parameter (Joint Task Force on Practice Parameters, 2005) states: 'Anaphylaxis is defined . . . as a condition caused by an IgE-mediated reaction. Anaphylactoid reactions are defined as those reactions that produce the same clinical picture as anaphylaxis but are not IgE mediated'.

Anaphylaxis may be fatal either because of shock or asphyxia. The shock may be either central, due to direct effects of anaphylactic mediators on the heart (commonest in hospital, in older people with diseased hearts), or peripheral, due to generalised vasodilatation (commonest in younger people, in reactions outside hospital). If the onset of shock is delayed, there may also be fluid loss into the tissues through angioedema; but by the time shock is established, there may be insufficient pressure in the venules to cause fluid to leak into the tissues. Anaphylactic shock inevitably causes myocardial ischaemia, both because of the low pulse pressure and arterial vasoconstriction in the coronaries or smaller vessels of the myocardium. Once shock is severe, the vena cava may become empty (particularly if the patient is made to sit up). No blood returns to the heart, and although pulseless electrical activity persists for a while, the lack of circulating blood soon leads to cerebral anoxia and death (Pumphrey, 2003).

The asphyxia may be due to severe asthma (often with mucous plugging) or angioedema of the upper airway with occlusion of the lumen. Food anaphylaxis is most commonly fatal due to asthma, whereas sting anaphylaxis is more commonly fatal because of shock.

There is a continuous spectrum of severity of reactions from trivial to fatal in patients seen in casualty or recounted by patients seen in clinic. Even the mildest reactions may be generalised (e.g. a mild generalised urticarial reaction caused by food allergy), and fatal reactions may be due to a localised reaction in the throat. There is no agreed dividing line above which the reaction is regarded as anaphylactic and below which it is simply called an acute allergic reaction. These factors taken together make it difficult to define anaphylaxis to universal satisfaction.

Table 5.2 Non-allergic anaphylaxis and non–IgE-mediated anaphylaxis*

	Mediator	Similarity to IgE-mediated anaphylaxis
Opioid sensitivity	Mast cells	Complete
Contrast media	Mast cells (non–mast cell pathway?)	Complete
Autonomic	Mast cells or direct vascular effects	Complete
Modified gelatins	Basophils?	Complete
NSAID reactions	Leucotrienes	Rashes, asthma, angioedema
Scombrotoxin poisoning	Histamine	vomiting, flushing,
ACE inhibitors or acquired c1inh deficiency	Bradykinin	bronchospasm angioedema
Dextran reactions	IgG, complement	Shock, rashes, bronchospasm
Cremophore (epoxylated castor oil used as solvent for vitamin K, Taxol, etc).	Complement	Shock, rashes, bronchospasm
Vancomycin	Not histamine	Rash ('red man')

*Many agents that can cause non-allergic reactions can also cause IgE-mediated in other patients – thus, vancomycin can cause IgE-mediated anaphylactic reactions as well as the commoner 'red man syndrome,' which will affect anyone given too rapid an infusion of vancomycin. It is possible that those that cause non-allergic anaphylaxis will sometimes also synergistically enhance the severity of IgE-mediated anaphylaxis. (C1inch = C1 esterase inhibitor.)

Non-allergic anaphylaxis and non-IgE–mediated anaphylaxis

Another complication comes from the multiplicity of pathogenic pathways that can cause reactions with some similarity to IgE-mediated anaphylaxis (Table 5.2. For some agents, there is conflicting evidence about the mechanism: reactions to modified gelatins used for plasma volume expansion may be due to IgE antibodies, and there is often a positive weal-and-flare skin-test response. In other cases, there may be a rise in plasma histamine but not in mast cell tryptase, suggesting selective triggering of basophils rather than mast cells.

Anaphylactic sensitisation

In his first description of anaphylaxis in dogs, Charles Richet noted that there had to be a gap of 3 to 6 weeks between the first (sensitising) dose and the second (challenge) dose of actinotoxin when anaphylaxis was seen (Richet, 1913). A majority of patients seen in clinic following their first generalised reaction to a wasp sting will tell of a previous sting 3 to 8 weeks earlier. Most patients with antibiotic anaphylaxis will have safely had many previous courses. Severe milk allergy in infants most commonly causes eczema; but if this food is strictly avoided for months and the sensitisation persists, the next exposure can cause anaphylaxis – usually with a major asthmatic component. Sensitisation to latex may follow wearing latex gloves (particularly if the hands are affected by eczema) or repetitive surgery in young children such as those with spina bifida: the specificity of the latex antibodies differs between these groups. Most such patients have only limited reactions on re-exposure, but a few will develop anaphylaxis. Many (most?) people with hay fever would have anaphylaxis if injected with an extract of the pollen causing their seasonal rhinitis.

What distinguishes those who will have an anaphylactic reaction from those who will not? The answer is complex and will vary from one allergen to another. Genetic variants in the renin-angiotensin system (Hermann and Ring, 1993) and/or treatment with anti-hypertensive drugs (Ober, MacLean and

Hannaway, 2003) may predispose to shock reactions, an asthmatic tendency and/or poor daily control of asthma predispose to asthmatic anaphylaxis, but we have no understanding about what suddenly causes anaphylaxis to an antibiotic in someone who has taken the same drug for years without problems.

Fatal anaphylaxis

Since most acute allergic reactions recover spontaneously with no lasting after effects, those reactions that may be fatal are of greatest concern. In the UK over the last 10 years, about half the recognised fatal reactions have been iatrogenic (reactions to drugs or contrast media) and one-quarter each were due to sting reactions and food allergy (Pumphrey, 2000). Rare additional causes have included spontaneous rupture of a hydatid cyst, allergy to hair dye, and latex allergy. One in five patients with non-fatal acute attacks with features of an allergic reaction have idiopathic urticaria/ angioedema or idiopathic anaphylaxis: such patients commonly attribute their symptoms to food allergy, but allergy tests and food challenge tests prove negative. It is not known how many sudden deaths may be due to such idiopathic reactions, as they may be misinterpreted as asthma or falsely attributed to food allergy.

The spectrum of fatal anaphylaxis has changed over the years. Between 1890 and 1950, passive immunity conferred by transfusion of immune globulin from repeatedly immunised animals (commonly horses) was used to treat a variety of infections such as tetanus and diphtheria. Allergic reactions were common. Mostly these occurred about 10 days after an injection, when the primary immune response to the horse serum formed antibodies that reacted with the horse proteins still in the circulation. These were therefore non-IgE–mediated allergy due to antigen plus IgG antibody complexes, with subsequent activation of complement. When horse serum was injected into someone who had already had IgG antibodies circulating, the immediate reaction (including flushing, difficulty breathing, and shock) would now be classified as non-IgE–mediated anaphylaxis. Alternatively, those already

allergic to horses through equestrian activities may have IgE-mediated anaphylaxis to injected horse serum (Demoly et al., 2002).

The introduction of penicillin reduced the use of antisera, but penicillin was soon recognised as the commonest cause of fatal anaphylaxis (Welch et al., 1957). Cephalosporins are equally allergenic and also cause fatal anaphylaxis. Fatal iatrogenic anaphylaxis is now most commonly reported during induction of anaesthesia; muscle relaxants are usually blamed for these reactions, but often multiple drugs are given in quick succession and it may be difficult to tell which was responsible or whether the combination was synergistic in causing the reaction (Baldo, Pham, and Zhao, 2001). Contrast media also cause fatal reactions; for these, curiously, non-fatal reactions are commoner in females, but nearly all the recent fatal reactions have been in males.

Acute systemic allergic reactions to stings affect those without other allergies as commonly as they affect atopics. It seems likely that they have affected a similar proportion of the population throughout history. Occasionally these reactions may be fatal – on average four such fatalities have been recorded each year in the UK in recent years. In contrast, acute allergic reactions to foods are definitely becoming more common, in line with the increase in frequency of atopy and asthma (Sampson, 1999). The great majority of those suffering acute allergic reactions to foods are atopic, with inhalant as well as food allergy. Infantile atopic eczema is also very common in this group. In recent years an average of six fatalities each year have been recorded in the UK, but it is likely that this is an underestimate. Sixty times as many people die from acute attacks of asthma; because asthma is regarded as a natural cause of death, the cause of the attack is rarely investigated. When it has been, a cause has often been obvious – either a food to which the deceased was known to be allergic such as milk or nuts, a drug such as aspirin, or an inhalant such as horse dander.

For around one-quarter of fatal drug or sting reactions, there has been no previous history of allergy at all; half had only minor reactions to previous exposure, and the remaining quarter had previous moderate or severe reactions; in the case of stings, these have usually recovered without any treatment. While those dying from food allergy usually have a history of previous reactions, only 1 in 4 has had a reaction severe enough to be given treatment before the one that proved fatal.

Both age at death and time course of reaction are characteristic of the cause.

Milder reactions

One-third or more of the UK population will have an IgE-mediated allergic reaction at some time in their lives (ISAAC, 1998). Such reactions are commonly mild and the sensitivity may be brief. At least 1 person in 5 is atopic, and perhaps 1 in 100 has had a moderately severe acute allergic reaction. Although some accounts highlight a tendency to increasing severity of reactions with repeated exposure, this does not generally seem to be the case; the severity of a series of reactions commonly follows a random pattern.

Local type I responses

Local responses may be due to the tiny amount of allergen – as when grass pollen causes allergic conjunctivitis in hay fever. Larger quantities of the same allergen in the same individual can cause anaphylaxis, such as following injection of too high a dose of grass pollen extracts during hyposensitisation.

The stability of the allergen may also determine whether the reaction can become generalised. Some food allergens are acid-labile and therefore tend to cause local symptoms on the lips and in the mouth. Different proteins from the same source may be more stable, so the symptoms depend on which the subject is sensitive to. For example, in northern Europe, peach allergy is commonly associated with birch pollen sensitivity, and the cross-reactive protein in the peach is heat- and acid-labile. Thus it is only the fresh fruit that will cause symptoms, and only in the mouth (fresh fruit syndrome, oral allergy syndrome) (Sicherer, 2001). In southern Europe, on the other hand, peach allergy is more commonly due to IgE antibodies reactive with a small heat- and acid-stable protein (lipid transfer protein) (Zuidmeer *et al*, 2005), which is more likely to cause generalised symptoms and is thought to have been responsible for fatal reactions.

Investigating allergic reactions

A transient acute illness with features of a reaction raises several questions: was it an allergic reaction? What triggered the reaction? What was the mechanism? It is not easy to prove that an acute illness was due to allergy; mediators released during a reaction are mostly unstable and difficult to measure. An exception is mast cell tryptase: α tryptase is secreted by mast cells all the time and the level of this protein in the serum may be used to monitor mastocytosis (a variable condition with greatly increased numbers of mast cells that tends to progress over years). Beta tryptase is stored in the mast cell granule and is released during allergic reactions. Only small rises in serum level may occur in asthmatic reactions, and raised levels have been measured post-mortem in some cases where an allergic reaction seems unlikely; one possible reason is sampling from the wrong site: distal limb veins are ideal, as central samples may be contaminated by tryptase released from mast cell–rich viscera. Histamine and its metabolite methylhistamine are other markers of allergic reactions, but raised levels may be due to dietary histamine. Leucotrienes also are excreted in the urine and may be measured: they are less stable than methylhistamine, and great care is needed in collecting the sample and in its analysis.

The next question is what triggered the reaction? Other than challenging a patient with the allergen by the same route that is thought to have provoked the reaction, there are two main ways of investigating allergy. If the reaction was IgE-mediated, the presence of IgE antibodies can be detected by measuring the binding of IgE to allergen extracts *in vitro* or by skin-prick tests, where minute quantities of an allergen extract are introduced by pricking through a drop of extract placed on the skin. Both types of testing are variably liable to false-positive and false-negative outcomes.

False-negative tests are commonly due to lack of the specific allergenic epitope (the three-dimensional structure on the surface of the allergen that the IgE antibody binds to), either because the extraction process failed to include the protein or because the protein became denatured during extraction or subsequently. Because of this, "prick-prick" tests, where the lancet is first inserted just under the skin of the fruit or vegetable under test and then into the skin of the patient, may be needed to reduce the chance of a false-negative test, particularly for labile proteins in those foods that cross-react with pollen allergens.

False-positive skin-prick tests are due to non-specific histamine release by a variety of agents including drugs (codeine, morphine, atracurium), lectins, saponins and other naturally occurring detergents, and many others. 'False-positive' IgE antibodies include those that bind to determinants that behave as though they were univalent (such as cross-reactive carbohydrate determinants) and therefore cannot trigger mast-cell activation because this depends on bridging between IgE molecules held on two different high-affinity IgE receptors on the mast cell membrane.

Management of acute hypersensitivity reactions

The three themes in the management of patients with allergies are allergen avoidance, reduction of risk of a severe reaction, and rescue from the effects of a reaction.

Allergen avoidance

Some allergens are easier to avoid than others, and many factors affect the risk of exposure. For example, those with wasp sting allergy are at very high risk of a sting if they interfere with a wasp nest and at very low risk in mid-winter. It may be worth wearing protective clothing at times of highest risk – for example, for pest-control officers who have become allergic to wasp stings through exposure at work. For others, wasp stings occur almost at random, with as high a chance of being stung in bed as when walking in the garden. Because sting reactions can (rarely) be fatal and even careful avoidance cannot guarantee that there will never be an accidental sting, other measures such as desensitisation and self-treatment with adrenaline (epinephrine) should be considered.

Nut allergy may also cause fatal reactions, and successful nut avoidance requires great care on the part of the consumer. The greatest risk comes from restaurant food, where labelling is unregulated. Much packaged food is defensively labelled 'this product may contain traces of nuts' to avoid litigation in the event of a reaction, but this makes shopping difficult for those attempting strict nut avoidance. Even with great care, occasional accidental consumption seems inevitable (Sicherer, Burks and Sampson, 1998), and if reactions might be severe, those with nut allergy should carry rescue medication.

Reduction of risk of a severe response

Hyposensitisation
Repeated injection of increasing doses of allergen has been used to reduce allergic sensitivity – a procedure termed allergen-specific immunotherapy. This is well established as management of sting anaphylaxis, and after 5 years of maintenance injections every 4 to 6 weeks, patients will tolerate one sting without severe reaction for many years (Golden, 2001). Immunotherapy probably works for most IgE-mediated anaphylaxis, but the risk of severe reaction during the 'updosing' (the initial series of injections with increasing doses of allergen) has proved too high for this to be widely accepted as standard management for food allergy.

Good daily control of asthma
Most fatal anaphylactic reactions to foods have been due to difficulty breathing and have occurred in those taking daily treatment for asthma. There is evidence that their daily treatment had been

suboptimal, and that discontinuation of daily inhaled steroid was a risk factor for the severity of the reaction. Overuse of a short-acting β-2 agonist is associated with severe and fatal asthma (Spitzer *et al.*, 1992); in such patients adrenaline may not relieve bronchospasm in the event of an allergic reaction to food.

Rescue from the effects of reactions

Reactions can rapidly cause shock or asphyxia. Treatment must equally quickly rescue the patient from these, and the best option is the immediate use of adrenaline (epinephrine). In the airways, the β-2 activity will relax bronchospasm. In the microcirculation, α activity tightens the pre-capillary sphincters and beta activity reduces the leakiness of the venules, thus preventing angioedema. β-1 activity increases the force of the ventricular contractions. Taken together, these activities oppose the most dangerous effects of anaphylaxis. Unless the patient has already collapsed, the correct initial adult dose of adrenaline is 0.5 mg, given into the thigh muscle on the anterolateral aspect at the midpoint of the thigh (Simons *et al.*, 2000). Adrenaline is not well absorbed if given as a subcutaneous injection or if injected into the muscles of the arm.

Histamine is one of the major mediators of anaphylaxis, and antihistamines are helpful in reducing the effects of IgE-mediated allergic reactions. Histamine is not the only mediator; therefore by itself, an antihistamine is inadequate to rescue a patient from a severe reaction. Reactions may be biphasic (Brazil and MacNamara, 1998). Adequate treatment including steroids at the time of the onset of the reaction may be helpful in preventing these later effects.

Basic life support may fail when asphyxia is due to complete occlusion of the airways. Attempts to inflate the lungs cause inflation of the stomach instead. Shock is best managed by having the patient lie down with the legs raised and giving adrenaline before the shock is so advanced that the adrenaline is not circulated around the body. External cardiac massage is doomed to failure once anaphylactic shock has emptied the vena cava.

Because anaphylactic reactions are acute medical emergencies that often happen away from access to medical care, self-treatment with adrenaline is recommended (Sicherer and Simons, 2005) for anyone thought to be at risk of a life-threatening reaction. Auto-injectors are available, but their success depends on careful training (Sicherer, Forman, and Noone, 2000). Their use should be specifically avoided when non-allergic hypersensitivity is related to panic, when adrenaline will exacerbate the attack.

Clinical scenarios

Scenario 1

A 38-year-old English woman married to a Greek complains of allergy to olives, garlic bread and onions: within 5 min of eating these foods, her mouth becomes dry, her vision blurred and her fingers stiff; she becomes paralysed and is unable to talk or walk for several minutes. She has a previous medical history of tetany– possibly associated with hyperventilation. Forced hyperventilation in the clinic does not reproduce her symptoms. Skin-prick tests and specific IgE antibodies are negative to the suspected foods, but open food challenge causes a typical attack. Her tendon reflexes are extremely brisk during the attack.

Multiple-choice questions

Q1

Reactions to these particular foods are most likely due to what?
  a. IgE antibodies to cross-reactive oligosaccharides determinants.
  b. Separate IgE antibodies to each of the foods are causing reactions.
  c. By association with a stressful meal at which these foods were eaten.
  d. Direct pharmacological effects of absorbed metabolites of the foods are affecting the peripheral nerves.
  e. Direct pharmacological effects of absorbed metabolites of the foods are affecting the central nervous system.

Answer

a. No; cross-reactive IgE antibodies cause false-positive results and the text says these tests were negative.
b. No; symptoms were not those of an allergic response.
c. Yes.
d. No.
e. No.

Q2

Appropriate further investigations would be
a. Double-blind placebo-controlled food challenge.
b. Prick-prick testing with the suspected foods.
c. Tests for gluten sensitivity.
d. Nerve conduction studies during open challenge.
e. In-depth psychiatric assessment to discover the cause of her behaviour.

Answer

a. Yes.
b. No; this is for labile allergens.
c. No; coeliac disease would not cause these symptoms.
d. No; at least not until the DBPCFC has been shown to be positive, which it won't be.
e. Yes.

Q3

The correct management of this case is by
a. Cognitive behavioural therapy.
b. Strict avoidance of the implicated foods.
c. Giving the patient an adrenaline pen to self-treat if she has a reaction.
d. Maintenance treatment with carbamazepine.
e. Hypnotherapy by an appropriate expert practitioner.

Answer

a. Yes.
b. No; although this may work, it is not satisfactory, as the list of implicated foods may grow.
c. No; this may compound panic symptoms.

d. No.
e. Possibly.

Q4

Her previous attacks of tetany had been thought possibly to be due to involuntary hyperventilation. In the clinic, voluntary hyperventilation failed to reproduce the symptoms. Why?
a. It is difficult to persuade patients to hyperventilate voluntarily to the same extent as in an involuntary attack.
b. As with her spastic reaction to food, there were other CNS factors inducing her tetany.
c. We have misjudged this patient: all her symptoms have been due to a parathyroid adenoma.
d. Her food avoidance had led to vitamin D deficiency; hence the hypocalcaemic tetany.
e. She really did have coeliac disease, and her tetany was due to hypocalcaemia and hypomagnesaemia.

Answer

a. True.
b. Probably.
c. No; this would cause hypercalcaemia, not tetany.
d. No; with a Greek husband, it is unlikely that she would have had so little sun exposure.
e. No; there are no other suggestions of coeliac disease in her history.

Scenario 2

A 46-year-old pest-control officer has no previous history of allergies. He is stung by a wasp while attempting to treat a wasps' nest with insecticide. He suffers nothing more than immediate local swelling at the site of the stings but asks the occupational health nurse for advice. He is given antihistamine tablets to help with the itching from the stings and his symptoms quickly subside. Three weeks later, he has a similar accident and is stung by seven wasps. He rapidly becomes unwell, with sweating and pallor. He sits in the van, where his colleague supports him with a safety belt in a sitting position while he phones for help. The patient's breathing becomes noisy and then stops. An ambulance arrives within 5 min, and the paramedic finds the patient to have no pulse, with the ECG changes of a myocardial ischaemia and ST-segment elevation. He diagnoses myocardial infarction but resuscitation is unsuccessful. The autopsy shows only mild coronary atheroma with no thrombus; there are no macroscopic or histological abnormalities suggesting a specific cause of death.

Multiple-choice questions

Q1

He had no reaction to the first 3 stings, but 3 weeks later he died following 7 stings. What does this indicate?
a. This proves that his death could not have been due to allergy to wasp stings.
b. The first stings caused an allergic immune response with a brief peak of IgE to wasp venom; unfortunately he was stung again during this peak.
c. Although it is possible to develop new allergy following a sting, 3 weeks is too short a time.
d. He was mildly allergic, and although 3 wasps were not enough to cause a reaction, 7 were.
e. He had no previous history of allergies, so this is most unlikely to have been an allergic reaction.

Answer

a. No.
b. Yes.
c. No.
d. Possible, but in that case one would have expected some minor allergic symptoms from the first stings.
e. No; wasp sting reactions occur equally in those with no previous allergies.

Q2

Which of the following is plausible as a cause of death?
a. Coincidental myocardial infarction.
b. Accidental insecticide poisoning.

c. Asphyxial anaphylaxis to wasp venom allergy causing respiratory obstruction.
d. Anaphylaxis to the sting, causing shock, together with postural obstruction of venous return to the heart.
e. Toxic death from multiple wasp stings.

Answer

a. No; autopsy findings preclude this.
b. No; incorrect time course, no typical symptoms.
c. No; autopsy findings preclude this.
d. Yes.
e. No; he had had almost as many stings earlier without harm. Deaths due to toxic stings in adults usually involve in excess of 200 stings and take days to become fatal.

Q3

Which of the following are reasonable proposals for improved management?
a. He should have been given adrenaline for self-treatment following the first stings.
b. He should have been wearing full protective clothing when treating wasps' nests.
c. He should have been placed lying down with his legs raised when he felt faint following the second sting.
d. This may be achieved by a massive infusion of fluid. Paramedic protocols *do not* make provisions for this.
e. He should have been desensitised to wasp venom because of his occupational exposure.

Answer

a. No; there was no particular reason to think that he would become so sensitised after years as a pest-control officer.
b. Yes; this should be standard practice.
c. Yes; whatever the cause of his shock, this would have been good first aid.
d. No; by this stage the treatment would be the same – intravenous adrenaline to correct the profound shock. No treatment would have been effective until the vena cava had been refilled.

This might have been achieved by a massive intravenous infusion of fluid with measures to ensure centripetal venous drainage (e.g. military anti-shock trousers or lithotomy position for postural drainage). No paramedic protocols make provision for this.

e. No; same reason as given in (a). There are risks to unwarranted allergen–specific immunotherapy, and it is expensive.

Q4

The serum mast cell tryptase level at autopsy was extremely high, and the total IgE level was 15KIU/l with 3KU$_A$/l wasp venom–specific IgE antibodies.

which of the following are possibilities?

a. The paramedic was correct in his diagnosis; the raised tryptase was due to incorrect sampling at autopsy.

b. The low IgE and wasp-specific IgE suggest that this was not an anaphylactic death because up to 17% of the adult male population may have a similar level of wasp-specific IgE antibodies.

c. The presence of wasp venom–specific IgE raises the probability that his death was due to an allergic reaction.

d. The tryptase level is sufficiently high to make an anaphylactic reaction probable.

e. Tryptase levels may be this high following untreated myocardial infarction.

Answer

a. No; the autopsy findings do not support a thrombotic or embolic cause for the ischaemia – otherwise this would be a possibility.

b. No; the circumstances suggest that this was anaphylaxis, and even though the specific IgE was low, it was a significant proportion of the total.

c. Yes.

d. Yes.

e. No.

Scenario 3

A 35-year-old non-asthmatic man (A) has had increasing hay fever over the last few years. His symptoms start in April and persist until September. He has strongly positive skin-prick tests for birch and grass pollens. He has recently developed severe itching and swelling in his mouth after eating a peach and 3 weeks later had similar symptoms after eating a cherry. His skin-prick test with commercial peach extract is negative, as is his blood test for specific IgE to peach.

In the clinic, he finds himself sitting next to a 35-year-old woman (B) who also had an allergic reaction after eating a peach. In her case, this comprised generalised urticaria, angioedema of the face and throat with stridor, and asthma, for which she received emergency treatment with adrenalin, antihistamine, and steroid. This patient differed in that her IgE to nectarine was strongly positive.

Multiple- choice questions

Q1

Which of these statements is true for A, which for B, which for both, and which for neither?

a. The allergy arose from eating peaches.

b. The allergy arose from exposure to birch pollen.

c. The reaction was due to a labile protein allergen.

d. The reaction was due to lipid transfer protein sensitisation.

e. Histamine release played a part in causing the symptoms.

Answer

a. B, not A.

b. A, not B.

c. A, not B.

d. B, not A.

e. Both A and B.

Q2

The first treatment for B's reaction should have been

a. Intravenous adrenaline 1ml, 1:1000 bolus

b. Intramuscular adrenaline 0.5 ml.

c. Chlorpheniramine (antihistamine) 10 mg IV.

d. Hydrocortisone 100 mg IV.

e. Intravenous adrenaline 1:10,000 IV titrated against response.

Answer

a. No; this is very dangerous in a conscious patient.
b. Yes.
c. No; not first drug.
d. No; not first drug.
e. Yes; provided that the patient is fully monitored.

Q3

A's reaction is best described as

a. Type I hypersensitivity is an old term for this condition which should now preferably be called IgE-mediated allergy.
b. An anaphylactoid reaction.
c. Food intolerance.
d. Non-allergic food hypersensitivity.
e. IgE-mediated food allergy.

Answer

a. No; the Gell and Coombs classification is no longer used.
b. No; this term should no longer be used.
c. No; the term 'intolerance' is no longer used in this context.
d. No; this was clearly IgE-mediated.
e. Yes.

Q4

The following genes may have contributed to A's tendency to asthma and peach allergy. Match the gene product with the chromosomal location and functional activity:

a.	CD14	1	5q	i	Allergic antibody library
b.	IL-13	2	12q	ii	Promotes IgE production
c.	IL4-R	3	16p	iii	Disease modifier for bronchospasm
d.	IgE			iv	Favours Th1 over Th2 responses
e.	β2-AR			v	Increases sensitivity of mast cells

Answer

a. 1 iv
b. 1 ii(v)
c. 3v
d. 2i
e. 1 iii

Scenario 4

A boy is stung three times in 3 weeks by wasps. As a result, he had symmetrical, generalised facial swelling, with eyes closed by the periorbital angioedema, and grossly swollen lips. Most of the swelling had settled by the next morning.

Scenario 5

A girl had three previous attacks of swelling over the course of a year; this, the fourth attack, was the first time it affected her face. There was symmetrical,generalised swelling, with eyes closed by the periorbital angioedema, and grossly swollen lips. Each attack followed minor trauma. Each time the swelling took a day to reach its maximum and 2 days to settle.

Multiple-choice questions

The following questions are to be used for both cases 4 and 5.

Q1

The time course and distribution of the girl's swellings is typical of

a. a large local (non–IgE-mediated) wasp sting reaction.
b. Idiopathic angioedema associated with a viral infection.
c. Hereditary angioedema.
d. Nephrotic disease.
e. An acute reaction due to IgE-mediated wasp sting allergy.

Answer

a. No; this has a slower time course (case 4) and wasps were not known to be involved (case 5).
b. No; no urticaria.

c. Case 5, yes.

d. No.

e. Case 4, yes.

Q2

The most likely mediators for these reactions is

a. Histamine.

b. Prostaglandin PGD2.

c. Bradykinin.

d. Interleukin-2.

e. Leucotriene C4.

Answer

a. Case 4, yes; case 5, no.

b. Case 4, yes; case 5, no.

c. Case 5, yes, case 4, no.

d. No.

e. Case 4, yes; case 5, no.

Q3

The angioedema is due to

a. Fluid leaking from arterioles.

b. Lymphatic obstruction.

c. Fluid leaking from capillaries.

d. Fluid leaking from venules.

e. Protein loss from the kidney.

Answer

a. No.

b. No.

c. No.

d. Yes.

e. No.

Q4

You might expect the following investigation results:

a. Negative wasp-specific IgE.

b. Low C1 esterase inhibitor functional activity

d. Low C4 level.

e. Raised mast cell tryptase.

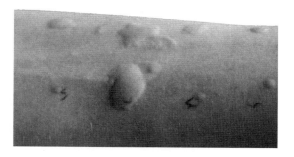

Answer

a. Case 5, yes; case 4, no.

b. Case 4, yes; case 5, no.

c. Yes.

d. Case 4, no; case 5, yes.

e. Case 4, yes; case 5, no.

FURTHER READING

Alvarez, G. G,, Schulzer, M., Jung, D., Fitzgerald, J. M. (2005). A systematic review of risk factors associated with near-fatal and fatal asthma. *Canadian Respiratory Journal* **12**, 265–70.

Arruda, L. K., Sole, D., Baena-Cagnani, C. E., Naspitz, C. K. (2005). Risk factors for asthma and atopy. *Current Opinion in Allergy and Clinical Immunology* **5**, 153–9.

Bacharier, L. B., Jabara, H., Geha, R. S. (1998). Molecular mechanisms of immunoglobulin E regulation. *International Archives of Allergy and Immunology* **115**, 257–69.

Baldo, B. A., Pham, N. H., Zhao, Z. (2001). Chemistry of drug allergenicity. *Current Opinion in Allergy and Clinical Immunology* **1**, 327–35.

Bethune, C. A., Gompels, M. M., Spickett, G. P. (1999). Physiological effects of starvation interpreted as food allergy. *British Medical Journal* **319**, 304–5.

Brazil, E., MacNamara, A. F. (1998). "Not so immediate" hypersensitivity – the danger of biphasic anaphylactic reactions. *Journal of Accident and Emergency Medicine* **15**, 252–3.

Cerutti, A., Qiao, X., He, B. (2005). Plasmacytoid dendritic cells and the regulation of immunoglobulin heavy chain class switching. *Immunology and Cell Biology* **83**, 554–62.

Christie, P. E., Henderson, W. R. Jr. (2002). Lipid inflammatory mediators: leukotrienes, prostaglandins, platelet-activating factor. *Clinical Allergy and Immunology* 16, 233–54.

Corrigan, C. J, Kettner, J., Doemer, C. *et al.* (2005). Efficacy and safety of preseasonal-specific immunotherapy with an aluminium-adsorbed six-grass pollen allergoid. *Allergy* **60**, 801–7.

Dale, H. H. (1953). Adventures in Physiology. London: Pergamon Press.

Davies, D. E., Wicks, J., Powell, R. M. *et al.* (2003). Airway remodeling in asthma: new insights. *Journal of Allergy and Clinical Immunology* **111**, 215–25.

Demoly, P., Botros, H. G., Rabillon, J. *et al.* (2002). Anaphylaxis to antitetanus toxoid serum. *Allergy* **57**, 860–1.

EAACI (2001). A revised nomenclature of allergy: an EAACI position statement from the EAACI nomenclature task force. *Allergy* **56**, 813–24.

Gell P. G. H., Coombes R. R. A. (eds). (1962). Clinical aspects of immunology. Oxford, UK: Blackwell.

Golden, D. B. (2001). Discontinuing venom immunotherapy. *Current Opinion in Allergy and Clinical Immunology* **1**, 353–6.

Hagel, I., Di Prisco, M. C., Goldblatt, J., Le Souef, P. N. (2004). The role of parasites in genetic susceptibility to allergy: IgE, helminthic infection and allergy, and the evolution of the human immune system. *Clinical Review of Allergy and Immunology* **26**, 75–83.

Halstead, L. A. (2005). Extraesophageal manifestations of GERD: diagnosis and therapy. *Drugs Today (Barcelona)* **41(Suppl B)**, 19–26.

Hanzlik, P. J., Karsner, H. A. T. (1920). Anaphylactoid phenomena from the intravenous administration of various colloids, arsenicals and other agents. *Journal of Pharmacology and Experimental Therapy* **14**, 379.

Hermann, K., Ring, J. (1993). The renin angiotensin system and hymenoptera venom anaphylaxis. *Clinical and Experimental Allergy* **23**, 762–9.

Holgate, S. T., Davies, D. E., Lackie, P. M. *et al.* (2000). Epithelial-mesenchymal interactions in the pathogenesis of asthma. *Journal of Allergy and Clinical Immunology* **105**, 193–204.

Hoshino, M., Fujita, Y., Saji, J. *et al.* (2005). Effect of suplatast tosilate on goblet cell metaplasia in patients with asthma. *Allergy* **60**, 1394–400.

Houghton, L. A., Whorwell, P. J. (2005). Towards a better understanding of abdominal bloating and distension in functional gastrointestinal disorders. *Neurogastroenterology and Motility* **17**, 500–11.

Inomata, N., Osuna, H., Yanagimachi, M., Ikezawa, Z. (2005). Late-onset anaphylaxis to fermented soybeans: the first confirmation of food-induced, late-onset anaphylaxis by provocation test. *Annals of Allergy, Asthma, and Immunolology* **94**, 402–6.

Johansson, S. G. O., Bieber, T., Dahl, R. *et al.* (2004). Revised nomenclature for allergy for global use: report of the Nomenclature Review Committee of the World Allergy Organization, October 2003. *Journal of Allergy and Clinical Immunology* **113**, 832–36.

Joint Task Force on Practice Parameters. (2005). The diagnosis and management of anaphylaxis: an updated practice parameter. *Journal of Allergy and Clinical Immunology* **115**, S483–523.

Julia, J. C., Martorell, A., Armengot, M. A. *et al.* (1999). Vocal cord dysfunction in a child. *Allergy* **54**, 748–51.

Kaplan, A. P., Joseph, K., Silverberg, M. (2002). Pathways for bradykinin formation and inflammatory disease. *Journal of Allergy and Clinical Immunology* **109**, 195–209.

Lilly, C. M. (2005). Diversity of asthma: evolving concepts of pathophysiology and lessons from genetics. *Journal of Allergy and Clinical Immunology* **115**, S526–31.

MacQueen, G., Marshall, J., Perdu, M. *et al.* (1989). Pavlovian conditioning of rat mucosal mast cells to secrete mast cell proteinase II. *Science* **243**, 83–5.

Metcalfe, D. D., Baram, D., Mekori, Y. A.. (1997). Mast cells. *Physiology Review* **77**, 1033–79.

Mills, E. N., Jenkins, J. A., Alcocer, M. J., Shewry, P. R. (2004). Structural, biological, and evolutionary relationships of plant food allergens sensitizing via the gastrointestinal tract. *Critical Reviews in Food Science and Nutrition* **44**, 379–407.

Nikpoor, B., Duan, Q. L,, Rouleau, G. A. (2005). Acute adverse reactions associated with angiotensin-converting enzyme inhibitors: genetic factors and therapeutic implications. *Expert Opinion in Pharmacotherapy* **6**, 1851–6.

Ober, A. I., MacLean, J. A., Hannaway, P. J. (2003). Life-threatening anaphylaxis to venom immunotherapy in a patient taking an angiotensin-converting enzyme inhibitor. *Journal of Allergy and Clinical Immunology* **112**, 1008–9.

Okabe, T., Hide, M., Koro, O. *et al.* (2001). The release of leukotriene B4 from human skin in response to substance P: evidence for the functional heterogeneity of human skin mast cells among individuals. *Clinical and Experimental Immunology* **124**, 150–6.

Oliver, J. M., Pfeiffer, J. R., Surviladze, Z. *et al.* (2004). Membrane receptor mapping: the membrane topography of Fc(epsilon)RI signaling. *Subcellular Biochemistry* **37**, 3–34.

Pumphrey, R. S. H. (2000). Lessons for management of anaphylaxis from a study of fatal reactions. *Clinical and Experimental Allergy* **30**, 1144–50.

Pumphrey, R. S. H. (2003). Fatal posture in anaphylactic shock. *Journal of Allergy and Clinical Immunology* **112**, 451–2.

Pumphrey, R. S., Nicholls, J. M. (2000). Epinephrine-resistant food anaphylaxis. *Lancet* **355**, 1099.

Richet, C. R. (1913). L'anaphylaxie. Paris, 1909. Available only in the English translation: Murray, B. J. (1913). Anaphylaxis. Liverpool: Liverpool University Press, pp. 1–2.

Russell, M., Dark K. A., Cummings, R. W. *et al.* (1984). Learned histamine release. *Science* **225**, 733–4.

Sampson, H. A. (1999). Food allergy: Part 1. immunopathogenesis and clinical disorders. *Journal of Allergy and Clinical Immunology* **103**, 717–28.

Sampson, H. A. (1999). Food allergy: Part 2. Diagnosis and management. *Journal of Allergy and Clinical Immunology* **103**, 981–9.

Shimizu, T., Shimizu, S., Hattori, R., Majima, Y. (2003). A mechanism of antigen-induced goblet cell degranulation in the nasal epithelium of sensitized rats. *Journal of Allergy and Clinical Immunology* **112**, 119–25.

Sicherer, S. H., Burks, A. W., Sampson, H. A. (1998). Clinical features of acute allergic reactions to peanut and tree nuts in children. *Pediatrics* **102**, e6. Available at http://www.pediatrics.org/cgi/content/full/102/1/e6

Sicherer, S. H. (2001). Clinical implications of cross-reactive food allergens. *Journal of Allergy and Clinical Immunology* 108, 881–90.

Sicherer, S. H., Simons, F. E. (2005). Quandaries in prescribing an emergency action plan and self-injectable epinephrine for first-aid management of anaphylaxis in the community. *Journal of Allergy and Clinical Immunology* 115, 575–83.

Sicherer, S. H., Forman, J. A., Noone, S. A. (2000). Use assessment of self-administered epinephrine among food-allergic children and pediatricians. *Pediatrics* **105**, 359–62.

Simons, F. E., Gu, X., Simons, K. J. (2001). Epinephrine absorption in adults: intramuscular versus subcutaneous injection. *Journal of Allergy and Clinical Immunology* **108**, 871–3.

Simon, R. A. (2004). Adverse respiratory reactions to aspirin and nonsteroidal anti-inflammatory drugs. *Current Allergy and Asthma Reports* **4**, 17–24.

Spitzer, W. O., Suissa, S., Ernst, P. *et al.* (1992). The use of beta-agonists and the risk of death and near death from asthma. *New England Journal of Medicine* **326**, 501–6

Staudenmayer, H., Binkley, K. E., Leznoff, A., Phillips, S. (2003). Idiopathic environmental intolerance: Part 2. A causation analysis applying Bradford Hill's criteria to the psychogenic theory. *Toxicology Review* **22**, 247–61.

Suzuki, A., Suzuki, R., Furuno, T. *et al.* (2004). N-cadherin plays a role in the synapse-like structures between mast cells and neurites. *Biological & Pharmaceutical Bulletin* **27**, 1891–4.

Tarlo, S. M., Poonai N., Binkley K. *et al.* (2002). Responses to panic induction procedures in subjects with multiple chemical sensitivity/idiopathic environmental intolerance: understanding the relationship with panic disorder. *Environmental Health Perspectives* **110(Suppl 4)**, 669–71.

The International Study of Asthma and Allergies in Childhood (ISAAC) Steering Committee. (1998). Worldwide variation in prevalence of symptoms of asthma, allergic rhinoconjunctivitis, and atopic eczema: ISAAC. *Lancet* **351**, 1225–32.

Umetsu, D. T., McIntire, J. J., DeKruyff, R. H. (2005). TIM-1, hepatitis A virus and the hygiene theory of atopy: association of TIM-1 with atopy. *Journal of Pediatric Gastroenterology and Nutrition* **40(Suppl 1)**, S43.

Vertigan, A. E., Theodoros, D. G., Gibson, P. G., Winkworth, A. L. (2005). The relationship between chronic cough and paradoxical vocal fold movement: a review of the literature. *Journal of Voice* [Epub ahead of print].

Ward, C., Walters, H. (2005). Airway wall remodelling: the influence of corticosteroids. *Current Opinion in Allergy and Clinical Immunology* **5**, 43–8.

Waser, M., Schierl, R., von Mutius, E. *et al.* (2004). Determinants of endotoxin levels in living environments of farmers' children and their peers from rural areas. *Clinical and Experimental Allergy* **34**, 389–97.

Young, E., Stoneham, M., Petruckevitch, A. *et al.* (1994). A population study of food intolerance. *Lancet* **343**, 1127–30.

Valent, P., Ghannadan, M., Hauswirth, A. W. *et al.* (2002). Signal transduction-associated and cell activation-linked antigens expressed in human mast cells. *International Journal of Hematology* **75**, 357–62.

Yamanishi, R., Yusa, I., Miyamoto, A. *et al.* (2003). Alum augments the experimental allergenicity of Kunitz-type soybean trypsin inhibitor independent of the antigen-adsorption. *Journal of Nutritional Science and Vitaminology (Tokyo)* 49, 409–13.

Welch, H., Lewis, C. N., Weinstein, H. I., Boeckman, B. B. (1957). Severe reactions to antibiotics; a nationwide survey. *Antibiotic Medical and Clinical Therapy* **12**, 800–13.

Zuidmeer, L., van Leeuwen, W. A., Budde, I. K., et al. (2005). Lipid transfer proteins from fruit: cloning, expression and quantification. *International Archives of Allergy and Immunology* 137, 273–81.

6

Infection – bacterial

Stephen D. Lawn and George E. Griffin

Introduction

Infectious pathogens may cause disease by two principal means: (1) direct toxic effects of organisms and their secreted exotoxins and (2) indirect pathology resulting from the host inflammatory response to organisms and their shed antigens. While some infectious pathogens cause disease by direct effects on host cells and physiological processes (e.g. tetanus and cholera), this chapter specifically focuses on aspects of disease that arise from immune-mediated effects.

Infection is the major cause of the inflammatory process – a phenomenon that has been recognised for centuries. Contemporary knowledge of the inflammatory process and its mediation now provides insight into the pathophysiology of many infectious disease. The immune system is a two-edged sword. Although immunological activation is essential to mount an effective host response to invading pathogens, paradoxically the host inflammatory response may cause much of the pathology associated with infection. Such injury arising from the effects of the immune system may be referred to as 'immunopathology'. The relative contribution of pathogen-associated toxicity and immune-mediated damage differs greatly between different infectious diseases and also between genetically different humans infected with the same organism.

The initial inflammatory response to an invading organism is independent of antigen recognition and comprises the innate immune response. Sub-sequent specific acquired immune responses are those inflammatory responses that result from antigen recognition; they include cell- and antibody-mediated (humoral) arms of the immune system. Both innate and specific acquired immune responses may contribute to the immunopathology of infection (Fig. 6.1), and this chapter reviews the underlying mechanisms. The examples of tuberculosis (TB) and human immunodeficiency virus type 1 (HIV-1) infection have been chosen to illustrate the central role of immune responses in the pathology associated with these infections as well as to illustrate how the important bi-directional interaction of these diseases is mediated by their respective effects on the immune system.

Innate immune responses

Multiple cell populations and inflammatory pathways are non-specifically activated as part of the innate immune response. The five cardinal signs of inflammation – redness (rubor), swelling (tumor), heat (calor), pain (dolor) and loss of function (fonctio laesa) – reflect the major processes underlying this response – namely, vasodilatation, increased capillary permeability and influx of phagocytes. These events are initiated and effected by a complex cascade of chemical mediators released in response to the presence of infectious organisms or to tissue damage. Together these pathways serve to facilitate recruitment and activation of effector cells to sites of infection as well as to initiate systemic responses.

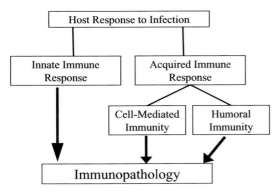

Figure 6.1 The arms of the immune response involved in immunopathology of infection.

Inflammatory mediators

Lipid inflammatory mediators

Following changes in the membranes of various cell types – including monocytes, macrophages, neutrophils and mast cells – phospholipase enzymes release membrane phospholipids. These are used to synthesize a range of potent inflammatory mediators, including platelet activating factor (PAF), leukotriene B4 (LTB4), slow-reacting substance of anaphylaxis (SRS-A), prostaglandins and thromboxanes. These mediators have wide-ranging inflammatory effects, including platelet aggregation, leucocyte chemotaxis, neutrophil activation, vasodilatation and increased vascular permeability.

Complement system

Cell-wall constituents of pathogenic organisms may directly activate the complement system in plasma via the alternative pathway. The complement cascade generates a number of important mediators of inflammation in the circulation. Anaphylatoxins (C3a, C4a and C5a) bind to mast cells to induce release of histamine and other mediators that increase vascular permeability. C3a and C5a also facilitate monocyte and neutrophil extravasation and chemotaxis to sites of infection.

Kinin, clotting and fibrinolytic systems

The kinin system is an enzymatic cascade in the circulation that is triggered when Hageman factor (a plasma clotting factor) is activated following endothelial damage. Bradykinin, the key product of this cascade, is a basic peptide that increases vascular permeability and causes vasodilatation and contraction of smooth muscle. Endothelial damage also leads to activation of the clotting and fibrinolytic systems. Products of these pathways include fibrinopeptides, which cause vasodilatation and neutrophil chemotaxis, and plasmin, which activates the complement system.

Chemokines

Chemokines are small polypeptide cytokines that chemotactically attract different leucocyte sub-populations to sites of infection (described further below). They are produced by a variety of cells, including monocytes, macrophages, neutrophils, endothelial cells, fibroblasts and platelets. Chemokines induce the expression of various adhesion molecules at the surface of various leucocyte populations, enabling them to bind to the vascular endothelium (margination). Following diapedesis (extravasation into the tissues), the leucocytes migrate along a chemokine gradient to the infection site where they are active.

Proinflammatory cytokines

Tumour necrosis factor alpha (TNF-α), interleukin-1 (IL-1) and IL-6 are collectively termed proinflammatory cytokines; their critical role in inflammation is considered in greater detail later in this chapter. These cytokines are produced at the site of infection primarily by macrophages. They play a pivotal role in the innate inflammatory immune response, inducing fever, stimulating synthesis of acute-phase proteins in the liver, increasing vascular permeability, promoting proliferation of fibroblasts, and subsequently also playing a key role in acquired immune responses.

Triggers of acute inflammation

As described above, invading organisms and their products activate many inflammatory pathways by causing changes in immune cell membranes, directly triggering enzymatic cascades in the circulation. A further very important mechanism of immune activation is the interaction of bacterial endotoxin with the macrophage expressed CD14 receptor and toll-like receptors (TLRs); these are pattern-recognition receptor that bind a range of conformationally related molecules. It acts as a high-affinity receptor for bacterial cell wall lipopolysaccharide (LPS), and engagement leads to marked cellular activation, upregulation of adhesion molecules, and release of proinflammatory cytokines. In this way, CD14 receptor and TLR play a key role in the host physiological response to bacterial endotoxin.

The inflammatory process

Local response

Activation of the wide range of inflammatory pathways described above leads to a rapid increase in blood flow and vascular permeability at the site of infection and hence to erythema and oedema as well as increased extravasation of leucocytes. Neutrophils play a central role in the early inflammatory process, responding to chemokines, such as interleukin-8 (IL-8), by adhering to activated endothelial cells and migrating into the tissues. Neutrophils phagocytose pathogens and release inflammatory mediators and chemokines, which attract macrophages to the site of infection. Activated neutrophils also produce and release reactive oxygen intermediates (ROIs), reactive nitrogen intermediates (RNIs) and degradative enzymes, such as metalloproteases, which contribute to tissue damage. Activated macrophages also engage in phagocytosis and secrete proinflammatory cytokines, which induce many of the local and systemic changes of the acute inflammatory process. Other leucocyte populations – including lymphocytes, monocytes, eosinophils, basophils and mast cells – may, in turn, be recruited to the inflammatory site.

Systemic acute-phase response

Local inflammatory responses are often accompanied by a systemic response known as the acute-phase response. This is stimulated by release of pro-inflammatory cytokines (TNF-α, IL-1 and IL-6) into the systemic circulation. These cytokines induce fever by acting on the hypothalamus; they also cause weight loss, increase production of white cells and stimulate synthesis of a wide range of acute-phase proteins in liver. This includes rapid secretion of high concentrations of C-reactive protein (CRP) into the circulation by hepatocytes. C-reactive protein binds to many microorganisms, promoting opsonization by complement. In addition, plasma albumin falls rapidly due to a combination of reduced synthesis in the liver and extravasation into interstitial fluid.

Immunopathology of innate immune responses

Innate immune responses may lead to both local and systemic immunopathology. The local inflammatory response at sites of infection, although essential to combat invading pathogens and limit their spread, may nevertheless lead to critical compromise of the organ involved (Table 6.1a). Thus, for example, massive acute inflammation of the epiglottis in response to *Haemophilus influenzae b* may lead to asphyxia and death. Similarly, inflammation triggered by *Streptococcus pneumoniae* may lead to extensive pneumonic consolidation in the lungs and respiratory failure.

The systemic acute-phase response, while facilitating various immune functions and inhibiting microbial replication, also results in many of the systemic symptoms of infection, such as fever, anorexia, and weight loss. A particularly serious innate systemic inflammatory response is that seen in individuals with systemic bacterial sepsis. Lipopolysaccharide (LPS) derived from the cell wall of gram-negative bacteria may cause intense activation of monocytes and macrophages mediated by binding to CD14 receptors. The resultant massive release of proinflammatory cytokines together with other vasoactive

Table 6.1 Examples of the immunopathology of infectious diseases mediated by (a) innate and (b) specific acquired immune responses

Organism	Disease	Important immunopathological process
a. Innate immune response		
Haemophilus influenzae b	Epiglottitis with asphyxia	Massive acute inflammation of epiglottis
Streptococcus pneumoniae	Pneumonia with respiratory failure	Extensive acute inflammation of lung parenchyma
Gram-negative bacteria	Septic shock	Lipopolysaccharide activation of macrophages principally via CD14 receptors and toll-like receptors (TLRs)s, leading to massive systemic proinflammatory cytokine secretion
b. Specific acquired immune responses		
Viruses		
HIV	AIDS	Immune destruction of infected CD4+ cells and widespread activation-induced CD4+ cell apoptosis
Epstien-Barr virus	Infectious mononucleosis	Massive CD8+ T lymphocyte proliferation and cytolysis of EBV-infected cells
Bacteria		
Group A Streptococcus	Acute rheumatic fever	Anti-streptococcal antibodies cross-react with host cell antigens (type II hypersensitivity)
Gram-positive bacteria	Glomerulonephritis associated with endocarditis	Immune complexes deposition in the kidneys (type III hypersensitivity)
Mycobacterium leprae	Tuberculoid leprosy	Type IV hypersensitivity with granuloma formation
	Erythema nodosum leprosum	Type III hypersensitivity with immune complex deposition and systemic pro-inflammatory cytokine action
Borrelia recurrentis	Relapsing fever	Systemic pro-inflammatory cytokine action, which may be exacerbated by antibiotic treatment (Jarisch-Herxheimer reaction)
Fungi		
Aspergillus fumigatus	Allergic bronchopulmonary aspergillosis	Type III hypersensitivity
Parasites		
Echinococcus granulosus	Anaphylaxis following hydatid cyst rupture	Type I hypersensitivity
Schistosoma mansoni	Periportal hepatic fibrosis	Type IV hypersensitivity, granuloma formation, fibrosis

inflammatory mediators derived from activation of enzymatic inflammatory cascades in blood leads to overwhelming vasodilatation and increased vascular permeability. These processes result in septic shock.

A further important innate systemic inflammatory reaction is the Jarisch-Herxheimer reaction, which is also mediated by massive proinflammatory cytokine release. Such a reaction may occur shortly after commencing antibiotic treatment of spirochaete infections such as syphilis (*Treponema pallidum*), relapsing fever (*Borrelia recurrentis*) and leptospirosis (*Leptospira* spp.). The reaction is characterized by the development of fever, head-ache, malaise and hypotension and is associated with systemic secretion of TNF-α, IL-6 and IL-8. The triggering mechanism for cytokine release is not fully understood. However, since the reaction corre-lates with rapid removal of spirochaetes from the peripheral blood, it is possible that widespread phagocytosis of the organism due to its disruption in the presence of antibiotic leads to overwhelming activation of macrophages. It is interesting that the Jarisch-Herxheimer reaction of relapsing fever can be blocked by pretreatment with antibody directed against TNF-α.

Specific acquired immune responses

Following innate inflammatory immune responses, antigen presentation and expansion of a CD4+ T-helper (T_H) lymphocyte clone lead to the devel-opment of specific acquired immunity. This may encompass both cell-mediated and humoral arms of the immune system, the predominance of which is directed by the pattern of cytokine secretion by the T_H lymphocyte clone. The key cellular interac-tions involved in this process are summarized in Figure 6.2.

Antigen presentation

TCR-CD3 complex

The central event in the generation of a specific acquired immune response is activation and pro-liferation of an antigen-specific clone of CD4+ T_H lymphocytes. Antigen specificity is determined by the T-cell receptor (TCR), which is expressed at the T_H lymphocyte cell surface. The TCR has a heterodimeric structure composed of either α and β chains or γ and δ chains (as described in Chapter 4, on autoimmune mechanisms). Unlike antibody, the TCR does not bind soluble anti-gen but rather processed peptide antigen epitopes expressed by antigen-presenting cells (APCs) in association with major histocompatibility complex

(MHC) self antigen. The TCR comprises variable and constant domains, and the variable region has three hypervariable complementarity-determining regions (CDRs) that determine antigen specificity. Although the TCR is solely responsible for antigen recognition, it has a very short cytoplasmic tail with little capacity for signal transduction. However, the TCR is closely associated with CD3 – a complex molecule consisting of invariant polypeptide chains arranged as three dimers. CD3 forms a complex with the TCR and serves in signal transduction following antigen recognition.

Co-receptors and co-stimulatory signaling

In addition to signaling by the TCR-CD3 complex, a second signal is required for T_H lymphocyte acti-vation. This is mediated by various co-stimulatory molecules that are also expressed on the surface of APCs (Table 6.2). The most important of these is B7, expressed by APCs, which interacts with either CD28 or CTLA-4 on the T_H cell. The resulting co-stimula-tory signal permits the activation and clonal expan-sion of T cells, whereas TCR–CD3 signaling in the absence of a co-stimulatory signal results in anergy of the T_H clone. In addition to these receptors, a num-ber of other co-receptors play important accessory roles in APC–T-lymphocyte interaction (Table 6.2). These may be adhesion molecules, strengthening the physical association of the two cells or they may act as signal transducers, augmenting cellular acti-vation. For example, binding of ICAM-1 to LFA-1 results in signal transduction and kinase activation at the T-cell membrane. This leads to the liberation of active nuclear factor κB (NF-κB) within the cyto-plasm, which then translocates to the nucleus, where it activates various genes including the IL-2 gene.

Cytokines and inflammation

The development of an effective acquired immune response involves complex coordinated interac-tions between a wide variety of cells within the immune and haemopoietic systems. These inter-cellular interactions are mediated by a group of

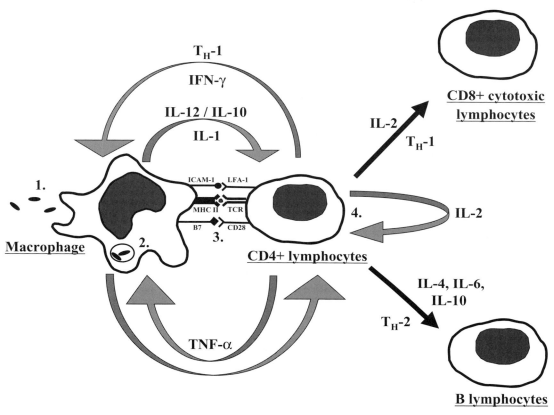

Figure 6.2 Diagram of the macrophage–T_H lymphocyte interaction illustrating antigen presentation, clonal proliferation of T lymphocytes and subsequent activation of immune effector cells. Macrophages phagocytose an invasive pathogen (1), process antigens (2), and present soluble epitopes at the cell surface in association with MHC (3). The antigen–MHC complex is recognized by the T-cell receptor (TCR); ICAM-1 and B7 provide costimulatory signals via LFA-1 and CD28 receptors at the T-cell surface. Antigen-specific CD4+ T lymphocytes proliferate under the effects of IL-1 and IL-2 (4). Simultaneous stimulation by IL-12 promotes expansion of T_H-1 cells, whereas IL-10 promotes expansion of T_H-2 cells. Subsequent T_H-1 or T_H-2 cytokine secretion by this expanding CD4+ clone drives a cell-mediated immune response by activation of macrophages and CD8+ cells (T_H-1) and/or a humoral immune response by activation of B cells (T_H-2).

low-molecular-weight regulatory proteins collectively termed cytokines. These are predominantly secreted by macrophages and lymphocytes and their effects are mediated by specific receptors expressed on the surface of target cells, leading to altered gene expression. Cytokines typically act in an autocrine fashion (action on the secreting cell) or paracrine fashion (action on other cells in close proximity) but may also exert effects on cells at a distance via the circulation (endocrine effects) (Fig. 6.3). Because of their role as messengers between leucocytes, many cytokines are referred to as interleukins (ILs); at present more than 30 interleukins are described. Numbers of other cytokines still retain their original descriptive names, including tumour necrosis factors alpha and beta (TNF-α and β) and the interferons (IFNs). The so-called pro-inflammatory cytokines, mentioned earlier (TNF-α, IL-1 and IL-6),

Table 6.2 Major costimulatory and adhesion molecules involved in T lymphocyte–macrophage interactions

Receptor	Ligand	Signal transduction	Adhesion
CD28	B7	+	
CTLA-4	B7	+	
LFA-1 (CD11a/CD18)	ICAM-1 (CD54)	+	+
LFA-2 (CD2)	LFA-3 (CD58)	+	+
CD4	HLA-DR (MHC II)	+	+
CD8	HLA A/B/C (MHC I)	+	+
CD45R	CD22	+	+

play a central role in the development of an inflammatory response. Further cytokines – including IL-8, MIP-1α, MIP-1β and rantes – are collectively termed chemokines in view of their chemoattractant properties.

Cytokines have a wide variety of effects, regulating cellular recruitment, differentiation, activation, and proliferation (Table 6.3). Indeed, many cytokines have multiple functions (pleiotropic cytokines) and do not have a single ascribable action. Different cytokines may have synergistic and antagonistic actions and may also serve to regulate the secretion of other cytokines and their receptors. By these means, the cytokine network can effectively orchestrate the inflammatory host response to infection as well as finely regulate its intensity and duration. TNF-α plays a central role in the host inflammatory

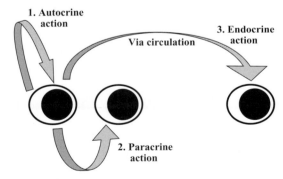

Figure 6.3 Cytokine action may be (1) autocrine (action on the cytokine-producing cell), (2) paracrine (action on cells in close proximity to the cytokine-producing cell) or (3) endocrine (acting via the circulation on distant cells).

response and has extremely wide-ranging effects (Table 6.4).

T$_H$1 and T$_H$2 cytokines

The host response to a particular pathogen must induce appropriate immune effector functions. A cell-mediated cytotoxic response is required to kill intracellular pathogens such as *Mycobacterium tuberculosis* (MTB) or viruses, whereas a humoral response is required to neutralize bacterial toxins and kill extracellular pathogens including parasites. Following antigen presentation, T$_H$ cells differentiate into two main subsets, T$_H$1 and T$_H$2, depending upon the cytokine environment in which they develop. Antigen-driven T-cell proliferation in the presence of IL-12 favours the development of a T$_H$1 lymphocyte clone, whereas antigen-driven T-cell proliferation in the presence of IL-4 favours the development of a T$_H$2 clone.

The functional distinction between T$_H$1 and T$_H$2 clones is, in turn, based upon their pattern of cytokine secretion (Table 6.3). This functional distinction was first described in mice and is much less clear-cut in humans. T$_H$1 cells predominantly secrete IL-2 and IFN-γ, which activate macrophages and antigen-specific CD8+ cytotoxic lymphocytes that have recognized antigen presented together with MHC class I. T$_H$1 cells thus drive a cell-mediated immune response. In contrast, T$_H$2 cells predominantly secrete IL-4, IL-5, IL-6 and IL-10, which activate B lymphocytes and antibody secretion. T$_H$2 cells thus drive a humoral immune response. There is

Table 6.3 Some of the principal cytokines and their actions

Cytokine	Principal sources	Principal functions
Pro-inflammatory cytokines		
IL-1 (IL-1(and IL-1()	Macrophages, fibroblasts, endothelial cells	Activation of lymphocytes and NK cells, acute-phase response, induces fever
IL-6	Macrophages, T_H lymphocytes	B-cell differentiating factor, stimulates antibody production and acute-phase response
TNFα	Macrophages	(See Table 2.3)
TNFβ	Lymphocytes	Similar to TNFα
T_H1 cytokines		
IL-2	CD4+ lymphocytes	T and B lymphocyte and macrophage activation, T-cell growth factor
IFNγ	CD4+/CD8+ lymphocytes	Induces MHC I and II, promotes antigen presentation, macrophage activation, antiviral action
IL-12	Macrophages	T_H1 lymphocyte differentiation, IFNγ production by T and NK cells
T_H2 cytokines		
IL-4	CD4+ lymphocytes	B- and T-cell activation
IL-5	CD4+ lymphocytes	B-cell and eosinophil growth and differentiation
IL-6 (see above)		
IL-10	Macrophages, CD4+ lymphocytes	T_H2 lymphocyte differentiation, B-cell activation, downregulates MHC class II, suppression of T_H1 cytokine secretion
Other		
IFNα	Leucocytes	Inhibits viral replication
IL-7	Bone marrow and thymus	Lymphoid stem cell differentiation, upregulates IL-2 receptor
TGFβ	Platelets, lymphocytes, Macrophages, mast cells	Inhibits lymphoid cell proliferation/inflammation, promotes IgA secretion
Chemokines		
IL-8	Macrophages, endothelial cells, neutrophils	Neutrophil and T-cell migration
Rantes	T lymphocytes, platelets	Monocytes, T cells, eosinophils, basophil migration
MIP-1α, MIP-1β	Macrophages, monocytes, endothelium, neutrophils	Monocytes, macrophages, B and T cells, eosinophil migration

cross-regulation between cytokines produced by T_H1 and T_H2 subsets, each inhibiting either the expansion or cytokine secretion of the other cell subset. Thus the functional type of immune response can be regulated according to the specific pathogen present.

The progression of certain diseases may be associated with the balance between T_H1 and T_H2 cytokine responses as measured in peripheral blood mononuclear cells *in vitro*. The clearest example of this in humans is leprosy. Since *Mycobacterium leprae* is an intracellular pathogen, it is most effectively combated by a strong cell-mediated (T_H1) immune response. Indeed, individuals with leprosy who have a strong T_H1 cytokine response have marked

Table 6.4 Diverse biological effects of tumour necrosis factor alpha (TNF-α)

Fever
Weight loss
Acute-phase response
Induction apoptosis
Induction reactive oxygen species
Antiviral activity
Cytotoxicity for tumour cells
Chemotaxis
Induction GM-CSF
Monocyte differentiation
Adhesion molecule expression
MHC I and II expression
Induction IL-1 and IL-6
Enhanced phagocytosis
Haematopoiesis
Proliferation fibroblasts
Induction procoagulant activity

granuloma formation, few organisms present in cutaneous lesions, slow disease progression and high rates of survival (tuberculoid leprosy). In contrast, individuals with a predominant T_H2 cytokine response show little evidence of cell-mediated immunity and tend to have more widely disseminated progressive, multi-bacillary disease (lepromatous leprosy).

TNF-α, IFN-γ and chronic inflammation

Chronic antigenic stimulation resulting from failed clearance of microbes, and microbial antigens may lead to the development of a chronic inflammatory state. IFN-γ and TNF-α play central roles within such a process. CD4+ T_H1 lymphocytes, CD8+ lymphocytes, and natural killer (NK) cells secrete IFN-γ, which activates macrophages by inducing expression of MHC class II, promoting antigen presentation and leading to increased microbicidal activity and cytokine secretion. Chronic inflammation is characterized by the accumulation of activated macrophages that secrete large amounts of TNF-α, which has both local and systemic effects. Activated macrophages and TNF-α are responsible for much

of the immunopathology associated with chronic inflammation as described in greater detail below, where we consider the immunopathology of TB.

Immunopathology of acquired immune responses

Similar to innate immune responses, proinflammatory cytokines in the circulation mediate many of the systemic symptoms of infection during specific acquired immune responses. The mechanisms of specific tissue injury associated with infections are diverse; a range of examples is listed in Table 6.1b. In the case of viral infections, the immunopathology often relates to the development of cytotoxic CD8+ lymphocytes. It has been postulated that virus-induced antibodies may also cause tissue damage – for example, mediating the maculopapular rash of measles. In the case of bacterial, fungal and parasitic diseases, many of the immunopathological processes are closely linked to the four classic patterns of hypersensitivity reaction.

Type I reactions

Type I hypersensitivity reactions are rapid and short-lived anaphylactic reactions that do not cause chronic tissue injury. Prior antigenic exposure to certain antigens leads to IgE synthesis, which serves as antigen receptor on the surface of mast cells. Binding of antigen to IgE triggers mast cell degranulation, releasing histamine and other acute inflammatory mediators. For example, hydatid cyst rupture can cause anaphylaxis. This is not, however, a common means of immunopathology in infectious processes.

Type II reactions

Tissue damage associated with type II hypersensitivity reactions are mediated by antibodies to microbial antigens that cross react with host cell antigens. For example, certain M serotypes of the Lancefield group A *Streptococcus pyogenes* stimulate high titres of immunoglobulin G (IgG) that cross-react with host cell antigens in the heart, joints and neural tissue, leading to the carditis, arthritis and Sydenham's chorea, whch characterize rheumatic fever.

Type III reactions

Type III hypersensitivity reactions to infectious diseases are also mediated by antibodies. Immune complex formation between antigens and antibodies results in activation of complement and chemotaxis of neutrophils that release tissue-damaging enzymes. Aggregation of platelets also causes formation of micro-thrombi and release of vasoactive amines. Many different tissues may be affected and polymorphonuclear infiltration, oedema and vasculitis characterize lesions. The natural history of such reactions is commonly persistent and chronic. Examples include glomerulonephritis associated with bacterial endocarditis, erythema nodosum leprosum (a hypersensitivity reaction to persistent *M. leprae* antigens in the skin) and allergic bronchopulmonary aspergillosis (which causes pulmonary infiltration and airflow obstruction in response to *Aspergillus fumigatus*).

Type IV reactions

Type IV reactions cause cell-mediated tissue pathology in which there is delayed-type hypersensitivity (DTH). The accumulation of large numbers of highly activated macrophages and formation of granulomas characterize tissue lesions. This is the classical mechanism by which the host response may cause very extensive and chronic tissue damage. Examples include TB, tuberculoid leprosy and periportal hepatic fibrosis in *Schistosoma mansoni* infection. We shall now consider in more detail the immunopathology associated with TB.

Host response and the pathogenesis of tuberculosis

TB is a major cause of morbidity and mortality worldwide. Approximately one-third of the world's population (2 billion people) is infected with *M.*

tuberculosis. and a proportion of such individuals develop active TB at some stage during their lives. This organism is a slow-growing bacterium that is not known to produce any exotoxins mediating tissue damage. However, it is its remarkable capacity to persist within the human host and induce a chronic inflammatory immune response that results in disease. In this section we illustrate how the great majority of the clinical features of TB result from the host response to MTB.

Host response to *M. tuberculosis* (MTB)

Person-to-person transmission of MTB typically occurs via airborne microscopic droplet nuclei that contain small numbers of bacilli. After being inhaled, the bacilli reach the terminal pulmonary airways and alveoli. Although pulmonary innate immune defence mechanisms to MTB remain poorly defined, scavenging alveolar and blood-derived macrophages clearly play a central role within the initial lesion, ingesting the bacilli and transporting them to regional lymph nodes. The major cell wall glycolipid of MTB, lipoarabinomannan (LAM), acts in a similar way to bacterial LPS, activating macrophages via TLRs following binding of LAM to the CD14 component of the CD14-TLR membrane complex. This results in secretion of proinflammatory cytokines. Depending on the relative microbicidal power of the macrophages and the virulence of the organism, the bacteria may either be killed and effectively eliminated by the initial inflammatory process or they may persist and replicate within the intracellular environment of macrophages.

Macrophages subsequently process antigen from persistent mycobacteria and present it to CD4+ T_H lymphocytes, leading to the development of cell-mediated immune responses and delayed-type hypersensitivity (DTH) within 2 to 4 weeks of initial infection. Interleukin (IL)-12 directs the clonal expansion of T-helper type 1 (T_H1) lymphocytes, resulting in secretion of interferon gamma (IFN-γ), which is essential for the activation of macrophages. The important role of IFN-γ in the host response to mycobacteria has been demonstrated in knockout

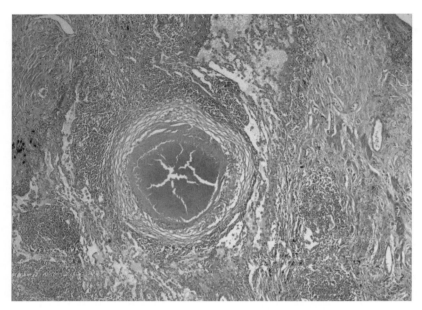

Figure 6.4 Histological section showing a typical TB granuloma with central caseous necrosis, mononuclear cell infiltrate and fibrosis. (Kindly supplied by the Department of Anatomical Pathology, Faculty of Health Sciences, University of Cape Town.) (See colour plate section.)

mice lacking IFN-γ. Whereas normal mice survive infection with an attenuated strain of bacille Calmette-Guérin (BCG), knockout mice that lack IFN-γ succumb to infection and die. Similarly, humans with a congenital deficiency in the IFN-γ receptor have a greatly heightened susceptibility to mycobacterial infections.

Release of chemokines such as IL-8 facilitates mononuclear cell recruitment, and secretion of pro-inflammatory cytokines, especially TNF-α, induces cellular activation. Macrophages and lymphocytes are subsequently orchestrated into granulomas, which provide the critical environment within which the host limits MTB infection by suppressing bacterial replication and facilitating intracellular killing. The TB granuloma (Fig. 6.4) is characterised by activation and epithelioid differentiation of macrophages and by the development of multinucleate Langhans giant cells. CD4+ T_H lymphocytes located within the periphery of the granuloma play a key role in orchestrating cell-mediated

immune function and secrete high levels of IFN-γ, which activates macrophages. In turn, highly activated macrophages parasitised by mycobacteria release lytic enzymes, reactive oxygen intermediates (ROIs) and reactive nitrogen intermediates (RNIs) at the site of infection. These destroy nearby healthy cells, resulting in the formation of a central area of caseous necrosis within the granuloma. This caseous material serves to inhibit extracellular bacillary growth.

In the majority of MTB-infected individuals, the granulomatous immune response restricts mycobacterial replication and maintains the infection in a clinically and microbiologically latent state. However, in individuals in whom the immune system becomes compromised, such latent TB may become activated. The infection progresses to active TB in approximately 10% of HIV-noninfected individuals at some stage of their lives, but this rate is much higher in individuals with HIV-1 infection. Failure to limit MTB replication leads to an increasing mycobacterial antigen burden that results in marked activation of macrophages and the macrophage–T lymphocyte immune axis. High concentrations of lytic enzymes cause the caseous centres of granulomas to change in composition during the process of liquefaction. In contrast to caseous necrosis, liquefied necrotic material provides a rich medium that supports rampant, uninhibited extracellular bacterial replication and spread. Active TB then results.

The immunopathology of tuberculosis

The majority of the clinical features of TB are directly attributable to the effects of the immune system rather than to direct toxic effects of the organism. Intense immune activation results in the considerable immunopathology of active TB, which is summarized in Figure 6.5. Circulating proinflammatory cytokines (TNF-α, IL-1 and IL-6) mediate systemic features such as fever, anorexia and weight loss, resulting in the classical wasted phenotype or 'consumption'.

Granulomas normally play a key protective role in MTB-infected individuals. However, in those in whom there is failure to contain mycobacterial proliferation, expanding granulomatous inflammatory lesions actually become destructive and lead to erosion and necrosis of surrounding structures. Within granulomas, dying macrophages release enzymes and toxic mediators that cause cellular necrosis, and high levels of TNF-α trigger activation-induced apoptosis of mononuclear cells. This chronic inflammatory response also leads to proliferation and activation of fibroblasts. While deposition of fibrous tissue may help to limit mycobacterial spread, fibrosis also leads to chronic impairment of normal tissue functioning.

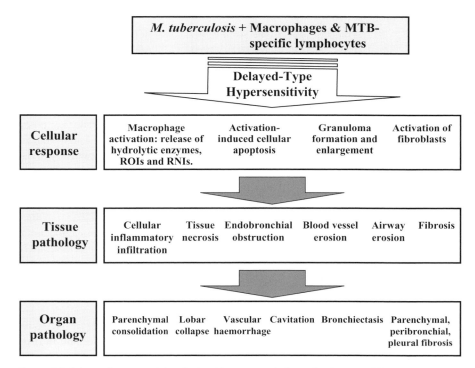

Figure 6.5 Schematic summarising the local immunopathology of pulmonary TB.
ROI = reactive oxygen intermediates; RNIs = reactive oxygen intermediates.

In individuals with pulmonary disease, the most common form of TB, the host response leads to lung parenchymal inflammation, consolidation and tissue necrosis. This may result in respiratory failure and permanent destructive changes to the airways (bronchiectasis). Mass inflammatory lesions, such as parenchymal foci of infection and intrathoracic tuberculous lymphadenitis, may cause (1) endobronchial obstruction with lobar collapse, distal abscess formation or bronchiectasis; (2) erosion of an airway, leading to discharge of liquefied necrotic material into the airway, which permits airway dissemination of mycobacteria and airborne spread of the disease; (3) erosion of a blood vessel, causing haemoptysis or haematogenous dissemination of mycobacteria. The florid inflammation resulting from rupture of a sub-pleural focus of infection into the pleural space may lead to the local accumulation of many litres of exudate. Fibrosis of lung parenchyma and pleura may cause chronic restrictive ventilatory defects, and peribronchial fibrosis may contribute to the pathology of bronchiectasis.

In addition to pulmonary TB, considerable immunopathology arises from TB at other anatomical sites, with both short and long-term complications (Table 6.5). Although TB remains an eminently curable disease using appropriate multi-drug therapy, a proportion of patients who are microbiologically cured nevertheless have permanent tissue damage resulting from the host inflammatory response.

Immunomodulating drugs and tuberculosis

In order to reduce the acute and chronic complications of TB that result from the host inflammatory response, immunosuppressant drugs may be co-administered with anti-tuberculosis drugs. It has been well documented that patients with advanced TB may deteriorate clinically during the first 2 weeks of treatment. Commencement of antituberculosis therapy causes the release of a huge mycobacterial antigen load, exacerbating the host inflammatory response. In part, this is likely to be due to liberation of a high concentration of LAM that activates macrophages via CD14 receptor signalling and in

Table 6.5 Immunopathology of tuberculosis

Site of disease	Complication/symptom
1. Systemic effects	
	Fever/anorexia/weight loss/anaemia/lassitude
2. Local effects	
Pulmonary	Consolidation/cavitation/lobar collapse/parenchymal fibrosis/endobronchial fibrosis/bronchiectasis/pleural thickening/haemoptysis
Pleural	Effusion/fibrosis
Pericardium	Pericardial effusion/pericardial tamponade/chronic constrictive pericarditis
Renal tract	Hydronephrosis/hydroureter
Central nervous system	Meningitis/cranial nerve palsies/cerebral infarction/hydrocephalus

many ways is analogous to the Jarisch-Herxheimer reaction discussed earlier. Steroid therapy in individuals with extensive tuberculous consolidation of the lungs may prevent critical deterioration in respiratory function during the first 2 weeks of antituberculosis treatment. Such glucocorticoid therapy is known to have anti-inflammatory activity, including the inhibition of TNF-α secretion by macrophages. Prednisolone is also often prescribed in those with TB of the central nervous system so as to prevent or minimise the neurological deterioration that may arise during the early stages of TB treatment as well as to decrease the risk of longer-term sequelae. Furthermore, steroids are also used with anti-mycobacterial drugs in the treatment of TB pericarditis, pleural TB, or renal TB to reduce the inflammatory response and associated acute and chronic complications, especially fibrosis. More specific immunomodulating drugs have also been used in clinical trials. For example, in view of the central role of TNF-α in the immunopathology of TB, thalidomide (a drug that reduces the TNF-α secretion) has been used and found to improve the rate of weight gain during treatment of pulmonary TB.

Host immune response and HIV-1 pathogenesis

Mechanisms of immunopathology associated with HIV-1 infection are very different from those resulting from TB. Simplistically, one might assume that the pathology of HIV-1 infection is due to infection and subsequent virus-induced or immune-mediated lysis of CD4+ T_H lymphocytes, resulting in immunodeficiency. However, it is quite apparent that the number of CD4+ cells actually infected by HIV-1 at any given time in an infected person is far too small to account for the degree of CD4+ lymphocytopenia that results. It is now understood that the systemic inflammatory response to HIV-1 infection plays an important role in the natural history of HIV-1 infection, both stimulating viral replication and promoting CD4+ cell loss by apoptosis (programmed cell death).

scriptional processes in order to complete its life cycle (Fig. 6.6). The rate of HIV-1 replication is intimately related to the activation state of those host cells. It is estimated that approximately 10^{10} virus particles are produced daily in an infected individual. Such high rates of viral replication induce a CD8+ T cell response that is able to maintain a state of clinical latency for long periods. However, although this antiviral response is aimed at suppressing HIV-1 replication and eliminating infected cells, it may also paradoxically play an important role in supporting the high rates of HIV-1 replication that occur throughout the course of HIV-1 infection. The mechanisms underlying this are reviewed below. Furthermore, immune activation resulting from the host response to other exogenous stimuli, such as co-infections, may also cause immune activation and increased HIV-1 replication by a variety of mechanisms (Table 6.6) described below.

HIV-1 life cycle

HIV-1 is a retrovirus that principally replicates within CD4+ lymphocytes and macrophages. It is dependent on many of the host cell metabolic and tran-

HIV-1 cellular entry

HIV-1 typically enters host cells through the interaction of the viral envelope protein gp120, with CD4 and a chemokine co-receptor (typically CCR5 or

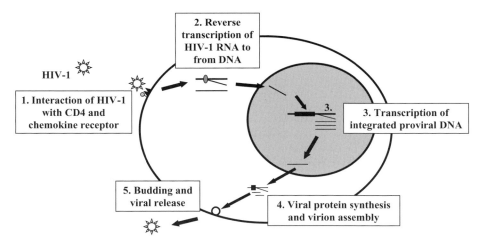

Figure 6.6 The HIV-1 life cycle. (1) Cellular uptake, (2) reverse transcription and (3) HIV-1 proviral transcription stages of the HIV-1 life cycle may be facilitated and accelerated by cellular activation signaling in the presence of coinfections.

Table 6.6 Mechanisms by which immune-activating stimuli may lead to increased HIV-1 replication

1. Upregulation of chemokine receptors favours HIV-1 cellular entry.
2. Cellular activation facilitates completion of reverse transcription, mediated by eg. NF-ATc.
3. Proinflammatory cytokines increase HIV-1 transcription mediated by the binding of transcriptional activators (e.g. NF"B) to the HIV-1 promoter.
4. Intercellular transmission of HIV-1 is facilitated by cell–cell contact during antigen presentation.
5. CD4+ lymphocyte proliferation provides a pool of cellular targets susceptible to HIV-1 infection.
6. Certain stimuli induce a T_H2 response, which favours HIV-1 replication.

CXCR4) on the host cell surface (Fig. 6.6). The relative expression of these co-receptors determines the relative susceptibility of cells to HIV-1 infection. In general, chemokine receptor expression is strongly linked to cellular activation. Immune activation resulting from the presence of opportunistic infections, other inflammatory stimuli or the antigenic stimulus of HIV-1 infection itself, may affect cell surface expression of these coreceptors by uninfected mononuclear cells, thereby modulating their susceptibility to HIV-1 infection. For example, *Mycobacterium avium* infection is associated with upregulation of CCR5 expression by peripheral blood mononuclear cells *in vivo*, facilitating cellular entry by HIV-1 strains using this receptor.

Reverse transcription

Following cellular entry to the cell, the HIV-1 RNA exists in a very labile form in the cytoplasm until reverse transcription is completed to form DNA. However, in the absence of sufficient cellular activation, reverse transcription may be incomplete and the virus may subsequently lose its capacity to initiate productive infection. Through induction of the intracellular transcription factor pathways such as those that generate NF-AT (nuclear factor of activated T cells), for example, proinflammatory

cytokine signaling enables completion of reverse transcription and progression of the viral life cycle. The presence of opportunistic infections and other inflammatory stimuli in the host may therefore facilitate completion of the afferent HIV-1 life cycle. Reverse-transcribed DNA subsequently translocates to the nucleus and integrates into the host genomic DNA, in which form it is termed a provirus (Fig. 6.6).

Proviral transcription

HIV-1 proviral transcription is greatly influenced by the state of host cell activation and is regulated by sequences in the 5′ long terminal repeat (LTR) of the viral genome (Fig. 6.7). A number of these viral regulatory sequences resemble those regulating human cellular genes and are able to specifically bind a variety of host cell transcription factors. In this way, HIV-1 is able to harness the host cellular transcriptional machinery in order to replicate. On exposure of the cell to various activating stimuli, including TNF-α, IL-1, LPS and phorbol esters, physiologically active NF-κB is generated in the cytoplasm, which then translocates to the nucleus. Here, as well as activating host cell gene transcription, NF-κB binds to specific recognition sequences in the enhancer region of the HIV-1 LTR, greatly increasing HIV-1 transcription. This results in the tight coordination of viral transcription and cellular activation. The NF-κB pathway thus represents an important mechanism by which bacteria, viruses and other inflammatory stimuli enhance HIV-1 replication by activating the immune system.

Cytokines and HIV-1 transcription

Since HIV-1 replication is closely regulated by the host cell transcriptional machinery, it comes under the influence of a complex network of pro-inflammatory and immunoregulatory cytokines. TNF-α plays a pivotal role in HIV-1 pathogenesis, inducing HIV-1 transcription in both macrophages and T lymphocytes via the NF-κB pathway. Other inflammatory cytokines (IL-1, IL-2 and IL-6) also promote HIV-1 replication.

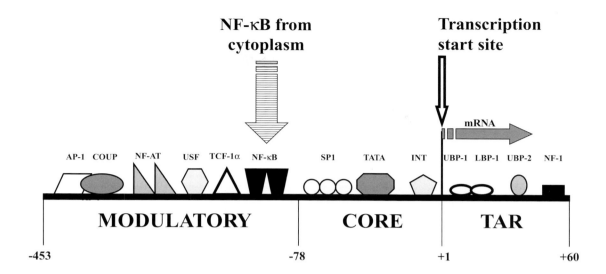

Figure 6.7 Cellular transcription factors that bind to the HIV-1 long terminal repeat (LTR). The HIV-1 promoter is functionally divided into the modulatory enhancer region and the core promoter region, both of which lie upstream of the transcription start point and the transactivation response region (TAR), which lies downstream. Following cellular activation, the interaction of these cellular transcription factors, such as NF-κB, with receptors in the HIV-1 promoter, results in marked upregulation of HIV-1 replication. (Adapted from Lawn, Butera and Folks, 2001.)

HIV-1 replication during antigen presentation

Macrophages serve as long-lived reservoirs of HIV-1 infection. Lymphocytes intimately associate with macrophages during antigen presentation (Fig. 6.8), and the resulting activation of both macrophages and CD4+ T-lymphocytes during cell contact leads to marked upregulation of pro-inflammatory cytokine secretion and intercellular signaling via adhesion molecules. As a result, HIV-1 transcription is greatly increased, and the microenvironment of highly activated mononuclear cells, proinflammatory cytokines and HIV-1 particles is ideal for viral propagation. By these mechanisms, co-infections may greatly increase HIV-1 replication and propagation at sites of co-infection and antigen presentation.

Immune activation and HIV-1 pathogenesis

As discussed above, immune activation results in increased HIV-1 replication and viral load. However, immune activation also has other important effects on the biology of HIV-1, host lymphocyte populations and potentially on the progression of HIV-1 infection to AIDS and on HIV-1 transmission (Fig. 6.9). Reverse transcription is highly error-prone and accelerated rates of HIV-1 replication are therefore associated with increased viral genotypic diversification. This increases the chance of the expression of more virulent quasi-species and therefore may favour disease progression. The number of CD4+ cells infected by HIV-1 is far too small to account for the profound CD4+ lymphocytopenia resulting from HIV-1 infection. However, it is now clear that the state of immune activation in HIV-1–infected individuals triggers widespread lymphocyte death by apoptosis. This depletes both HIV-infected and non-infected bystander cells. There is also evidence that chronic immune activation also suppresses haematopoietic regeneration of T-cell populations. Thus, CD4+ lymphocytopenia is multifactorial in aetiology and is closely linked to the host inflammatory response.

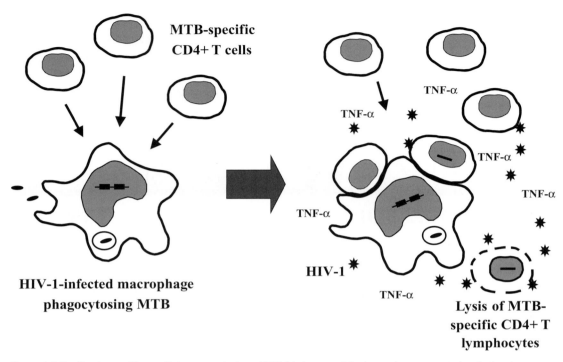

MTB-specific CD4+ T cells

HIV-1-infected macrophage phagocytosing MTB

TNF-α

TNF-α

TNF-α

TNF-α

TNF-α

HIV-1

TNF-α

Lysis of MTB-specific CD4+ T lymphocytes

Figure 6.8 Replication and intercellular transmission of HIV-1 is increased during antigen presentation. Intimate intercellular apposition, activation signaling and proinflammatory cytokine secretion during antigen presentation provides the perfect microenvironment rampant replication and intercellular spread of HIV-1. (Reproduced with permission from Lawn, S. D. *et al.*, 2002). Tuberculosis unleashed: the impact of human immunodeficiency virus type 1 coinfection on the host granulomatous response to *M. tuberculosis*. (From Lawn, Butera and Shinnick, 2002.)

Together, these diverse effects of immune activation on HIV-1 and on the host lymphocytes may potentially enhance disease progression in HIV-infected persons and may ultimately out-weigh the beneficial aspects of antiviral immune responses. This may be particularly important for those living in developing countries, where there is little or no access to antiretroviral drugs and frequent co-infections sustain a chronically heightened state of immune activation. Moreover, local immune activation associated with sexually transmitted diseases in the male and female genital tract accelerate local HIV-1 replication, increasing the viral concentration in genital secretions and promoting sexual transmission of HIV-1.

Copathogenesis of tuberculosis and HIV-1 infection

Having reviewed the mechanisms of immunopathology underlying TB and HIV-1 infection, we are now in a position to understand the very important interactions between these two diseases in co-infected individuals. Early in the HIV-1 epidemic, it became clear that HIV-1 infection greatly increased the risk of developing TB. Indeed, HIV-1 infection has emerged as the dominant risk factor for developing active TB, and in some cities in sub-Saharan African, over 80% of individuals with TB are coinfected with HIV-1. However, it has also become clear that the interaction between these two diseases is bi-directional, with

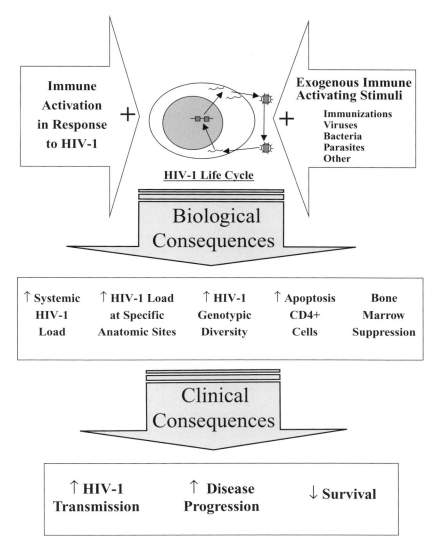

Figure 6.9 The consequences of immune activation in HIV-1 infection *in vivo*. This conceptual diagram highlights the broad consequences of immune activation on the biology of HIV-1 and on lymphoid cell populations *in vivo* and their subsequent impact on HIV-1 transmission, disease progression and survival in HIV-1–infected persons. (Adapted from Lawn, Butera and Folks, 2001.)

each infection promoting the pathogenesis of the other. Clearly the virus and bacterium do not directly interact. Rather, their respective effects on the host inflammatory response mediate this two-way interaction, each infection promoting the replication and modulating the immunopathology of the other.

Impact of HIV-1 on tuberculosis

As discussed earlier, the pathology of TB in immuno-competent individuals is almost entirely attributable to the host immune response. However, HIV-1 co-infection leads to CD4+ T_H lymphocytopenia and thereby critically impairs host cell–mediated immunity and granuloma formation in response to MTB. The impact of this is evident at histological, clinical, and epidemiological levels.

Histological effects

Histological studies of tissue specimens from individuals with TB and HIV-1 co-infection reveal a spectrum of appearances that reflect the degree of immunosuppression. Three histological stages of cellular immune response that correlate with depletion of the peripheral blood CD4+ lymphocyte count have been described: (1) in immunocompetent individuals with HIV-1 infection, TB granulomas are normal, being characterized by abundant epithelioid macrophages, Langhans giant cells, peripherally located CD4+ lymphocytes and a paucity of bacteria; (2) in individuals with moderate HIV-associated immunodeficiency, Langhans giant cells are not seen, epithelioid differentiation and activation of macrophages are absent, there is CD4+ lymphocytopenia, and acid-fast bacilli (AFBs) are more numerous; and (3) in individuals with advanced HIV-associated immunosuppression and AIDS, there is a striking paucity of granuloma formation with little cellular recruitment, very few CD4+ lymphocytes, and even larger numbers of AFBs. Thus HIV-1 coinfection profoundly impairs the granulomatous host response to MTB.

Clinical effects

As a result of impaired host cell immunity, HIV-1 co-infection alters the clinicopathological manifestations of the disease in co-infected individuals (Table 6.7). Clinically, the features of TB in HIV-1–infected individuals with well-preserved CD4+ lymphocyte counts are indistinguishable from those of individuals with TB but no HIV-1 coinfection. However, progression of immunodeficiency in HIV-infected persons diminishes the host inflammatory response to TB, increasing the likelihood of cutaneous anergy to purified protein derivative (PPD) and decreasing the immunopathology nor-

Table 6.7 The effects of HIV-1 on the clinical, radiological, and histopathological features of tuberculosis

Clinical features
Extrapulmonary and miliary disease
Mycobacteremia
Cutaneous anergy to PPD
↑ Mortality
Chest radiology
↓ Consolidation, ↓ pleural thickening
↓ Cavitation, ↓ upper lobe disease, ↓ fibrosis
Post-mortem studies
Disseminated multi-organ involvement
Occult, disseminated MTB infection in people who
   died with AIDS
Histology
↓ Langhans giant cells
↓ Epithelioid differentiation of macrophages
CD4+ lymphocytopenia, ↓ CD4+ activation
↓ Granuloma formation
Numerous and disseminated AFB

mally associated with TB. Thus, the radiographic appearances of pulmonary TB in patients with HIV-1–associated immunodeficiency reflect impaired tissue inflammatory response to infection with decreased parenchymal consolidation, cavitation, and fibrosis (Fig. 6.10). The reduced inflammatory response limits tissue containment of mycobacteria, permitting bloodstream dissemination. Extrapulmonary disease is therefore more common and autopsy specimens from patients who died of TB and the acquired immunodeficiency syndrome (AIDS) also show a high frequency of extrapulmonary and disseminated disease with multi-organ involvement.

The marked reduction in the immunopathology of TB in those with HIV-1 coinfection is vividly illustrated by case reports of HIV-infected individuals with occult, asymptomatic pulmonary TB, who have been observed to develop acute respiratory failure following commencement of highly active anti-retroviral treatment (HAART). In such individuals, advanced immunosuppression prior to antiviral

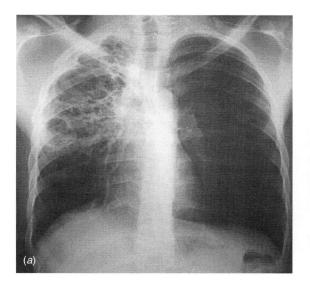
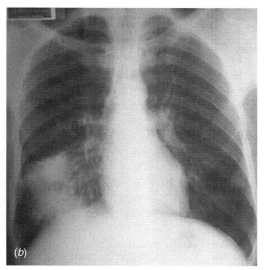

Figure 6.10 Chest radiographs of (a) an HIV-negative individual with pulmonary TB showing marked right-upper-lobe destruction with cativation, volume loss and fibrosis and (b) an individual with pulmonary TB and marked HIV-1–associated immunodeficiency, showing atypical lower lobe disease and hilar lymphadenopathy with no cavitation or fibrosis.

treatment abrogated any inflammatory response within the lungs. However, subsequent immune reconstitution during antiretroviral therapy restored anti-mycobacterial immune responses, resulting in acute interstitial inflammation in response to mycobacteria and respiratory failure.

Epidemiological effects

The lifetime risk of developing active TB in individuals with latent *M. tuberculosis* infection is estimated to be approximately 10%. However, among HIV-1–infected persons with latent infection, the risk is many-fold higher and is estimated to be approximately 10% per year. Thus, infection with HIV-1 has now emerged as the single strongest risk factor for the development of active TB. The HIV-1 pandemic has consequently fueled a resurgence in the incidence of TB over the past decade, contributing to the approximately 8 to 10 million new cases of TB and 2 million deaths from TB occurring worldwide each year.

Impact of tuberculosis on HIV-1 infection

Although the impact of HIV-1 on TB is quite evident both clinically and epidemiologically, the interaction of these two diseases is bi-directional, with TB having a number of important effects of HIV-1 infection in co-infected individuals (Table 6.8). By the mechanisms described earlier, the marked proinflammatory immune response associated with active TB results in increased HIV-1 replication. Thus, a rise in plasma HIV-1 load is seen in individuals who develop active pulmonary TB. In HIV-infected persons with TB meningitis, viral load in

Table 6.8 The effects of tuberculosis co-infection on HIV-1

Increased HIV-1 replication at the site of TB
Increased systemic HIV-1 load
Increased genotypic diversification of HIV-1
Accelerated decline in immune function
Shortened patient survival

cerebrospinal fluid is higher than that present in blood; in those with pulmonary TB, HIV-1 load is greater in diseased lung segments compared to segments that are not inflamed; and in those with pleural TB, HIV-1 load is greater in pleural fluid compared to blood. These findings indicate that HIV-1 replication is compartmentalized within the body and that local inflammatory processes result in increased viral replication at such affected sites. Active TB coinfection is also associated with increased HIV-1 genotypic diversification. Furthermore, as a result of increased viral replication, HIV-1-infected individuals successfully treated for TB have an accelerated decline in immune function compared to individuals who have not had TB, possibly leading to leading to more rapid progression to AIDS.

The co-factor effect of TB on the progression of HIV-1 may be more marked than that associated with other co-infections for several reasons. The course of the disease is prolonged; TB induces marked proinflammatory cytokine secretion, especially of TNF-α, and TB causes both local and systemic immune activation. To date, trials of immune-modulating drugs to reduce the co-factor effect of TB on HIV-1 infection have not revealed beneficial effects on HIV-1 load. Substantial reversal of these phenomena is currently achievable only by using HAART, emphasizing the need for access to effective antiretroviral treatment of coinfected persons.

Conclusions

In this chapter, we have demonstrated that the host inflammatory response to infection may have pathophysiological effects that result in acute, chronic, and irreversible organ damage. The immune system is usually assumed to provide protection against infectious organisms and their potentially harmful effects. However, it is clear that many – and in the case some infections, virtually all – the symptoms and pathology of the infectious process are actually attributable to the host inflammatory response to the organism. Understanding these mechanisms, we realize that

in some instances treatment of infectious diseases may require not only drugs that directly target the invading pathogen but also drugs that modulate the host inflammatory response so as to diminish these adverse effects.

Summary

Infectious pathogens cause disease by two principal means: (1) the organisms themselves or secreted exotoxins have direct toxic effects on the host and (2) the organisms and their shed antigens trigger host inflammatory responses that cause pathology. The immune system is a two-edged sword; although immunological activation is essential to mount an effective host response to invading pathogens, paradoxically the host inflammatory response may cause much of the pathology associated with infection. Injury arising from the effects of the immune system may be referred to as 'immunopathology' and is the focus of this chapter.

Over the past two decades, advances in our knowledge of the host inflammatory process and its mediation have provided great insights into the immunopathology of infectious diseases. In this chapter, we have reviewed how both innate and specific acquired immune responses may contribute to disease. By way of example, we described how host responses to *M. tuberculosis* and HIV-1 are central to the pathogenesis of these infections. We also illustrated how the important bi-directional interaction of these diseases results from their respective effects on the immune system.

Acknowledgements

Dr. Stephen D. Lawn is funded by the Wellcome Trust.

Clinical scenarios

Glandular fever

A 19-year-old male presented with a 5-day history of severe sore throat, fever and marked malaise.

Clinical examination revealed large exudative tonsils, cervical lymphadenopathy and mild hepatosplenomegaly. A peripheral blood film revealed a lymphocytosis and atypical mononuclear cells. IgM to Epstein-Barr virus was detected in serum, confirming a suspected diagnosis of glandular fever. The swelling of the lymphoreticular organs in this disease is due to massive proliferation of CD8+ cytotoxic lymphocytes in response to the virus.

Jarisch-Herxheimer reaction

A 35-year-old man living in rural Ethiopia was admitted to hospital with a biphasic febrile illness. He described an abrupt onset of fever, rigors, myalgia, and headache 7 days previously, which initially resolved but recurred on the day of admission. Blood film examination revealed the presence of spirochaetes. A diagnosis of louse-borne relapsing fever due to *Borrelia recurrentis* was made. Ninety minutes after the commencement of treatment with intramuscular penicillin the patient's temperature rose by 2°C to 41°C and a fall in blood pressure necessitated rapid intravenous fluid therapy. The patient had developed a Jarisch-Herxheimer reaction (JHR). A massive release of proinflammatory cytokines in response to rapid killing of spirochaetes is responsible for this reaction.

Erythema nodosum leprosum

A 37-year-old Indian man presented with facial cutaneous nodules and patchy anaesthesia in the hands. A skin biopsy revealed the histological features of lepromatous leprosy. After 18 months of multi-drug treatment, examination of slit-skin smears revealed a good response to treatment with only a very low level of persistent viable bacteria. However, he was subsequently admitted with an acute onset of widespread raised cutaneous erythematous lesions 1 to 3 cm in diameter. These were associated with marked fever and an acute-phase response. A clinical diagnosis of erythema nodosum leprosum (ENL) was made and symptoms settled over several days with thalido-

mide treatment. ENL is an immunological reaction to *M. leprae* antigens that may persist in the skin for many years despite effective multi-drug treatment. It is thought that this reaction is due to type III hypersensitivity together with systemic secretion of high levels of proinflammatory cytokines, especially TNF-α. Thalidomide is an immune-modulating drug that decreases the secretion of TNF-α and leads to rapid improvement in the symptoms of ENL.

Pulmonary tuberculosis

A 47-year-old male smoker from India presented with a 5-month history of productive cough, for which he received several courses of antibiotics for presumed chronic bronchitis. However, he subsequently developed fever, weight loss, increasing volumes of sputum production and exertional dyspnoea and was finally admitted to hospital. Sputum smears were positive for acid-fast bacilli. A chest radiograph revealed widespread patchy consolidation in both lungs and cavities throughout the left lung, together with extensive volume loss and pleural thickening. He received antituberculosis multi-drug treatment for 6 months, during which he improved clinically, and follow-up sputum samples were all smear- and culture-negative. Despite microbiological cure of his TB, he had persistent sputum production and dyspnoea. The chronic inflammatory response to TB had caused extensive parenchymal necrosis, pulmonary and pleural fibrosis, and airway damage with bronchiectasis.

HAART and immune reconstitution TB

A 35-year-old homosexual man presented with weight loss, intermittent fever and a previous episode of herpes zoster. Clinical examination revealed lymphadenopathy, oral candidiasis and mild wasting. The CD4+ T-cell count was 80 × 10^6/l and plasma HIV-1 load of RNA copies was 800 000/ml. Highly active anti-retroviral treatment was started, leading to a rapid fall in viral load and a rise in CD4+ lymphocyte count. However, after 4 weeks of treatment, the patient was admitted to hospital with fever, cough and breathlessness. A chest radiograph revealed widespread alveolar shadowing. Examination of bronchoalveolar lavage fluid revealed acid-fast bacilli. The patient had had an occult disseminated *M. tuberculosis* infection which, prior to antiretroviral treatment, had remained asymptomatic due to the lack of a host inflammatory response. However, following immune reconstitution during antiretroviral treatment, the patient developed a diffuse tuberculous alveolitis as a recovery in CD4+ T_H lymphocyte function resulted in an inflammatory response to the organism.

Multiple-choice questions (true or false)

1. The following cytokines induce fever:
   a. IFN-γ
   b. TNF-α
   c. IL-8
   d. IL-1
   e. IL-10
2. Concerning administration of thalidomide to individuals being treated for tuberculosis, the following effects are typically seen:
   a. A rise in serum IFN-γ concentration
   b. A decrease in serum TNF-α concentration
   c. Increased macrophage activation
   d. Increased TB cure rates
   e. Increased weight gain
3. Immune activation associated with coinfections in HIV-infected persons increases HIV-1 replication by the following mechanisms:
   a. Increased HIV-1 uptake
   b. Activation of the HIV-1 LTR
   c. Increased HIV-1 transcription
   d. Increased IL-8 secretion
   e. Increased TNF-α secretion
4. Concerning the effects of HIV-1 coinfection on pulmonary tuberculosis, the following are true:

   a. There is reduced granuloma formation.
   b. There is an increased frequency of mycobacteraemia.
   c. There is increased chest radiographic shadowing.
   d. There is an increased systemic level of TNF-α.
   e. There is increased clonal expansion of MTB-specific T lymphocytes.

Answers

1. T T F T F
2. F T F F T
3. T T T F T
4. F T F T F

FURTHER READING

Alfano, M., Poli, G. (2002). The cytokine network in HIV infection. *Current Molecular Medicine* **2**, 677–89.

Bentwich, Z., Maartens, G., Torten, D. *et al.* (2000). Concurrent infections and HIV pathogenesis. *AIDS* **14**, 2071–81.

Bloom, B. R. (ed.). (1994). Tuberculosis, Pathogenesis, Protection and Control. Washington, DC: ASM Press.

Dannenberg, A. M. Jr. (1991). Delayed-type hypersensitivity and cell-mediated immunity in the pathogenesis of tuberculosis. *Immunology Today* **12**, 228–33.

Goletti, D., Weissman, D., Jackson, R. W. *et al.* (1996). Effect of *Mycobacterium tuberculosis* on HIV replication. Role of immune activation. *Journal of Immunology* **157**, 1271–8.

Goldsby, R. A., Kindt, T. J., Osbourne, B. A., Kuby, J. (2003). Immunology, 5th ed. New York: Freeman.

Havlir, D. V., Barnes, P. F. (1999). Tuberculosis in patients with human immunodeficiency virus infection. *New England Journal of Medicine* **340**, 367–73.

Lawn, S. D., Butera, S. T., Folks, T. M. (2001). Contribution of immune activation to the pathogenesis and transmission of human immunodeficiency virus type 1 infection. *Clinical Microbiology Reviews* **14**, 753–77.

Lawn, S. D., Butera, S. T., Shinnick, T. M. (2002). Tuberculosis unleashed: the impact of human immunodeficiency virus type 1 coinfection on the host granulomatous response to *Mycobacterium tuberculosis*. *Microbes and Infection* **4**, 635–46.

Lawn, S. D., Pisell, T. L., Hirsch, C. S., Wu, M., Butera, S. T., Toosi, Z. (2001) Anatomically compartmentalized human immunodeficiency virus replication in HLA-DR+ cells and CD14+ macrophages at the site of pleural tuberculosis coinfection. *Journal of Infectious Disease* **184,** 1127–33.

Mims, C. A., Nash, A. (2001). Stephen J. Mims' Pathogenesis of Infectious Disease, 5th ed. London: Academic Press.

Shelburne, S. A. III, Hamill, R. J. (2003). The immune reconstitution inflammatory syndrome. *AIDS Reviews* **5,** 67–79.

Whalen, C. C., Nsubuga, P., Okwera, A. *et al.* (2000). Impact of pulmonary tuberculosis on survival of HIV-infected adults: a prospective epidemiologic study in Uganda. *AIDS* **14,** 1219–28.

7

Infection – parasitic

Malcolm E. Molyneux

Malaria

The plasmodia responsible for malaria are protozoan parasites distinguished by their largely intracellular location in the human host and their dependence upon a vector both for completion of their life cycle and the transmission necessary for their survival. Unlike many of the larger metazoan parasites, plasmodia can multiply within the human host, so that a single infection can lead to an overwhelming parasitic burden.

Malaria is the most important human parasitic disease in terms of the morbidity and mortality for which it is responsible. Of the four major species of plasmodia infecting humans (*P. falciparum, P. vivax, P. malariae* and *P. ovale*) one – *P. falciparum* – is responsible for nearly all the severe disease and mortality due to malaria (1 million to 2.5 million deaths every year), while the other species cause febrile illness, sometimes leading to anaemia but rarely to death.

The exploration of disease mechanisms is beginning to contribute to our understanding of some of the characteristics of malarial disease in populations and individuals. Even in the absence of antimalarial treatment, *P. falciparum* infections can cause a range of clinical effects, from asymptomatic to fatal, depending on the interplay of a variety of host and parasite factors.

Relevance of the plasmodial life cycle to disease manifestations

Various stages of the parasite cause no symptoms. These include *sporozoites, hepatic-stage parasites,* circulating *intra-erythrocytic* asexual parasites, *gametocytes* and *hypnozoites* (the latter develop in *P. vivax* and *P. ovale* only). Three processes fundamental to the parasite's life cycle result in disease: (1) the release of merozoites and other red cell contents when mature blood-stage schizonts rupture; (2) the accompanying destruction of infected erythrocytes; and (3) the adherence of parasitized erythrocytes to vascular endothelia, leading to the sequestration of parasitized erythrocytes in microvascular beds (this process of cytoadherence and sequestration is peculiar to *P. falciparum*).

The febrile illness

Fever – with its accompanying malaise, anorexia, headache, chills, sweating and rigors – is a cytokine-mediated host response that is common to infections by almost all pathogens (see Chapter 6). Monoclonal antibody to tumour necrosis factor (TNF) has been shown to reduce fever in West African children suffering from severe malaria. What triggers the host cytokine response in malaria is unknown but is likely to be a toxin, or possibly several toxins, released from the rupturing schizont. Glycosylphosphatidylinositol (GPI) of parasite origin is one candidate for the role of a 'malaria toxin'. Administered as a vaccine to mice, a *P. falciparum* GPI conjugated to a suitable carrier prevents complications and death in animals challenged with a subsequent *P. falciparum* infection. A comparable effect is yet to be demonstrated in human malaria. It is probable that the 'antitoxic immunity' that is characteristic of older children and adults in endemic areas (less fever and illness, for a given density of parasitaemia, than in non-immune people) may result from immune mechanisms directed against some such parasite 'toxin'.

Malarial fever is not usually distinguishable clinically from fever due to other agents. A periodicity of fever may develop that becomes highly suggestive of malaria, but this is usually in prolonged untreated infections. Periodicity results from synchronisation of the parasite population, which may be due to the fact that elevated body temperature differentially slows the growth of late-stage parasites, allowing younger parasites to 'catch up'.

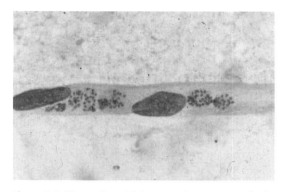

Figure 7.1 *Plasmodium falciparum* schizonts in cerebral venule, from post-mortem brain smear in child with cerebral malaria. (See colour plate section.)

Severe malaria

Plasmodium falciparum infections may progress, especially in the non-immune and untreated, to cause possibly life-threatening organ or tissue dysfunction. In children in endemic areas, the common complications are severe anaemia, acidosis, prostration, hypoglycaemia and encephalopathy (convulsions and altered consciousness); these may occur singly or in any combination. Non-immune adults may suffer the same complications but are also liable to develop acute renal failure, acute respiratory distress syndrome (ARDS), disseminated intravascular coagulation and intravascular haemolysis. In endemic areas, children suffer most of the severe disease, adults being protected by a combination of innate and acquired immunity. Even in children in endemic areas, it is only a minority of infections that progress to severe disease.

Pathogenesis of complicated disease

Cytoadherence and sequestration

Erythrocytes containing mature stages of *P. falciparum* adhere to microvascular endothelium and thereby accumulate in capillaries and venules of deep tissues (*sequestration*) (See Fig. 7.1). Several lines of evidence suggest that the process of seques-

tration may be important in the pathogenesis of severe disease: (1) sequestration is peculiar to *P. falciparum*, which is the only plasmodial species causing severe disease; (2) histological samples from various tissues in fatal malaria commonly reveal intense sequestration of parasitised erythrocytes; (3) sequestration is maximal in those tissues or organs that are most susceptible to functional impairment in severe falciparum malaria – brain, bone marrow, intestinal mucosa, lung.

Cytoadherence involves a specific linkage between proteins expressed on the surface of the infected red cell and receptors on host tissues. As the parasite matures in the infected erythrocyte, a family of highly variable parasite genes ('var' genes) begin to encode proteins that pass to the surface of the cell, where they are collectively known as *P. falciparum erythrocyte membrane protein 1 (PfEMP-1)*. Other parasite-derived proteins are similarly expressed on the red cell surface but remain to be characterised. Variability in the PfEMP-1 expressed by a particular population of parasites has been estimated at around 2% per parasite life cycle, a property that may enable the parasite to evade some of the host's specific acquired immune responses directed at these proteins. When studied in an *in vitro* culture, PfEMP-1 expression and specific cytoadherence are accelerated and enhanced with elevation of the surrounding temperature from 37° to 40°C, suggesting that fever may have a similar effect *in vivo*.

Host receptors capable of mediating cytoadherence include CD36, ICAM-1, chondroitin sulphate A, hyaluronic acid, e-selectin, V-CAM-1 and thrombospondin. ICAM-1 may be the principal receptor mediating cytoadherence in the brain, CD36 in most other tissues and chondroitin sulphate A in the placenta. Cytoadherence of parasitised erythrocytes resembles that of host leucocytes in that there are rolling and static components, and it is likely that different receptors mediate each of these processes. Cytokines such as TNF-α upregulate the expression of host endothelial receptors, providing another mechanism by which a malaria infection enhances its own sequestration.

Parasitised erythrocytes cytoadhere not only to endothelial cells but also to *other parasitised erythrocytes*, a process leading to 'autoagglutination' of infected red cells. In some (not all) instances, platelets appear to be a necessary intermediary between adjacent cells. Autoagglutination may account for the appearance of heavily sequestered venules and capillaries, in which parasitised cells towards the centre of the vessel lumen are some distance from the vascular endothelium and unlikely to be adherent to it.

Parasitised erythrocytes may also adhere to *uninfected erythrocytes*, resulting in the formation *in vitro* of 'rosettes', each consisting of a parasitised red cell surrounded by several uninfected erythrocytes. Although some studies have shown that parasites with a capacity to form rosettes are more likely than others to be associated with severe disease, this has not been found in all surveys, and rosettes have not been identified in human tissues from patients dying of falciparum malaria, so that the contribution of rosetting to sequestration is uncertain.

There is still no incontrovertible evidence that sequestration mediates tissue or organ dysfunction, but the circumstantial evidence is strong. Several mechanisms are plausible and require continued research: (1) actively metabolising parasites may 'rob' local tissues of ingredients essential to their viability, such as glucose and micronutrients; (2)

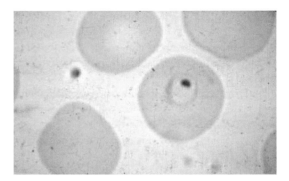

Figure 7.2 Thin blood film (Field's stain) with ring-stage asexual *P. falciparum* trophozoite in apparently normal erythrocyte (×4000). (See colour plate section.)

the perfusion of tissues may be impaired by the mass of stationary parasitised red cells; (3) damage can be demonstrated to junctions between adjacent endothelial cells, with loss of integrity of the vessel wall (which in the brain constitutes the 'blood-brain barrier'); (4) the eventual rupture of *P. falciparum* schizonts, with the local discharge of merozoites, 'toxins' and haemozoin (pigment resulting from the parasite's digestion of haemoglobin) must provide a large additional local stimulus. Consequences of this include demonstrable recruitment of leucocytes, deposition of fibrin and platelets, and the induction of nitric oxide synthase (iNOS), which suggests that nitric oxide may be generated locally.

It is clear that sequestration commonly has no detectable adverse effect on tissue or organ function, because sequestration is also a feature of uncomplicated falciparum malaria (no late-stage parasites are visible in the peripheral blood). (See Fig. 7.2.) It remains to be determined whether impaired tissue function results when there is an overwhelming mass of sequestered parasites or from a crucial distribution or quality of the sequestered cells.

Cytokine responses

Cytokines mediate the characteristic fever of malaria, as of other infections (discussed above). Whether cytokines are essential to the pathogenesis of severe and fatal disease remains a subject of important inquiry. Several studies have demonstrated an association between circulating cytokine concentrations (TNF, IL-1, IL-6, IL-8) and disease severity, but whether this association is causal and if so in which direction remains to be elucidated. A large randomised controlled trial of recombinant anti-TNF in West African children with malarial coma demonstrated an anti-fever effect but no benefit to survival. (This does not disprove a role for TNF in pathogenesis of fatal disease, as the intervention may have been too late or in other ways ineffectual.) Studies of drugs that ameliorate cytokine responses, such as pentoxyfilline, have so far failed to provide evidence that such drugs prevent or reverse severe disease.

Several problems make it difficult to study the role of cytokines in the pathogenesis of fatal malaria. There is no readily available animal model of severe falciparum malaria; malarias in common animal models have different pathology; trials of anti-cytokine treatments in patients with severe malaria may enrol subjects after crucial damage has already been done; and important cytokine effects may occur locally in tissues not accessible to study during life. Similar problems surround the study of other mediators and downstream effects of cytokine activity.

Severe anaemia

A degree of anaemia develops in most malaria infections, and severe anaemia (packed cell volume 15% or less, haemoglobin concentration 5 g/dl or less) is a common and important single complication, especially in infants and toddlers in endemic areas (see Fig. 7.3). Mechanisms that may contribute to the development of anaemia include (1) the destruction of red cells by parasites at schizont rupture; (2) reduced life span of unparasitised erythrocytes, possibly resulting from cross-reacting antibodies developed against the surface of parasitised cells – increased splenic clearance of unparasitised red cells can be demonstrated during malaria; and (3) impaired bone marrow function, as dyserythro-

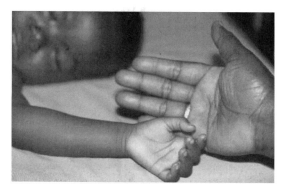

Figure 7.3 Pallor of palm of an infant with severe malarial anaemia. (See colour plate section.)

poiesis is visible on light microscopy of bone marrow smears and reticulocytes are absent from the peripheral blood even when anaemia is severe. Sequestration of parasitised erythrocytes in bone marrow sinusoids is a common finding, and it seems likely that dyserythropoiesis is mediated by altered local cytokine secretions. Some studies suggest that in severe anaemia there is a relative deficiency of the IL-10 response that normally modulates TNF activity. It is possible that haemozoin, released with rupture of schizont-infected red cells, is toxic to the macrophages that consume it, with consequent deficient secretion of IL-12, leading to impaired generation of a T_H1 host response. This impairment of macrophage function may partially explain the increased occurrence of non-typhoid salmonella infections observed in children with severe malarial anaemia.

Coma and convulsions

In an individual with altered consciousness and *P falciparum* parasitaemia, several possibilities must be considered: (1) the illness may have another cause, with incidental parasitaemia – this is a strong possibility in populations having a high prevalence of asymptomatic parasitaemia; (2) the patient may be having a seizure – sometimes extraneous movements are not obvious, and the true nature of the event is revealed by electro-encephalography: malarial fever

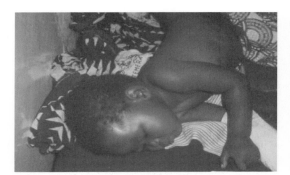

Figure 7.4 Child with cerebral malaria; coma and opisthotonos.

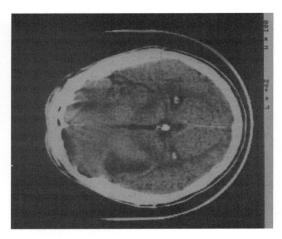

Figure 7.5 Temporal lobe infarction in an adult recovering from cerebral malaria who then had severe residual amnesia.

is particularly likely to precipitate a febrile convulsion in infants and young children, and more complex seizures are also common in malaria – in this circumstance consciousness may be regained within a few minutes or hours after the seizure stops or is treated; (3) the patient may be in the post-ictal phase after a recent convulsion – again, recovery of consciousness may then be imminent; (4) there may be a metabolic complication of malaria, such as hypoglycaemia; or (5) the disease may have none of the foregoing explanations and be directly due to *P. falciparum* infection (see Fig 7.4).

Mechanisms by which intracerebral sequestration may contribute to encephalopathy have been discussed above. In considering the likely pathophysiology of malarial coma, two observations must be recognized: (1) about 90% of children and 95% of adults who recover from a malarial coma do so without detectable neurological sequelae: whatever the principal mechanisms of coma, they do not generally produce irreversible damage to brain tissue; (2) conversely, 10% of children and 5% of adults who recover consciousness have detectable neurological sequelae, and these are often accompanied by areas of infarction demonstrable by computed tomography of the brain (see Fig. 7.5). It is likely that coma is usually the result of a diffuse impairment of cerebral function related to sequestration and that sequelae result in a minority of cases when a vessel or group of vessels become secondarily obstructed by parasites,

pigment and fibrin deposition, leading to localised infarction.

In the majority of children with 'cerebral malaria', the opening pressure of the cerebrospinal fluid is high. Papilloedema is occasionally found and is associated with a poor prognosis. At autopsy, brain weights tend to be higher than appropriate for the child's age and weight, and flattened gyri and filled sulci suggest that the brain has been swollen within the skull. All these features suggest that cerebral oedema is a common component of the pathology of fatal cerebral malaria. Frank herniation of brain between compartments is, however, rarely found at autopsy in a patient dying of malarial coma.

Hypoglycaemia

Children with malarial coma commonly have hypoglycaemia, but correction of the plasma glucose concentration with a dextrose infusion rarely restores consciousness, suggesting additional causes of coma. Hypoglycaemia in these circumstances may be due to a combination of reduced hepatic glycogen reserves, inhibition of hepatic glucuronyl transferase (and therefore of gluconeogenesis) by cytokines and anaerobic glycolysis in hypoxic or underperfused tissues. Plasma insulin concentrations are appropriately low. Hypoglycaemia may also develop through a different mechanism in individuals – especially pregnant women – who are receiving treatment with quinine. This drug is a potent stimulus to the secretion of insulin from the pancreatic beta cells, which have increased activity and sensitivity in pregnancy, and plasma insulin concentrations in this circumstance are higher than appropriate for the plasma glucose concentration.

Acidosis

Often indicated clinically by the patient's characteristically deep breathing, acidosis may be largely the result of impaired tissue oxygenation through a combination of anaemia, hypovolaemia and impaired tissue perfusion and metabolism in the presence of sequestered parasites.

Acute renal failure

Rarely seen in children in malarious areas, acute renal failure is a grave and quite common complication of falciparum malaria in non-immune adults. It develops in the context of hypovolaemia and hypotension that may follow fluid losses through anorexia, vomiting, sweating and hyperventilation. Clinically and histopathologically the underlying event is acute tubular necrosis, and recovery is usual within a few days or weeks if the patient survives the illness and is appropriately dialysed.

Disseminated intravascular coagulation

An overt bleeding tendency in severe malaria is uncommon (rare in children), but some degree of activation of the coagulation cascade is usual and some degree of thrombocytopenia is almost invariable. In most patients with symptomatic malaria, plasma antithrombin III concentrations are low, in association with increased plasma levels of thrombin–antithrombin III. Platelet survival is reduced and bone marrow appearances suggest dyspoietic thrombogenesis. Intravascular deposition of platelets can

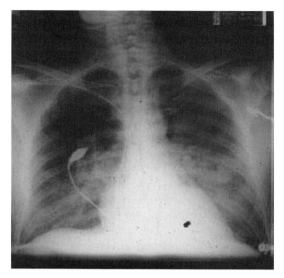

Figure 7.6 Acute respiratory distress syndrome in an adult with complicated *falciparum* malaria.

be demonstrated in sites of intense sequestration, sometimes in association with microthrombi.

Pulmonary oedema and acute respiratory distress syndrome (ARDS)

These two complications may resemble each other clinically and radiologically but have a different pathogenesis. (See Fig. 7.6.) Pulmonary oedema may follow excessive infusion of fluids, especially in the presence of impaired renal function. In ARDS, there has not been over-hydration, and pulmonary wedge pressures are low or normal. Histology indicates the presence of both parasitised red cells and leucocytes in pulmonary microvessels. This condition is uncommon in children and is often fatal when it occurs in adults.

Determinants of disease severity

What determines whether a particular individual infected with *P. falciparum* develops negligible, mild, moderate, severe or fatal disease? A particular illness is the result of an interplay of several parasite, host, vector and circumstancial factors.

Parasite factors

We know that the different species of plasmodia cause different degrees of illness, with only *P. falciparum* commonly causing severe and fatal disease. Even within the species *P. falciparum*, different parasite 'strains' have different capacities to cause disease, a fact well known to physicians who administered malaria parasites to generate fever for the treatment of syphilis early in the last century. Virulence in *P. falciparum* may depend on the parasite's growth (multiplication) rate, its PfEMP-1 expression (affecting its cytoadherence characteristics or tissue specificity), its capacity for agglutination or rosette formation, and its toxin-releasing and cytokine-inducing potential. Parasite mutations are known to affect susceptibility to drugs – for example, point mutations in the genes for parasite enzymes *dihydrofolate reductase* and *dihydropteroate synthetase* confer degrees of resistance to drugs, such as pyrimethamine and sulfadoxine respectively, that target these enzymes. While not affecting parasite virulence, these mutations may impair responses to initial treatment and thus influence disease severity.

Host factors

The most obvious host determinant of the severity of malaria is the level of *acquired specific antimalarial immunity*. Thus adults in an area of intense *P. falciparum* transmission tend to suffer few or mild symptoms while children in the same areas are at risk of severe and fatal disease. Immunity is directed against all stages of the parasite's life cycle in the human host (sporozoites, liver stages, blood stage asexual parasites and gametocytes) and probably also against 'toxins'. Both antibody and T cell–mediated mechanisms contribute to acquired specific immunity.

Humans are diverse both in their capacity to mount an effective specific immune response and also in components of most or all of the non-specific disease mechanisms described earlier in this chapter. Since *P. falciparum* can kill large numbers of peo-

ple before they reach reproductive age, it is likely that the parasite has exerted a selective pressure on many genes in populations in malarious areas. The most readily demonstrable example of such an effect is the gene mutation causing substitution of valine for glutamic acid at position 6 in the beta chain of haemoglobin. An individual inheriting this mutation from both parents suffers from sickle cell disease, with frequent haematological crises and a strong likelihood of dying in childhood. An individual inheriting the mutation from only one parent has almost no clinical disease from the mutation but is dramatically protected against severe and fatal malaria. A balanced polymorphism results in the population, accounting for much higher prevalences of the sickle mutation in malarious than other areas of the world, and the prevalence of the heterozygous sickle state among children with severe malaria is about one-tenth or less of its prevalence in the population as a whole. Similar, but usually less powerful and less consistent, host genetic contributions to malaria susceptibility are now being identified through large case-control and parent–child studies with carefully defined severe disease in the index patients. Mutations affecting HLA class I and II antigens, the promoter region of TNF genes, ICAM-1 expression on vascular endothelium and many other mutations have been reported to be under- or over-represented among children with severe or fatal malaria. Some of these effects are seen in some populations but not in others, and some are associated with certain malaria complications (e.g. coma or severe anaemia) and not others.

With the completion of sequencing of both human and *P. falciparum* genomes and with the increasing use of multicentre epidemiological studies, it is likely that more will be learned in the near future about parasite and host characteristics that determine disease severity and about particular combinations of host and parasite that may be critical for morbidity or mortality.

Influence of transmission pattern

Even within malarious areas, there are great geographical differences in the frequency and seasonality of infections. There is some evidence to suggest that although children bear the brunt of disease in all such areas, the patterns of disease in children differ. Where transmission of *P. falciparum* is intense year 'round, the commonest complication is severe anaemia in infants and toddlers, while in areas with restricted seasonal transmission, encephalopathy in toddlers and slightly older children is more common. Whether and how disease patterns will be affected by the introduction of measures that alter infection rates – such as impregnated bed nets – remains to be seen as these methods are increasingly widely introduced.

Circumstances

The impact of malaria in a population is partly determined by how quickly disease is recognized and how well it is treated. These are dependent upon the availability of health services, the quality of diagnostic and therapeutic falcilities, and the accessibility of these to all sectors of the population. The efficacy of drugs used in the first-line treatment of uncomplicated disease is also an important factor: there is epidemiological evidence of increasing malarial mortality associated with decreasing efficacy of chloroquine in parts of Africa over recent decades. Adequate drugs are an important but not a sufficient defence against severe malaria, however, as many fatal illnesses develop over a matter of hours and even the most immediate therapy could not be expected to rescue the patient. Malaria control must therefore advance along all fronts, and the development of a vaccine continues to be a priority.

Summary

The intracellular protozoon *P. falciparum* is the cause of enormous annual mortality, especially among children, in tropical areas. The pattern of disease and death in a population varies with the intensity of transmission, as frequent exposure leads to the acquisition of partial immunity.

Infection in a partially immune host may be asymptomatic or may lead to any of a variety of syndromes ranging from uncomplicated febrile illness to multi-organ failure. The severity of the illness depends on the interplay of many factors: parasite virulence, host immunity, the availability, efficacy and promptness of drug treatment, and host genetic and environmental risk factors that are incompletely understood.

The major complications of *P. falciparum* infection include encephalopathy, severe anaemia, acidosis, hypoglycaemia, acute renal failure, disseminated intravascular coagulation and ARDS, the last three in this list being uncommon in children. Mechanisms postulated to play a role in the development of severe disease include organ-specific or widespread sequestration of parasitised erythrocytes in microvascular beds and excessive host inflammatory responses. A combination of these mechanisms is likely to be important in the pathogenesis of many of the complicating syndromes.

Clinical scenarios

Scenario 1

A 2-year-old child is admitted in coma to a hospital in West Africa. The rectal temperature is 38.8°C. There is regular deep breathing (40/min) with indrawing of the lower chest wall, but auscultation of the chest is normal. The blood glucose concentration is 1.2 mmol/l. A thin blood film shows 1% *P. falciparum* parasitaemia (1% of red cells parasitised). The blood haemoglobin concentration is 6 g/dl.

True or false?

1. Hypoglycaemia is likely to be due to prior quinine treatment causing hyperinsulinaemia.
2. The blood film indicates that *P. falciparum* is the cause of the current illness.
3. Anti-TNF therapy, if available, would improve this child's chances of survival.
4. The deep breathing suggests acute respiratory distress syndrome (ARDS).

5. Only ring-stage parasites are likely to be seen in the peripheral blood, as the more mature parasite stages are sequestered in deep tissues.

Comments

1. False. Much more likely is hypoglycaemia due to severe infection, resulting from a combination of starvation and impaired hepatic gluconeogenesis.
2. False. In this endemic area, many children have incidental parasitaemia. The positive film suggests that malaria is a possible cause, but other diagnoses must be excluded.
3. False. Trials of anti-TNF have shown no survival benefit in this situation.
4. False. ARDS is a rare complication of malaria in children, while deep breathing in this child's circumstances strongly suggests acidosis.
5. True.

Scenario 2

A British woman aged 36 years returned yesterday from a 2-week visit to south Vietnam, during which she took no malaria prophylaxis. She had not been abroad before and flew direct to Vietnam via Singapore. Three days after arriving in Vietnam she had fever and vomiting, which settled without treatment. Today she complains of shivering, malaise, and headache. Her sublingual temperature is 39°C and pulse rate 96/min. There are no other abnormal signs. A thin blood film shows no malarial parasites.

True or false?

1. The fever on her third day in Vietnam was possibly the first indication of malaria.
2. The negative blood film rules out a diagnosis of malaria.
3. If the temperature is sustained (i.e. not periodic), malaria is unlikely.
4. The blood film should be repeated after 2 days to try to confirm or exclude malaria.
5. If she is pregnant and has malaria, there is a greater chance of severe disease.

Comments

1. False. Malarial parasites take at least a week to develop in the liver.
2. False. A thin blood film may fail to pick up a *P. falciparum* infection sufficient to cause symptoms and even severe disease in a non-immune individual.
3. False. Although periodic fever is characteristic of prolonged malaria, fever in the early stages is often sustained.
4. False. Two days is too long to wait: a *P. falciparum* infection could progress rapidly to severe disease.
5. True.

FURTHER READING

Beeson, J. G., Brown, G. V. (2004). *Plasmodium falciparum*–infected erythrocytes demonstrate dual specificity for adhesion to hyaluronic acid and chondroitin sulfate A and have distinct adhesive properties. *Journal of Infectious Disease* **189,** 69–79.

Chitnis, C. E. (2001). Molecular insights into receptors used by malaria parasites for erythrocyte invasion. *Current Opinion in Haematology* **8,** 85–91.

Grau, G. E., Mackenzie, C. D., Carr, R. A. *et al.*, (2003). Platelet accumulation in brain microvessels in fatal paediatric cerebral malaria. *Journal of Infectious Disease* **187,** 461–6.

Kwiatkowski, D. (1999).The molecular genetic approach to malarial pathogenesis and immunity. *Parasitologia* **41,** 233–240.

Maitland, K., Levin, M., English, M. *et al.*, (2003). Severe *P. falciparum* malaria in Kenyan children: evidence for hypovolaemia. *Quarterly Journal of Medicine* **96,** 427–34.

Miller, L. H., Baruch, D. I., Marsh, K., Doumbo, O. K. (2002). The pathogenic basis of malaria. *Nature* **415,** 673–79.

Taylor, T. E., Fu, W. N., Carr, R. A., Whitten, R. O., Mueller, J. G., Fosiko, N. M., Liomba, N. G., Molyneux, M. E. (2004). Differentiating the pathologies of cerebral malaria by post mortem parasite counts. *Nature Medicine* **10**(2): 143–145.

Warrell, D. A., Gilles, H. M. (eds.). (2002). Essential Malariology, 4th ed. London, New York, New Delhi: Arnold. .

World Health Organization. (2000). Severe falciparum malaria. *Transactions of the Royal Society of Tropical Medicine and Hygiene* **94(Suppl 1)**, S1–90.

8

The acute coronary syndrome

Anthony M. Heagerty

Introduction

The increased sophistication that now characterises the detection of cell damage and death has changed the perception of what constitutes an acute coronary syndrome from that of chest pain with or without tissue necrosis to one of a spectrum of problems comprising unstable angina, myocardial infarction without electrocardiographic ST-segment elevation, and myocardial infarction with ST-segment elevation. All demand an embarrassment of the blood supply to heart muscle, which can occur for a variety of reasons; but the most important cause is atherosclerotic disease of the epicardial coronary arteries. The mechanisms that lead to the development of an acute coronary syndrome are discussed below.

Unstable angina

Chest discomfort is the hallmark symptom most frequently although not invariably experienced when myocardial oxygen demand exceeds supply. The encroachment by an atheromatous plaque into the arterial lumen will cause a fixed stenosis so that, during episodes of stress or exercise, the downstream region of myocardium is rendered ischaemic. For many patients, the situations that bring about angina are recognised and constant for periods sometimes as long as many years, so much so that individuals can avoid circumstances that precipitate their problem. For others, symptoms develop more rapidly, with the situation worsening over a few weeks or even just several days. This is termed unstable angina and

occurs because of the fissuring or rupture of atheromatous plaque, followed by platelet aggregation at the site of the plaque breakdown. These processes of plaque rupture and platelet deposition form the major foci of research into our understanding of the molecular processes that generate acute coronary syndromes.

Until relatively recently, the formed atheromatous lesion was regarded as a fixed lipid core surrounded by a fibrous cap. The central core contains an abundance of lipid-laden macrophage foam cells, which are derived from peripheral blood monocytes. When situated in the arterial wall, these cells ingest lipid and are able to produce procoagulant stimuli that can promote thrombus formation. The fibrous cap has a major role in influencing whether a plaque ruptures; those with thin caps are more likely to do so than those with thicker ones, because the latter are more liable to withstand mechanically distorting stress.

The work of Libby has provided evidence that the cap is not a fixed entity; it can remodel and is the site of intense metabolic turnover. The structure is largely determined by the extracellular matrix constituents, including collagen subtypes I and II, elastin and other proteoglycans. The amount of collagen in the cap is influenced by inflammatory mediators that control synthesis and degradation. Inflammatory cytokines such as transforming growth factor β (TGF-β) and platelet-derived growth factor (PDGF) can promote collagen synthesis, whereas interferon γ (IFN-γ) can reduce the propensity of smooth muscle cells to express collagen when presented with

TGF-β; this is the main origin of collagen matrix arterial tissue. Matrix metalloproteinases can degrade collagen and weaken the cap. Therefore areas where plaques rupture generally have few smooth muscle cells: without the source of matrix molecules, there is an increased likelihood of weakening.

The development of an acute coronary syndrome is associated with the structural breakdown of the plaque. However, the successful use of agents that provoke fibrinolysis has implicated a major role for thrombus in the events that follow plaque rupture. In unstable angina, angiographic appearances suggesting non-occlusive thrombus is present in 85% of cases or more; the proven benefit of aspirin in such patients also suggests such a role. Therefore if the fibrous cap weakens and fractures, procoagulant factors in the blood have access to the thrombogenic lipid core; and if balance between thrombotic and fibrinolytic mechanism is disturbed, occlusion (partial or complete) can bring about an acute coronary syndrome. The main blood constituent initially responsible is the platelet: adhesion to exposed collagen occurs via glycoprotein type Ib receptors with thrombosis and arterial constriction reinforced by the local release of factors such as thromboxane A_2, serotonin, adenosine diphosphate, some leukotrienes, platelet activating factor, thrombin, free radicals and endothelin.

Most recently the role of inflammation in the generation of these syndromes has been highlighted. A number of studies have demonstrated that patients with raised serum C-reactive protein (CRP), fibrinogen, or interleukin 6 have an increased risk of further coronary episodes.

Acute myocardial infarction

This occurs when the myocardium is exposed to prolonged periods of ischaemia and there is irreversible damage to the ventricle. Infarction begins in the endocardium and may be confined there if an adequate supply of oxygenated blood is restored sufficiently quickly. Such an infarct is usually defined as non-Q wave on electrocardiography (ECG). However, periods of ischaemia beyond 1 hour lead to more myocardial damage, progressing further

towards the epicardium, and Q waves develop on the ECG (Q-wave infarction). Again, the pathological studies of Davies and Thomas demonstrated that virtually all fatal cases of myocardial infarction were related to rupture or fissuring of atheromatous plaques. The developing thrombus often spreads into segments of the coronary artery without significant disease. Reconstruction of the thrombus showed that the thrombus on the plaque is rich in platelets, whereas downstream it contains a high proportion of fibrin.

In all acute coronary syndromes there are factors that increase risk. Some are not modifiable, such as age, male sex and genetic predisposition; whereas others, such as hypercholesterolaemia, hypertension, diabetes and smoking, are (see below). As indicated, many individuals live asymptomatic lives despite having atheromatous disease; others have plaques that intrude upon the coronary artery, and anginal symptoms develop on a predictable and reproducible basis for many years without apparent progression of the disease. Human pathological studies have demonstrated that over much of its evolution, the growth of a plaque occurs by outward expansion, so that many plaques may cause no haemodynamic disturbance. Indeed it has been shown that the arterial wall itself can remodel, thereby increasing its external diameter to accommodate plaques and avoiding luminal narrowing, which may explain this phenomenon. The conundrum is that plaques destined to cause problems may grow and ulcerate rapidly. There is an increasingly widespread view that atheromatous plaques develop and regress in unstable situations, but why this should occur in susceptible individuals is not clear. Advanced plaques continue to possess a lipid core and fibrous cap. The core is acellular but surrounded by macrophages. The core remains the most active site for thrombus formation. It is important to point out that the number of macrophages in plaques varies greatly, and many individuals have plaques without a lipid core; also, a patient may have numerous coronary plaques that are all different in composition.

Thrombosis can occur first as a result of loss of endothelium over the surface of the plaque or as a result of disintegration or a tear in a lipid-rich plaque. It has been reported that advanced atherosclerotic lesions containing thrombi are frequently found from the fourth decade onwards. Small endothelial loss exposes collagen and tissue factor, and microde-posits of platelets form to stimulate repair by releas-ing appropriate factors. Larger areas of loss bring about the formation of larger thrombi containing fibrin, red cells and platelets; these can encroach upon the lumen and cause symptoms. Such endo-thelial loss is associated with inflammatory activity. Both processes may contribute to plaque enlarge-ment.

At the basis of acute coronary syndromes remains rupture of the fibrous cap and the direct contact of systemic blood with the lipid-rich core, collagen, and tissue factor. If the rupture is small, the plaque may be expanded by blood but not dramatically expanded in size. If the rupture is larger, there may be a rapid local distortion of the vascular wall with attendant luminal narrowing or occlusion.

In consequence, unstable angina implies that a patient has mural thrombus exposed to the arterial lumen for a prolonged period. The active surface is covered by platelets, and there is fibrin beneath. Fib-rinolytic drugs such as streptokinase are less effec-tive in treating the condition because the fibrin is not very accessible, whereas anti-platelet drugs such as aspirin are administered as quickly as possible because of their proven benefit.

It should be pointed out that this explanation for acute coronary syndromes would indicate that such events are always substantial and produce clin-ical symptoms. However, pathological studies have demonstrated that plaque rupture is common, with many episodes causing no problems. The variation in spectrum of disease and why particular patients present with acute coronary syndromes is proba-bly explained by demonstrable differences in plaque composition.

Risk factors for acute coronary syndromes

A number of genetic, environmental, dietary and lifestyle factors influence the potential development of acute coronary syndrome in an individual. In par-ticular, the evidence is overwhelming for an increase of heart disease in individuals with high blood cholesterol levels; with the introduction of powerful lowering agents, there is proof that good reduction is associated with reduced risk. However, this can-not be and is not the whole story: individuals with normal cholesterol levels sustain myocardial infarc-tion. We also know that for a total cholesterol/high-density-lipoprotein cholesterol (HDL-C) ratio of up to 7.4, men have more heart disease than women. This is lost at higher ratios. In other words, there is a gender difference in risk that is believed to be largely due to the protective ability of female sex hormones, because postmenopausal women rapidly attain male incidence rates for heart disease.

In addition, there is no question that diabetes and impaired glucose tolerance confers additional risk, as does the presence of hypertension. Add smoking to these, and that risk is multiplied by the combina-tion (Table 8.1). Readers are commended to larger expert texts for a comprehensive discussion of risk factors, but at this juncture it should be recognised

Table 8.1 Eight-year probability of cardiovascular events*

Risk factor	Rate per 1 000 men	Rate per 1 000 women
None	54	50
Hypertension[†]	139	117
Hypertension and hypercholesterolaemia[‡]	213	159
Hypertension, hyperc-holesterolaemia, and smoking	193	326
Hypertension, hyperc-holesterolaemia, smoking and ECG-LVH§	622	323

*Diabetes in patients above age 50 years, according to risk factor: Framingham Study, 26-year follow-up.

†Hypertension: systolic pressure > 165 mm Hg.

‡Cholesterol: > 6.6 mmol/l.

§ECG-LVH: left ventricular hypertrophy as demonstrated on ECG.

that the list above is not comprehensive: obesity, left ventricular hypertrophy, family history, high normal white cell count and fibrinogen are additional recognised influences, as are raised levels of plasma homocysteine and low levels of folate.

From the perspective of mechanisms, the actions of these risk factors are the subject of speculation; however, placed in the broadest context, they must either influence the development of atherosclerotic plaques or their destabilisation and thrombotic processes. In terms of hyperlipidaemia, there is evidence that serum cholesterol is associated with marked impairment of endothelium-dependent dilatation, and degrees of this are reported in populations even with normal lipid profiles. Also, restoration of cholesterol to acceptable levels by drugs restores functional endothelial integrity. The mechanism by which an abnormal lipid profile impairs vascular function has been the subject of considerable attention. There must be a reduced availability of nitric oxide: it seems that there is increased synthesis but also enhanced degradation. Potential mechanisms include reduced availability of L-arginine (the precursor of nitric oxide); down-regulation of the guanosine Giα subunit, which mediates activation of nitric oxide by biochemical stimuli; reduced expression of endothelial nitric oxide synthase; and inactivation of nitric oxide by superoxide anions or oxidised lipoproteins. Indeed, evidence exists for contributions from all of these. The exact lipid subfraction responsible would appear to be oxidised low-density-lipoprotein cholesterol(LDL-C). Recently it has been reported that oxidised LDL-C could attenuate endothelium-dependent relaxation *in vitro*, which could be overcome by HDL-C, and that HDL-C can ameliorate abnormal vasoconstriction in human coronary arteries. High levels of oxidised LDL-C may generate free radical species from endothelial cells; it is known that superoxide anions in particular are released from the vessels of hypercholesterolaemic animals and that these anions can inactivate nitric oxide.

An attack upon vascular endothelial integrity, especially when it involves reduced bioavailability of nitric oxide, would be expected to have profound effects upon circulatory haemodynamics as well as on the ability of the cell to repair itself and maintain a confluent level over the underlying smooth muscle cells. There is evidence that nitric oxide can influence basal vascular tone, and a recent trial has demonstrated a fall in blood pressure by the use of lipid-lowering drugs. If the reparative properties of the vasculature are embarrassed, atherosclerosis could be allowed to proceed more rapidly. The multiplicative effects of other risk factors, such as hypertension and diabetes, can be explained by the often associated dyslipidaemia reported in such conditions plus experimental data suggesting that high pressures can accelerate cholesterol deposition in the subendothelial layers of the vasculature.

In turn, any factor that influences thrombogenic mechanisms may be expected to affect adversely plaque stabilisation and the outcome following rupture. Therefore raised homocysteine or fibrinogen levels or low folate concentrates may play key roles in this regard. Then it becomes straightforward to understand how having more than one risk factor accelerates the risk of developing cardiovascular disease and stroke.

Symptoms and signs

The patient with an acute coronary syndrome presents with a constellation of symptoms and signs that reflects the degree of hypoxia and damage sustained by the myocardium. Some 45% of patients die within 1 h of the onset of symptoms: indeed, many experience no symptoms at all and succumb from a malignant cardiac dysrhythmia such as ventricular fibrillation. Those who survive this period predominantly present with chest pain. In unstable angina, this may be relieved by the administration of nitrate therapy and bed rest; patients with myocardial infarction have protracted pain often unrelieved by nitrate therapy. Such pains may radiate to the jaw and left arm. The other symptoms are explained by the severity of the insult to the myocardium and the degree of haemodynamic embarrassment that ensues. Subjects are often anxious and nauseated. This is exacerbated by the opiate analgesia often administered. Varying degrees of shock lead to low blood pressure, cutaneous vasoconstriction, and pallor; sweating as well as pump failure result in fluid congestions in the lungs. Clinical examination reveals soft heart sounds on auscultation and, where present, the signs of heart failure. Attendant complications of infarction are beyond the scope of a chapter dealing with mechanisms and represent severe myocardial necrosis.

The diagnosis of acute coronary syndrome

In unstable angina the 12-lead ECT may be normal during pain-free periods but change with symptoms. Ischaemic myocardium conducts poorly; as a result, the electrical vector across the heart alters. Typically there is ST-segment depression and/or T-wave flattening or inversion. Similar changes are often observed in non-Q-wave infarction; therefore distinguishing between these two entities may be difficult based solely on ECG changes. Acute full-thickness (Q-wave) infarction is associated with ST-segment elevation and T-wave inversion. Ischaemic myocardium is electrically unstable and irritable and may provoke sinister and often terminal rhythm disturbances. Such changes evolve if the healing process begins.

In recent years the distinction between angina and infarction has been blurred. This is because of the increasingly sophisticated assays for detecting myocardial cell damage. For some time the 'gold standard' for diagnosing myocardial infarction was to measure creatine kinase (CK) and its myocardium-specific isoenzyme CK-MB.

This enzyme can be detected by spectrophotometry, fluorometrically or by radioimmunoassay. It rises in the blood approximately 2 to 3 h after the onset of infarction, peaking at 12 h and falling to normal in 24 h, although it may stay high for longer if the damage sustained is continued or the initial myocardial insult is large. Assays of CK were often accompanied in the past by measurements of aspartate transaminase and lactate dehydrogenase. These rise and peak late after the onset of infarction (20 to 30 h) but are not myocardium-specific. Also, the emphasis

has been on diagnosing cell damage as early as possible because of the large number of interventional and therapeutic options available for re-establishing blood flow and reducing infarct size and complications. Against this background there is an awareness of the limitations of standard biochemical markers of cardiac cell injury. As a result, the cardiac troponins T and I (cTnT and cTnI) have achieved a prominent role.

The troponin complex is found on the thin filament of the striated muscle contractile system and includes cTnT (39 kDa), cTnI (26 kDa) and troponin C. They regulate contraction by modulating the calcium-dependent interaction of actin and myosin. Each is encoded by a single gene. Specific cardiac and skeletal muscle forms are recognised; they are mainly bound to myofibrils, with less than 10% of isoforms in the cytosol. After cellular injury, there is a rapid release from the cytoplasm followed by the more protracted loss from the myofibrils. Therefore concentrations rise at 4 to 8 h, peaking at 12 to 24 h. Both cTnT and cTnI can be used to detect myocardial cell death below the diagnostic threshold of CK-MB, which has meant that many patients previously labelled as having just angina are now being shown to have some irreversible damage. In addition, these enzymes (cTnT and cTnI) are useful in diagnosing traumatic myocardial injury and following coronary artery bypass surgery, angioplasty and heart failure. The sensitivity and specificity of troponin measurements are such that patients with high-risk clinical features on admission who are negative for cTnT and CK-MB at 0, 4, and 8 h have been shown to have a good in-hospital prognosis.

Against this background, patients who have had ischaemic ECG changes or cardiac troponin release or raised CK-MB enzyme demonstrated at any time during admission are now labelled as having a confirmed acute coronary syndrome.

As indicated above, a number of inflammatory markers acting independently of myocardial cell necrosis have been associated with atherosclerosis and acute coronary syndromes. Most widely investigated so far is CRP. Raised levels are linked to increased risk of recurrent events, whether there is evidence of myocardial cell damage or not. In line with the accumulating evidence that inflammatory processes are implicated in the generation of atheroma and subsequent plaque destabilisation, it is not surprising that CRP has been described as having a pro-atherothrombotic role; it can induce tissue factor production by monocytes, enhance low-density lipoprotein uptake by macrophages, and stimulate the expression of adhesion molecules by endothelial cells. In a further advance, it has been shown that pregnancy-associated plasma protein A (PAPP-A), which is a metalloproteinase and an activator of atherogenic insulin-like growth factor (IGF), is expressed in ruptured but not stable plaques. In consequence, blood levels of PAPP-A are elevated in acute coronary syndromes and appear to identify patients with unstable angina in the absence of raised cTnI or CRP. It is possible that this marker may identify patients with unstable angina in the absence of raised cTnI or CRP and that it may identify patients with unstable plaques before cell damage occurs.

Risk stratification

Because of the ever-expanding management options for acute coronary syndromes, strategies are being developed to identify patients at risk of developing further problems after initial presentation. As indicated above, patients with the largest infarcts have a worse prognosis, but even many unstable angina patients experience small amounts of myocardial cell damage. A typical approach to the acute coronary syndrome includes multiple treatments, such as aspirin, β-adrenoreceptor–blocking drugs, nitrates, unfractionated heparin, low-molecular-weight heparin, intravenous glycoprotein IIb/IIIa receptor inhibitors, clopidogrel, coronary artery angioplasty and stenting, thrombolytic drugs, acetyl co-enzyme, lipid-lowering agents (statins), angiotensin converting enzyme inhibitors and bypass surgery. This list will inevitably expand in the future. In consequence, in this time of scarce health care resources, we must try to identify the group of patients at highest risk of adverse future problems so as to treat them as aggressively as possible.

In this context, the clinical condition of the patient, ECG findings and levels of cardiac enzymes (e.g. CK-MB) and markers (e.g. troponins) are only partially useful. It is true that patients with unstable angina or non-Q-wave myocardial infarction who have a raised troponin have an increased mortality over a short period. Also, a panel of tests such as cTnI, CK-MB and myoglobin can enhance diagnostic accuracy beyond knowledge of a single such parameter. However, the search is still ongoing for a biomarker that is prognostic. Brain (B-type) natriuretic peptide is a 32–amino acid neurohormone synthesised in the ventricular myocardium and released into the circulation when the heart is dilated. It acts by causing natriuresis, vasodilatation, inhibition of the renin-angiotensin aldosterone cascade and inhibition of the sympathetic nervous system. After acute myocardial infarction, levels rise within 24 h and it has very recently been reported that a single measurement of B-type natriuretic peptide obtained a few days after the onset of ischaemic symptoms provides predictive information on risk of death in patients with non-Q-wave and Q-wave myocardial infarction as well as those with unstable angina. In addition, it gives an indication of the risk of new or progressive heart failure and new or recurrent myocardial infarction. This relationship appears to be independent of ECG changes, cTnI levels, renal function and the presence or absence of heart failure. Even in patients with unstable angina, an elevated level points to a worse prognosis.

Complications of acute coronary syndromes

The majority of patients who survive the onset of symptoms (see above) and receive treatment have an uncomplicated clinical course with demonstrable declines in in-hospital and long-term mortality and morbidity. These can be ascribed to restoration of blood flow to ischaemic regions of the myocardium and subsequent reductions in the amount of irreversible damage sustained. The life-threatening complications of myocardial infarction largely reflect the degree of necrosis: the more the heart is damaged, the more likely the patient is to

Table 8.2 Major complications of acute myocardial infarction

Ventricular dysrhythmias
Atrial dysrhythmias
Heart block (incomplete or complete)
Bradycardia
Extensive right ventricular infarction
Acute ventricular septal defect
Valvular rupture
Heart failure
Ventricular rupture
Systemic emboli from mural thrombus
Left ventricular aneurysm

develop these complications (Table 8.2). They are described in detail elsewhere.

Management of acute coronary syndromes

The immediate management of patients with the acute coronary syndrome has become more complex in recent years. Detailed therapeutics is outside the scope of this book; the reader is advised to consult the list of further readings at the end of this chapter (e.g. Smith et al., 2001). In short, the majority of patients require oxygen, analgesia and antiemetics. To interrupt the thrombotic process, the combination of aspirin and clopidogrel is now of proven benefit in unstable angina. Patients also receive heparin and nitrates intravenously as well as β-blockers and calcium channel blocking agents to prevent further attacks.

In addition, patients with infarction receive thrombolytic agents and are usually started on ACE inhibitors, β-blockers (where tolerated) and aspirin. All subjects should have their raised cholesterol levels lowered and their blood pressure controlled if elevated.

Against this background of increasing pharmaco-therapeutic options, interest in early investigation and revascularisation in acute coronary syndromes has arisen. Initial studies were disappointing: the Thrombolysis In Myocardial Infarction (TIMI) III B trial involved patients with unstable angina or non-Q-wave acute myocardial infarction but did not report clinically significant differences between the incidence of death, myocardial infarction, and recurrent reducible ischaemia between the invasively and conservatively treated groups. However, the incidence of re-hospitalisation at 6 weeks was 50% less in those who received revascularisation early. More recent studies of angioplasty and stenting have confirmed the superiority of the invasive management of acute coronary syndromes in conjunction with antithrombotic drugs and agents proven to be useful in secondary prevention. As a result, management is changing: waiting for pharmacological stabilisation is no longer advisable; early angiography and treatment of the culprit plaque is the watchword.

Summary

Coronary heart disease continues to be the major killer in many acculturated societies, and its importance is growing rapidly in developing nations. Our knowledge of how atheromatous narrowing of coronary arteries develops and what occurs when patients develop acute myocardial infarction is expanding rapidly. This view focuses on the acute coronary syndrome and the cellular and molecular mechanisms thought to be responsible for this clinical state, so that now, a picture is emerging of plaque rupture, material occlusion, cell injury and death associated with a clinical state involving chest pain, pump dysfunction and, occasionally, shock. In terms of therapeutic development, strategies directed towards preventing plaque rupture or the subsequent consequences thereof make rational sense and have already been demonstrated to improve outcomes in the short and long term.

Clinical scenario

A 48-year-old man with a history of hypertension was referred as an emergency to the local casualty department by his GP. He had developed central chest pain earlier in the day, which was gradually increasing in severity. Although he had initially thought that it might have been indigestion, he had called his GP when it did not ease with antacids.

On arrival to casualty, he was breathless and in pain. He was noted to be clammy and pale. His blood pressure was 190/110 and his heart rate was 105 and regular. The remainder of the clinical examination was normal. A 12-lead ECG showed ST-segment elevation across the anterior chest leads, with left axis deviation and voltage criteria for left ventricular hypertrophy.

Questions

1. What is the diagnosis?
2. What is the treatment?
3. What is the explanation for the clamminess and pallor observed in this patient?

Answers

1. The diagnosis is acute anterior myocardial infarction.
2. The first consideration in the treatment of this patient is resuscitation: he should receive oxygen, and intravenous access will be established. He should initially be treated in the resuscitation area of casualty before transfer to the coronary care unit. Soluble aspirin (300 mg) should be given with intravenous opiates for pain relief. At this point a decision needs to be taken with regard to his treatment: he can be treated with thrombolysis, in which case his blood pressure needs to be reduced to a safe level, or, if the facilities are available, he can undergo primary percutaneous coronary intervention.
3. These symptoms are representative of an enhanced sympathetic drive, which characteristically accompanies a myocardial infarction.

Multiple-choice questions (true or false)

1. Risk factors for acute coronary syndromes include:
    a. Cholesterol/HDL ratio
    b. Vitamin B12 levels
    c. Obesity
    d. Female gender
    e. Hypertension
2. Unstable angina is:
    a. Associated with ST-segment elevation on the ECG
    b. A cause of ventricular arrhythmias
    c. Treated with aspirin and clopidogrel
    d. Due to a non-occlusive thrombus in 85% of cases
    e. The result of white cell aggregation on a ruptured plaque)
3. Myocardial specific markers in acute coronary syndromes include:
    a. Creatine kinase
    b. cTnT
    c. Lactate dehydrogenase
    d. CK-MB
    e. cTnI
4. With regard to the atheromatous lesion:
    a. Foam cells in the lipid core are derived from lymphocytes
    b. The fibrous cap consists mostly of smooth muscle cells
    c. Matrix metalloproteinases cross-link and strengthen collagen
    d. Platelet-derived growth factor increases collagen synthesis
    e. Platelet adhesion to exposed collagen occurs via glycoprotein type IIa receptors

Answers

1: a, T; b, F; c, T; d, F; e, T
2: a, F; b, T; c, T; d, T; e, F
3: a, F; b, T; c, F; d, T; e, T
4: a, F; b, F; c, F; d, T; e, F

FURTHER READING

Aikawa, M., Libby, P. (2004). Atherosclerotic plaque inflammation: the final frontier? *Canadian Journal of Cardiology* **20,** 631–34.

Creager, M. A, Selwyn, A. (1997). When normal cholesterol levels injure the endothelium. *Circulation* **96,** 3255–7.

Davies, M. J., Thomas, A. C. (1985). Plaque fissuring – the cause of acute myocardial infarction, sudden ischaemic death and crescendo angina. *British Heart Journal* **53,** 363–73.

Davies, M. J. (1996). Stability and instability: the two faces of coronary atherosclerosis. The Paul Dudley White Lecture 1995. *Circulation* **94,** 2013–20.

Gonzi, G, Merlini, P. A., Ardissimo, D. (2001). Invasive coronary revascularisation is better than conservative treatment in patients with acute coronary syndromes. *Heart* **86,** 363–4.

Goode, G. K., Heagerty, A. M. (1995). In vitro responses of human peripheral small arteries in hypercholesterolaemia and effects of therapy. *Circulation* **91,** 2898–3.

Libby, P. (2001). Current concepts of the pathogenesis of the acute coronary syndromes. *Circulation* **104,** 365–72.

Lloyd-Jones, D., Kannel W. B. (2000). Coronary risk factors: an overview. In Willerson J. T., Cohn, J. N. (eds.). Cardiovascular Medicine. New York, Edinburgh, London, Philadelphia: Churchill Livingstone, 2193–215.

Smith, S. C. Jr., Dove, J. T., Jacobs, A. K. *et al.* (2001). ACC/AHA guidelines for percutaneous coronary intervention: executive summary and recommendations: a report of the American College of Cardiology/American Heart Assocation Task Force on Practice Guidelines (Committee to revise the 1993 guidelines for percutaneous transluminal coronary angioplasty). *Circulation* **103,** 3019–41.

Smith, S. C., Blair, S. N., Bonow, R. O. *et al.* (2001). Preventing heart attack and death in patients with atherosclerotic cardiovascular disease: 2001 update: consensus panel guide to comprehensive risk reduction for patients with coronary and other atherosclerotic vascular disease. *Circulation* **104,** 1577–9.

Stary, H. C., Bleakley, C. A., Dinsmore, R. E. *et al.* (1995). A definition of advanced types of atherosclerotic lesions and a histological classification of atherosclerosis. *Circulation* **92,** 1355–74.

Willerson, J. T., Maseri, A. (2000). Pathophysiology and clinical recognition of coronary artery disease syndromes. In Willerson J. T., Cohn, J. N. (eds.). Cardiovascular Medicine. New York, Edinburgh, London, Philadelphia: Churchill Livingstone, 528–68.

9

Heart failure

Ludwig Neyses and Mamta H. Buch

Introduction

The term 'heart failure' is solely reserved for the consequences of primary heart disease. Other diseases, such an anaemia or thyrotoxicosis, may lead to 'circulatory [or high-output] failure', but the heart is intact.

Two definitions of heart failure are used for clinical and research purposes respectively:

1. The pathophysiological (scientific) definition: heart failure is a state in which cardiac output is unable to meet the metabolic needs of peripheral tissues at rest or during exercise.

2. The clinical definition: heart failure is the combination of signs and symptoms of heart failure (if due to heart disease).

Neither of the definitions, however, acknowledges the crucial feature of the heart failure syndrome: its progressive nature. This is well illustrated in the clinical scenario at the end of this chapter with onset of overt failure 3 years after myocardial infarction and further slow progression.

Approximately 5% of western populations suffer from (at least mild) heart failure; it is one of the commonest causes of death. The incidence of heart failure increases rapidly with age, and progressive aging of the population makes it one of only two cardiovascular disease groups whose prevalence continues to rise, diabetes mellitus being the second.

Causes of heart failure

From the definitions above, it can be appreciated that heart failure is not a single disease entity but rather a haemodynamic state that may be caused by a variety of diseases. The medical definition of an entity termed heart failure is useful only because in all cases an initial disease damages the myocardium, which then responds in a uniform manner: the relentless progression of both healthy and diseased parts of the heart muscle towards failure. Figure 9.1 represents an example of dilated cardiomyopathy (DCM), a primary disease of the myocardium.

The most common diseases causing heart failure are (Table 9.1):

1. Coronary heart disease (either through myocardial infarction or chronic ischaemic alterations in the absence of large infarctions.

2. Arterial hypertension, which is associated with cardiac hypertrophy and either diastolic or systolic failure.

3. Aortic stenosis. Other valve disease is somewhat less frequent.

4. Dilated cardiomyopathy. Around 50% of DCMs are caused by mutations in cytoskeletal proteins, many other forms are induced by alcohol abuse and the pathogenesis of some remains uncertain. An example is shown in Figure 9.1.

5. Diabetes causes heart failure through associated macro- and microvascular disease and hypertension. It appears that, independent of reduced perfusion, diabetes has a direct negative influence on the myocardium.

6. Atrial fibrillation with rapid ventricular response. This may lead to tachycardia-induced heart failure and in most cases is entirely reversible by slowing the ventricular rate.

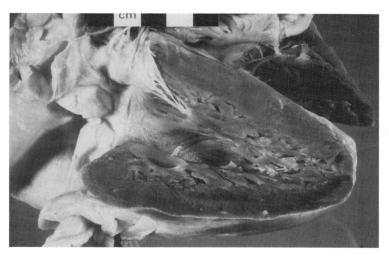

Figure 9.1 A post-mortem specimen from a patient with dilated cardiomyopathy demonstrating severe left ventricular dilatation in end-stage heart failure.

Naturally, several diseases may coexist in heart failure: for example, a patient with coronary heart disease may have uncontrolled hypertension and/or diabetes mellitus compounding and worsening his heart failure.

Symptoms of heart failure

It is useful and traditional to divide the symptoms and signs of heart failure into four categories: right or left ventricular failure; each ventricular chamber can then cause symptoms of forward failure (i.e. low output) or backward failure (i.e. reduced venous return and hence congestion). Table 9.2 lists these symptoms. It should be understood, however, that in the clinical scenario the most common forms of heart failure often show elements of all four categories, albeit to varying degrees. Often one or two symptoms dominate the clinical picture; for example, in clinical Scenario 2 (p. 189), the patient

Table 9.1 The most common causes of heart failure in clinical practice

	Examples	Affected chamber		
		LV	RV	Both
Ventricular contractile dysfunction	Coronary heart disease	+ + +	(+)	
	Cardiomyopathy			+ + +
Increased resistance to contraction and cardiac output	Hypertension	+ + +		
	Aortic valve stenosis	+ + +		
	Coarctation of the aorta	+ + +		
	Pulmonary hypertension		+ + +	
	Pulmonary valve stenosis		+ + +	
Cardiac dysrhythmias	Atrial fibrillation			+ + +
Inadequate cardiac filling	Constrictive pericarditis		+ + +	

Table 9.2 Signs and symptoms of heart failure*†

	Right ventricle	Left ventricle
Forward failure (= low output)	as left ventricle	fatigue, weakness, cyanosis, peripheral vasoconstriction, nocturia
Backward failure	ankle oedema, ascites, liver ↑, JVP ↑ pleural or pericardial effusion	pulmonary congestion, dyspnoea, cough, pleural or pericardial effusion

*Classically, signs and symptoms of heart failure are grouped into four categories, depending on which ventricle fails and whether it is its forward-pumping function or backwash of blood that prevails. In clinical practice, often one group of symptoms prevails, but associated signs from the other groups can be identified on close scrutiny. Nocturia is thought to occur when renal vasoconstriction resolves in recumbency. Late symptoms of severe heart failure include confusion (reduced cerebral bloodflow) and oliguria (reduced renal bloodflow). Cardiac cachexia is also a sign of advanced failure; it is thought to arise from increased levels of tumor necrosis factor alpha and reduced food intake.
†Upward-pointing arrows denote increases in size or pressure. JVP = jugular venous pressure.

complained of (1) decreased exercise tolerance and muscle fatigue (i.e. symptoms of low left ventricular output, which indicates forward failure; (2) breathlessness (dyspnoea) due to pulmonary congestion, indicating left ventricular backward failure; and (3) ankle oedema (i.e. right ventricular backward failure with increased venous capillary pressure). However, dyspnoea and pulmonary fluid overload were the predominant symptoms, and the patient was therefore classified for clinical and teaching purposes as having left ventricular backward failure.

The symptoms of right ventricular forward failure are indistinguishable from those of left ventricular forward failure.

The severity of symptoms has been classified by the New York Heart Association (NYHA) (see Table 9.3). It should be noted that there is only a loose correlation between symptoms and ventricular function (i.e. it is common to find patients with severely reduced ventricular function who are almost asymptomatic; on the other hand, less severe forms of ventricular dysfunction may cause severe oedema or breathlessness). The reasons for this discrepancy are unclear. It is a common clinical error to judge prognosis on the basis of left ventricular function alone.

The mechanisms underlying the symptoms of heart failure are explained in more detail below. Fluid retention (termed congestion) in the pulmonary and peripheral circulation is easily explained. The failing ventricle builds up a higher end-diastolic pressure because less blood is ejected; this leads to decreased filling and an increase in venous pressure, which is backwashed into the venous segment of the capillaries. Less fluid is reabsorbed from the venous segment of the capillaries. Interstitial pressure rises and more fluid is pressed back into the venous segment, until a new equilibrium is achieved characterised by an increase in interstitial fluid. This clinically manifests as peripheral oedema (ankle or sacrum on lying down), pulmonary congestion on chest X-ray or as crackles on auscultation. In its severest form, fluid collection in the pulmonary alveoli leads to pulmonary oedema, a dramatic and acutely life-threatening state.

Other symptoms of heart failure, such as breathlessness (i.e. dyspnoea) without pulmonary congestion or peripheral muscle fatigue, are more difficult to explain. Central nervous mechanisms are probably responsible for dyspnoea, and histological and biochemical alterations have been found in biopsies from peripheral skeletal muscle in patients with heart failure.

Table 9.3 New York Heart Association (NYHA) classification of heart failure*

Class	Characteristics
ClassI: minimal	Patients with cardiac disease without limitation of physical activity; ordinary physical activity does not cause undue dyspnoea or fatigue
ClassII: mild	Patients with cardiac disease resulting in slight limitation of physical activity; comfortable at rest; ordinary physical activity results in dyspnoea or fatigue
ClassIII: moderate	Patients with cardiac disease resulting in marked limitation of physical activity; comfortable at rest; less than ordinary physical activity causes dyspnoea or fatigue
ClassIV	Patients with cardiac disease resulting in inability to carry on any physical activity without discomfort; symptoms of heart failure may be present even at rest; if any physical activity is undertaken, discomfort is increased

*This represents a rough, but clinically useful grading of the symptoms of heart failure. 'Ordinary physical activity' (which differentiates class 2 and 3) is usually defined as walking one block (in a US city) or climbing one flight of stairs.

Pathophysiology of heart failure

Systolic versus diastolic heart failure

In most cases, the underlying disease leads to a reduction in systolic function of the heart and therefore to systolic failure. Most of the mechanisms outlined below refer to this form of failure. However, a number of patients have a reduction in cardiac output because of reduced filling of (generally the left) ventricle during diastole; this is termed 'diastolic failure'. It principally occurs in the senile heart and in severe hypertrophy, particularly because these conditions are associated with fibrosis. Up to 40% of all patients with systolic failure have a variable degree of diastolic failure. Diastolic failure can be well defined invasively using catheterisation techniques, but because these cannot easily be performed in large numbers of patients, little is known about its pathophysiology and treatment. In the following text we therefore refer to systolic failure unless stated otherwise.

The principal circulatory abnormalities of heart failure are:

1. A reduction in cardiac output (at rest or during exercise); this is the causative factor
2. Hypertrophy of myocardial cells and interstitial fibrosis in almost all instances
3. Peripheral vasoconstriction – i.e. constriction of the arterioles or metarterioles
4. Fluid and sodium retention
5. Progression – i.e. progressive weakening of the heart muscle, even of the parts of the heart that are primarily healthy, such as in the surviving myocardium after myocardial infarction

For clarity, it is useful to describe the historical development of the pathophysiological theories of heart failure. One mechanical and three molecular theories of how heart failure develops have been described over the last 100 years. These have supplemented – as opposed to supplanted – each other, and it should be clear that all processes described take place in parallel in a patient with heart failure. In addition, these processes influence each other in complex ways, which are only partly understood and are not described in detail here. Incidentally, heart failure is a fascinating example of how research into disease mechanisms develops in general: advances in technical and basic science are applied to medical problems and drive our understanding of the mechanisms of disease. Haemodynamic measurements started in the second decade of the twentieth century when reliable pressure measurements became available; neurohumoral activation was detected in the 1970s, after the introduction of the radio-immunoassay, allowing measurement of angiotensin II, norepinephrine, and so on. The application of modern molecular biology to heart muscle disease started in the late 1980s.

The mechanical (haemodynamic) description of heart failure based on the Frank-Starling mechanism

The overall contractile properties of the normal and failing heart are well described by a displacement of the so-called Frank-Starling curve (Fig. 9.2). These two investigators, Frank and Starling, showed that at constant aortic pressure the stroke volume of the heart depends on the filling pressure of the ventricle. This was an important finding because it distinguished the heart from a mechanical pump, the out-

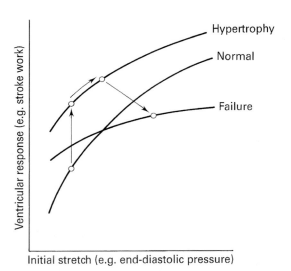

Figure 9.2 The Frank-Starling mechanism in heart failure. The Frank-Starling curves demonstrate the relationship between the ventricular response, as represented by stroke work, and the initial stretch of myocardial muscle fibres, as represented by end-diastolic pressure. The 'normal' curve describes an increased ventricular response with increased end-diastolic pressure. A larger response is seen when the whole ventricle undergoes hypertrophy. Myocardial dysfunction and consequent heart failure produce a flattening of the curve, so that the higher filling pressure is needed to produce stretch. This results in a poor ventricular response.

put of which remains constant over a wide range of filling pressures. Although the Frank-Starling curve was constructed using isolated hearts, it largely holds true in an *in situ* situation. In some instances, stroke volume remains constant, but resistance of the peripheral vessels (arterioles and metarterioles) increases. This results in an increase in stroke work, which also needs increased filling of the ventricle if output is to be maintained. Therefore it has become customary to describe the Frank-Starling curve as the dependence of stroke work on filling pressure. In the failing heart, the first task is to maintain stroke volume to guarantee perfusion of peripheral tissues despite an increase in peripheral resistance, which is a consistent feature of heart failure. This is achieved by an increase in filling pressure.

The downward displacement of the curve describes this complex situation: the failing heart needs a higher filling pressure in order to be able to maintain stroke work. In addition, the weaker the ventricle becomes over time, the more the curve takes a downward course and the higher the filling pressure needed to maintain output will be; the vicious cycle of heart failure is set in motion. The molecular basis of the Frank-Starling mechanism is still not quite clear.

Molecular theories of heart failure

The present molecular theory of heart failure is composed of three successive concepts corresponding to the three arms of the diagram in Figure 9.3.

A decrease in cardiac output is always the initiating event. It is brought about by a heart disease and leads to three different processes:
1. Hypo-perfusion of the kidneys
2. Neurohumoral activation and endothelial dysfunction
3. Alterations in the heart itself

These mechanisms are dealt with in the following paragraphs

Hypoperfusion of the kidneys

This leads to Na and H_2O retention and an increase in blood volume and cardiac preload (i.e. end-diastolic

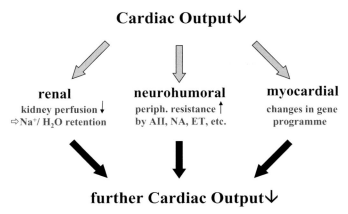

Figure 9.3 The three pathophysiological pathways leading to the development of heart failure. All three contribute to the progressive weakening of the heart muscle. They also correspond to the three major theories about heart failure developed over the last 100 years (in temporal order, from left to right). Upward- and downward-pointing arrows indicate increase or decrease, respectively. The pathways obviously interact (e.g. an increase in catecholamines will contribute to down-regulation of myocardial adrenoceptors and so on). AII = angiotensin II; NA = noradrenaline; ET = endothelin. (See colour plate section.)

pressure). Over long time intervals, this will lead to a further decrease in cardiac output and kidney perfusion; H$_2$O and Na retention will ensue, which will further decrease output, setting in motion a vicious cycle.

Symptoms of fluid retention will appear when capillary filtration exceeds reflux of tissue fluid into the capillaries (see above.)

Hypoperfusion of the kidneys leads to a fall in glomerular filtration, which activates renin secretion from the juxtaglomerular cells into the circulation.

Neurohumoral activation

When reliable radio-immunoassays became available and the importance of the renin-angiotensin system was elucidated, raised serum levels of angiotensin II, norepinephrine and later endothelin 1 and cytokines were detected. This is termed 'neurohumoral activation' because raised norepinephrine blood levels result from norepinephrine spill-over from peripheral sympathetic neurons (hence the word 'neuro') and the renin-angiotensin system was thought to be exclusively operative in the blood, hence 'humoral' ('humor' being Latin for 'fluid'). We now know that the heart contains a local renin-angiotensin system and that endothelin is produced in all vessels. The local paracrine action (i.e. from one cell to its neighbours) is probably equally or more important than the activation in the bloodstream, but the term 'humoral' has remained.

The cause of raised renin levels in the blood is under-perfusion of the kidney, which leads to reduced glomerular filtration. The compensatory response of the renin-producing cells from the zona glomerulosa is renin secretion into the bloodstream, which in turn leads to activation of the renin–angiotensin cascade. The resulting increase in angiotensin II leads to constriction of the efferent glomerula vessels and hence to restitution of glomerular filtration.

The mechanisms by which sympathetic stimulation and hence increased norepinephrine secretion are brought about are less clear. The sum effect of these vasoconstrictors is to constrict peripheral resistance vessels (arterioles and metarterioles). The increased afterload imposed on the heart will then result in a further decrease in cardiac output and augment neurohumoral activation, setting in motion the vicious cycle depicted in Figure 9.3.

Cytokines

A series of molecules named cytokines, which have a physiological function in the paracrine communication of cells, originally had been shown to have a role in immunological neoplastic disease. Of the many such molecules, tumour necrosis factor α (TNF-α), interkeukin beta (IL-β) and IL-6 have been shown to be increased in approximately 30% of patients with heart failure, usually in severer forms. They are in part responsible for endothelial dysfunction and apoptosis of cardiac myocytes (see below). TNF-α appears to be responsible for the severe catabolic state seen in some patients with advanced heart failure (termed 'cardiac cachexia').

Endothelial dysfunction

An important mechanism contributing to the peripheral vasoconstriction in heart failure has been detected in recent years: endothelial dysfunction. Increases in blood flow (e.g. during exercise) normally lead to production of nitric oxide (NO) from the endothelium and relaxation of smooth muscle cells in the media of the arterioles. In heart failure, NO secretion is reduced and vasodilatation less complete; this is termed endothelial dysfunction. It is at least in part caused by increases in angiotensin II, endothelin and cytokines.

Cardiac alterations in cardiac hypertrophy and failure

The intimate relationship between cardiac hypertrophy and failure has long been known: cardiac hypertrophy (most commonly in the setting of essential hypertension) frequently leads or contributes to heart failure (e.g. failure is more common in patients with myocardial infarction who also have hypertension).

On the other hand, the failing myocardium almost invariably shows the features of hypertrophy outlined below. The exceptions to this general rule mostly relate to acute failure (e.g. acute myocarditis or acute aortic regurgitation). If the patient survives these conditions, there is, however, a rapid hypertrophic response. Cardiac hypertrophy may occur in two settings: physiological or pathological. Physiological hypertrophy occurs during training (e.g. in athletes). It is characterised by full reversibility and rarely has negative consequences. Here only the mechanisms of pathological hypertrophy are dealt with.

It is most useful to organise views of cardiac alterations in cardiac hypertrophy and failure according to the histological changes seen in these conditions. These are:

1. Hypertrophy (e.g. growth in cell size, not number) of the myocardium
2. Fibrosis leading to increased stiffness of the myocardium (i.e. decreased "compliance" and hence filling abnormality)
3. Cellular disarray (i.e. the normal array of myocardial cells is distorted and there is slippage of the alignment of the cells, leading to inefficient contraction)
4. Cell loss

Of course the term 'cell loss' refers to the loss of cells in the failing part of the myocardium, not to the primary loss brought about by, for example, a myocardial infarction. Probably some of the cell loss is caused by apoptosis (i.e. programmed cell death) as opposed to necrosis, which represents passive cell death.

Both forms of cell death can be distinguished by the electron microscopic appearance of the dying cell and by biochemical methods. The intellectual attraction of apoptosis, of course, is that a cascade of events programmed by nuclear gene expression may be amenable to therapeutic intervention. However, the extent of apoptosis and the events leading to it in heart failure are still largely unclear.

Molecular alterations and mechanisms of myocardial hypertrophy and failure

Of course, the histological alterations described above reflect underlying changes in gene expression. Therefore this discussion is organised as follows:

1. Descriptive alterations
2. Mechanisms leading to cardiac hypertrophy and failure of the heart muscle
3. The little which is known of the development of fibrosis in heart failure

Changes in the molecular phenotype of the hypertrophied and failing myocardium

Approximately 8 000 to 10 000 genes are expressed at the protein level in the myocardium. The overwhelming majority of these will increase in proportion with the amount of hypertrophy: for example, if the myocardium grows by 25%, so will the number of molecules of most proteins in the cell. This often occurs through an increase in translational efficiency; on average, 25% more protein molecules are translated from the given messenger RNA. Reduced degradation of proteins has also been demonstrated in some instances.

Much less than 1% of the expressed proteins will undergo an isoform switch – that is, a related but independent gene of the same family will be expressed. An approximately equal number of proteins will increase disproportionately in relation to overall hypertrophy or even show a decrease.

Qualitative changes in protein expression

The most prominent change in hypertrophy in rats (the most commonly used animal model of hypertrophy) is an isoform switch of the myosin heavy chain gene. The alpha isoform of the major histocompatibility complex (αMHC) confers fast contraction at the expense of high energy consumption. In the hypertrophied heart, the beta isoform is increased, which confers slower but energetically more efficient contraction. This is thought to be an adaptational response. Other contractile proteins include α cardiac actin, which is switched to alpha skeletal actin. The more slowly contracting human ventricle contains almost no αMHC and the major contractile protein is βMHC. However, in humans, the ventricular form of the essential light chain is partially replaced by the atrial isoform. The minor changes in amino acid composition are placed at strategic sites of the protein and hence confer increased contractility on the sarcomeres incorporating the atrial isoform.

Brain natriuretic peptide (BNP) and atrial natriuretic peptide (ANP) are not significantly expressed in the normal adult ventricle; their re-expression in hypertrophy is thought to lead to a limitation of the hypertrophic response through activation of the cyclic guanosine monophosphate (cGMP) formation.

Other modifications in isoform composition have been described in rodents and in humans, but their significance is less clear and they are therefore not discussed here.

It has been said that the hypertrophied heart reverts to a foetal phenotype because the hypertrophic gene expression pattern resembles the one in the foetal heart, which also expresses more beta than alpha MHC, BNP and so on. Naturally, it is difficult to say whether this adaptation is beneficial: evolution may not have optimized the expression of genes in hypertrophy because it occurs mostly long after the reproductive age, and whether or not an individual is well adapted to heart disease is hence irrelevant to evolution.

Quantitative changes in protein expression and phosphorylation

As explained above, a few proteins show isoform switches in the failing cell; the majority change only in proportion with the degree of hypertrophy. A third group of proteins, however, show alterations that are out of proportion with the degree of hypertrophy. The most prominent of these both in the rodent models and in humans are the following:

Calcium transport proteins
In heart failure, calcium uptake into the sarcoplasmic reticulum is reduced, while calcium release

from this compartment is increased. Changes in hypertrophy are largely similar but less pronounced.

With regard to uptake, by far the best-studied calcium transporter is the sarcoplasmic/endoplasmic reticulum calcium ATPase (SERCA), which pumps approximately 75% of the calcium released during systole back into the sarcoplasmic reticulum during diastole. In hypertrophy, there is only a slight decrease in the activity and protein expression of this pump, but in the failing heart, it is reduced by approximately 30%. This leads to slower calcium uptake in diastole and contributes to the delay in diastolic relaxation.

This quantitative decrease in SERCA protein expression is accompanied by important modifications of the phosphorylation (and hence activation) patterns of proteins participating in calcium transport.

Under normal conditions, phospholamban, the regulatory protein of SERCA, inhibits SERCA action; this inhibition is relieved by phosphorylation through the action of beta-adrenergic activation of protein kinase A (e.g. during exercise). This leads to increased efficiency of the SERCA and hence more rapid calcium uptake in diastole as well as an increase in calcium in the sarcoplasmic reticulum. In the failing heart, phospholamban is under-phosphorylated in relation to the needs of the heart muscle, resulting in an inordinate inhibition of SERCA and hence reduced calcium uptake into the sarcoplasmic reticulum.

Calcium release occurs through the calcium release channel (called the ryanodine receptor because the drug ryanodine binds and inhibits it). In heart failure, the chronic hyperadrenergic state (neurohumoral activation; see above) leads to chronic hyperphosphorylation of the ryanodine receptor. This leads to dissociation of a protein called FKB 12.6 from the ryanodine receptor. When bound to the receptor, FKB 12.6 reduces release of calcium. The ensuing exaggerated calcium release will entrain calcium depletion of the sarcoplasmic reticulum and eventually result in reduced contractility. Because FKB 12.6 is also implicated in orchestrating coordinated calcium release from the many release

channels in a single heart cell, its dissociation from the receptor will lead to uncoordinated calcium release and potentially be responsible for ventricular rhythm disorders and sudden death.

The abundance of the Na/Ca exchanger of the plasma membrane increases in heart failure. Because this system transports calcium out of the cell in exchange for sodium, this is thought to be a compensatory response to the reduction in SERCA in order to keep intracellular free calcium constant.

Expression of the L-type calcium channel current (which sets the process of excitation/contraction coupling in motion) has variously been described as reduced or normal in hypertrophy and failure.

The beta-adrenergic system

The second prominent alteration in quantitative gene expression in myocardial hypertrophy and failure concerns the beta-adrenergic system. Initially, neurohumoral activation (see above) and the increase in noradrenaline in particular leads to increased contractility of the myocardium, a compensatory response. As the heart fails, this compensation is limited by a down-regulation in the number of beta receptors on the myocardium and by changes in signal transduction from the receptor, mainly through phosphorylation and activation of the protein arrestin, which inhibits receptor activity. This mechanism limits contractile stimulation of the heart muscle by catecholamines. Treatment with beta blockers has recently been shown to improve the prognosis in heart failure; it restores the number of beta receptors in the heart, but it is unclear how this can be beneficial in the presence of blockers of this very same receptor.

Metabolic changes

In the hypertrophied and failing heart, metabolic changes take place. The normal myocardium uses free fatty acids and carbohydrates as substrates. In the failing heart, a marked increase in fatty acid utilisation takes place. Again, it is not known whether this change is adaptive (positive) or maladaptive (negative) for the progressive evolution of heart failure.

Molecular mechanisms of gene changes in the hypertrophied and failing heart

In the last paragraphs above, we have established the descriptive changes in the molecular composition (i.e. the gene programme) in the failing myocardium. A much more interesting question both in terms of understanding and of the development of novel treatment strategies is the question of the molecular mechanisms underlying these alterations.

Over recent years, many pathways that may contribute to the development of hypertrophy and subsequent failure have been identified. These are schematically depicted in Figure 9.4. It can be appreciated that most of the signal transduction pathways that have been identified to be operative in other cells (e.g. neurones, liver, neoplastic cells, etc.) have also been demonstrated in the myocardium, but often with different target molecules and hence leading to different functional changes compared to non-cardiac cells. Put otherwise, the actual signal transduction steps have largely been conserved by evolution, but their ultimate function varies greatly depending upon the organ and the developmental stage in which they are being used.

Here only two rather well-defined mechanisms that are most likely to have relevance in humans are discussed in detail. It should be noted, however, that it appears likely that one combination of the many pathways outlined in Figure 9.4 might cause hypertrophy in one pathological situation (e.g. aortic stenosis), whereas another combination may be relevant in other situations (e.g. essential or renal hypertension or volume overload, as in aortic regurgitation). The two major pathways are depicted in Figure 9.4.

In the 'calcineurin pathway,' a rise in cytosolic calcium occurs when stretch (e.g. a rise in blood pressure) or beta stimulation (e.g. neurohumoral activation – see above) act on the heart. This rise in calcium stimulates the phosphatase calcineurin, a calcium- and calmodulin-dependent enzyme, which leads to dephosphorylation of nuclear factor of activated T cells (NFAT), a name derived from their original description in lymphoid T cells.

Dephosphorylated NFAT is translocated to the nucleus and acts as a trancription factor on promoters of genes typical of cardiac hypertrophy, which are then transcribed. Glycogen synthase kinase can phosphorylate NFATs and so retain them in the cytoplasm and hence act as an antihypertrophic enzyme. It should be noted that much of the nomenclature in modern molecular biology derives from the days of classical biochemistry; hence the term 'glycogen synthase kinase' does not imply that the NFAT pathway of hypertrophy has anything to do with glycogen synthesis.

The second pathway (depicted in Fig. 9.4) has been directly derived from human genetic disease research. Mutations of many proteins along this pathway have been shown to lead to hereditary forms of dilated cardiomyopathy. In this pathway, stretch on the extracellular matrix (e.g. by a rise in blood pressure) leads to stretch on the laminin/sarcoglycan complex. This deformation is transmitted through the cell membrane and sets in motion a series of structural alterations and phosphorylations of downstream proteins, which ultimately lead to activation of nuclear transcription factors and hypertrophic genes.

Fibrosis

It cannot be overstated that fibrosis is an essential feature of pathological hypertrophy (and absent in physiological hypertrophy, e.g. in athletes). Pathological fibrosis is not only characterised by deposition of more collagen but also by a switch in collagen isoforms: physiological collagen I mediates tensile strength (i.e. resistance to tearing). Interestingly, collagen I has been shown to have a similar tensile strength to steel! Collagen III provides elasticity and can be compared to the meshes of a hammock. In pathological hypertrophy, there is increased deposition of collagen I; this is the essential component leading to reduced diastolic compliance of the heart and hence reduced diastolic filling in pathological hypertrophy and heart failure. Fibrosis is also largely

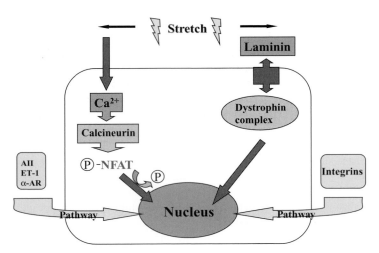

Figure 9.4 Simplified schematic of the molecular mechanisms leading to cardiac hypertrophy and failure. Stretch-dependent and independent pathways have been identified. Stretch usually results from mechanical overload (e.g. aortic stenosis, arterial hypertension) but may also stem from abnormal contractility of the myocardial cell itself (e.g. in hypertrophic cardiomyopathy). This latter condition mostly arises from a mutation in a contractile protein. Stretch may trigger one of two events: either an increase in intracellular calcium levels at each heartbeat (through as yet unknown mechanisms). This will activate the calcium/calmodulin-dependent phosphatase calcineurin in the cytosol. A protein of the transcription factor family NFAT, members of which reside in the cytoplasm in their phosphorylated form, will be dephosphorylated and translocate to the nucleus, where it induces the expression of genes typical of hypertrophy. In the other stretch-related pathway, stretch is thought to act on the extracellular matrix. This signal will be transmitted through the membrane via laminin (extracellular) and dystroglycan (dark square) or the integrin family of proteins. There are also molecular mechanisms that are conducive to hypertrophy independent of stretch. These are mostly thought to be mediated by receptors coupled to G proteins (largely Gq). Stimulation of the receptors for angiotensin II, endothelin and the alpha-adrenergic receptor by their cognate ligands is well documented to be sufficient for the induction of hypertrophy (and failure). The unresolved question is: which pathway(s) are relevant in human cardiac hypertrophy? It appears likely that distinctive mechanisms variably combine in different clinical situations. (See colour plate section.)

responsible for the clinical picture of diastolic heart failure, which is characterised by normal systolic function of the heart muscle but a severe decrease in diastolic filling. Indeed, most patients with systolic heart failure also have some degree of diastolic impairment, largely due to fibrosis.

Summary

Heart failure is a syndrome in which cardiac output is unable to meet the metabolic demands of peripheral tissues. It is a leading cause of morbidity and mortality in the western population. The most frequent underlying causes of heart failure are coronary heart disease, hypertension, valvular disease, and idiopathic dilated cardiomyopathy. Clinically, it is characterised by the signs and symptoms of left and/or right ventricular failure. Regardless of the underlying aetiology, there is fundamentally a significant loss of contractile function, which triggers a relentless, progressive decline to severe heart failure and eventually death. The complexity of this syndrome arises through the interplay of three pathogenetic theories that have emerged over the last 100 years: cardiorenal, neurohumoral and left ventricular remodelling. The close relationship between these processes leads to a vicious cycle with a progressive reduction in cardiac output. Central to the remodelling process is cardiac hypertrophy; and although this is conventionally regarded as an adaptive response, sustained cardiac hypertrophy represents a leading predictor of heart failure. The molecular mechanisms that underpin the transition from cardiac hypertrophy to heart failure remain incompletely understood. We have discussed recent major advances in this area with particular reference to the calcineurin/ NFAT pathway and the dystrophin complex pathway.

Clinical scenarios

Scenario 1

A 70-year-old man, a heavy smoker with hypercholesterolaemia, was admitted to an intensive care unit 10 h after the onset of chest pain. An acute myocardial infarction was diagnosed on ECG. Emergency coronary angiography revealed complete occlusion of his left anterior descending artery (LAD) by a thrombus at the level of a high-grade stenosis; blood flow was restored by dilatation of the stenosis and implantation of a stent. However, due to the delay in perfusion, a large scar of the anterior left ventricular wall persisted on echocardiography 3 months after the infarction. Three years later, this patient presented with increasing breathlessness due to pulmonary fluid congestion demon-

strated by chest X-ray. Repeat coronary angiography showed patent coronary vessels and a severely reduced ejection fraction of 25% (normal: 70%) with an anterior wall aneurysm. Therapy with diuretics, ACE inhibitors and beta blockers and later digitalis and spironolactone was instituted, but he died 3 years later of refractory heart failure while awaiting cardiac transplantation.

Scenario 2

A 75-year-old overweight woman with well-controlled non–insulin-dependent diabetes type IIb and untreated arterial hypertension complained of increasing breathlessness (dyspnoea) over 3 years. Recently, she found that she could not walk up one flight of stairs without stopping, and she noted swelling of both ankles in the evening. On examination, a lateralised apex beat and bilateral ankle oedema but no other abnormalities were noted. Electrocardiography showed uncertain signs of hypertrophy; echocardiography revealed globally moderately reduced left ventricular systolic function and diastolic filling defects (i.e. combined systolic and diastolic heart failure). Her blood pressure and symptoms were well controlled with a combination of a thiazide diuretic and an angiotensin converting enzyme inhibitor (ACE) inhibitor. Because she had to care for her grandchildren, whose parents were divorced, she also made an unusual effort to lose weight and control her diabetes well. She died at the age of 82 of ovarian cancer.

Questions

1. What are the clinical and pathophysiological definitions of heart failure?
2. Define the NYHA criteria for the severity of heart failure.
3. Give three examples of genes that show alterations in heart hypertrophy and failure over and above the quantitative changes in proportion to the increase in cell size seen in most proteins.

4. Define the Frank-Starling mechanism and the three major pathophysiological mechanisms leading to heart failure.
5. Describe four potential myocardial signalling pathways leading to myocardial failure.

FURTHER READING

Benjamin, I. J., Schneider, M. D. (2005). Learning from failure: congestive heart failure in the postgenomic age. *Journal of Clinical Investigation* **115,** 495–9.

Francis, G. S., Wilson Tang, W. H. (2003). Pathophysiology of congestive heart failure. *Reviews in Cardiovascular Medicine* **4(suppl** 2), S14–20.

Frey, N, Katus, H. A., Olson, E. N., Hill, J. A. (2004). Hypertrophy of the heart: a new therapeutic target? *Circulation* **109,** 1580–9.

Mann, D. L., Bristow, M. R. (2005). Mechanisms and models in heart failure. *Circulation* **111,** 2837–49.

Ritter, O., Neyses, L. (2003). The molecular basis of myocardial hypertrophy and heart failure. *Trends in Molecular Medicine* **9,** 313–21.

10

Acute neurodegeneration: cerebral ischaemia and stroke

Craig J. Smith, Jerard Ross, Nancy J. Rothwell and Pippa J. Tyrrell

Key Points

- Stroke is a major cause of mortality and morbidity. Cerebral infarction (ischaemic stroke) caused by arterial occlusion is the commonest type of stroke, but ischaemia also contributes to the pathophysiology of primary intracerebral and subarachnoid haemorrhage.
- The onset of cerebral ischaemia initiates a cascade of electrophysiological and molecular events (the ischaemic cascade) resulting in immediate and delayed neurodegeneration.
- Immediate cellular energy failure leads to loss of electrochemical gradients, calcium ion influx and accumulation of excitotoxic amino acids, particularly glutamate, resulting in rapid cellular death in the ischaemic core.
- Activation of an inflammatory response contributes to further ischaemic brain injury, mainly in the ischaemic penumbra. Key inflammatory events include activation of resident glial cells, expression of inflammatory mediators (including cytokines and adhesion molecules), and infiltration of blood leucocytes. The cytokine interleukin-1 (IL-1) is a major pro-inflammatory mediator and is strongly implicated in ischaemic brain injury.
- Aspirin is currently the mainstay of pharmacological treatment of acute ischaemic stroke, whereas intravenous thrombolysis with tissue plasminogen activator is an effective treatment for only a small minority of patients.
- Neuroprotection is a therapeutic strategy aiming to limit neuronal injury by targeting specific events

in the ischaemic cascade. There are currently no neuroprotective drugs that are both safe and efficacious in patients with acute ischaemic stroke.

Introduction

Stroke is defined as a syndrome of rapidly developing clinical symptoms and signs of focal, occasionally global loss of cerebral function lasting more than 24 h or leading to death, with no apparent cause other than of vascular origin. By contrast, a transient ischaemic attack (TIA) is characterised by acute loss of focal cerebral or monocular function, with symptoms resolving completely within 24 h. In the developed world, the annual incidence of stroke is around 0.2%, rising with increasing age. Stroke is the third leading cause of mortality worldwide, with case fatality around 30% at 1 month. In the UK, stroke accounts for around 6% of National Health Service (NHS) expenditure and is the leading cause of adult disability.

The commonest pathological type of stroke is cerebral infarction (ischaemic stroke), accounting for approximately 80%. A further 10% of strokes are due to primary intracerebral haemorrhage (PICH); 5% are due to subarachnoid haemorrhage (SAH) and the remainder are venous, of uncertain aetiology or non-vascular. In clinical practice, differentiating cerebral infarction from PICH and SAH is fundamental, as investigation, management and prognosis vary between these pathological subtypes.

Acute neurodegeneration involves rapid neuronal destruction, followed by delayed neuronal injury in response to a sudden insult such as acute stroke, brain haemorrhage or head injury. Cerebral ischaemia plays a role in the pathophysiology of both ischaemic and haemorrhagic stroke and can be considered as focal or global, depending on whether ischaemia affects part or all of a vascular territory or the entire cerebral cortex.

This chapter focuses mainly on neurodegeneration occurring after the onset of focal cerebral ischaemia in acute ischaemic stroke.

Neurovascular anatomy

The brain derives its blood supply (Fig. 10.1) from terminal branches of the paired internal carotid arteries (anterior system) and the paired vertebral arteries (posterior system), with anastomoses between these arteries at different levels. The cerebral circulation is a *dynamic system* with both inter- and intra-individual variation (i.e. between hemispheres and varying at different times).

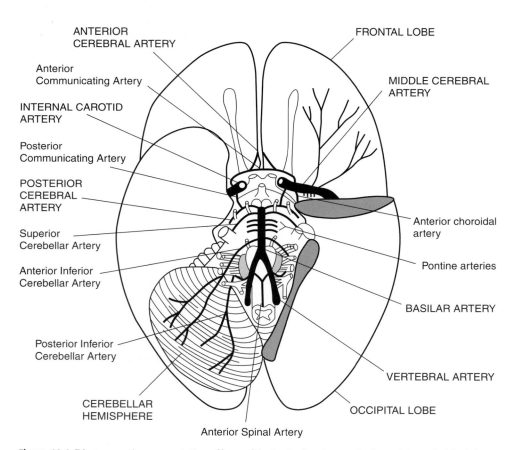

Figure 10.1 Diagrammatic representation of base of the brain showing cerebral arterial supply. The left temporal lobe and cerebellar hemisphere have been removed. (Reproduced with kind permission from *Neuroanatomy For Medical Students*, 3rd edn. Oxford, UK: Butterworth-Heinemann, Julia L Wilkinson (author), 1998.)

The anterior (carotid) system

The terminal branches of the internal carotid artery (ICA) are the middle cerebral artery (MCA), anterior cerebral artery (ACA) and the posterior communicating artery (PCoA). The MCA supplies most of the external surface of the hemisphere and gives off between six and twelve perforating vessels (perforators), supplying part of the internal capsule and basal ganglia. The ACA communicates with the contralateral ACA via the anterior communicating artery (ACoA). The paired ACAs supply the orbital part of the frontal lobe and parasagittal cortex, including the entire motor and sensory cortex of the lower limb.

The posterior (vertebrobasilar) system

The paired vertebral arteries (VAs) arise from the first part of the subclavian arteries and combine to form the basilar artery (BA). The vertebral and basilar vessels supply the brainstem and cerebellum (see Fig. 10.1). The BA bifurcates to form the posterior cerebral arteries (PCAs) supplying the occipital cortex and the inferomedial aspect of the temporal lobe, with penetrating vessels to the brainstem, thalamus and posterior internal capsule.

The circle of Willis is a series of anastomoses between the anterior and posterior systems. Anteriorly, the ACAs are joined by the ACoA, while the PCoA joins the ICA to the ipsilateral PCA. Anomalies of the circle of Willis are present in upwards of 50% of people and are more frequent in patients with cerebrovascular disease.

Clinical presentation and classification of ischaemic stroke

Ischaemic strokes differ in their aetiology, vascular territory affected, clinical presentation, severity and prognosis. Bearing this in mind, it is logical to subdivide or classify ischaemic stroke in order to rationalise approaches to investigation and therapy. For the purpose of this chapter we have chosen a simplified approach based on likely vascular territory and clinical presentation [the Oxfordshire Community Stroke Project (OCSP) classification; see Table 10.1], with particular emphasis on MCA territory infarction.

The anterior circulation syndromes

These clinical syndromes relate to lesions located in the cortical and/or subcortical territory of the anterior circulation, namely the ICA, MCA and ACA. Overall, MCA territory infarcts are the most commonly encountered ischaemic stroke subtypes.

Extensive or complete infarction in the territory of the MCA (cortical and subcortical) produces a major neurological deficit. This is described by the OCSP classification as total anterior circulation infarction (TACI; see Table 10.1), with the triad of contralateral hemiparesis (often with hemisensory loss), contralateral homonymous hemianopia and higher cerebral dysfunction (e.g. dysphasia, neglect). The computed tomography (CT) brain scan and clinical presentation of a patient with TACI is shown in Figure 10.2. The hemiparesis may affect predominantly the upper limb, as the lower limb motor representation is typically supplied by the ACA. In addition, patients with a TACI may also present with contralateral gaze paresis and impaired level of consciousness.

Infarction in a superficial or deep branch of the MCA results in more restricted cortical or subcortical infarction, described by the OCSP classification as partial anterior circulation infarction (PACI; see Table 10.1). Isolated ACA territory infarction is much less common and usually presents as a PACI; for example, restricted infarction in the frontal lobe (cortical branch of ACA) presenting with contralateral monoparesis of the lower limb.

Infarction in the territory of the ICA can produce a variable clinical picture including TACI, ipsilateral monocular visual disturbance or various manifestations of PACI.

In clinical practice, distinction between PACI and TACI is important, as patterns of recovery and recurrence are different. TACI is generally associated with a poor prognosis, with mortality in the order of 40% in the first month. By contrast, patients with PACI

Table 10.1 The Oxfordshire community stroke project (OCSP) classification of ischaemic stroke

OCSP subgroup	Clinical syndrome(s)	Frequency (%)	Mortality at 1 year (%)
TACI	*All of the triad*: hemiparesis/hemisensory loss • Contralateral hemiparesis (αhemisensory loss) • Contralateral homonymous hemianopia • New disturbance of higher cerebral function	17	60
PACI	*Any of the following*: • Contralateral hemiparesis/hemisensory loss and homonymous hemianopia • Contralateral hemiparesis/hemisensory loss and new higher cerebral dysfunction • New higher cerebral dysfunction and contralateral homonymous hemianopia • New higher cerebral dysfunction alone • Restricted contralateral hemiparesis/hemisensory loss (e.g. monoparesis)	34	16
POCI	*Any of the following*: • Ipsilateral cranial nerve palsy (ies) and conralateral hemiparesis/hemisensory loss • Bilateral hemiparesis/hemisensory loss • Disorder of conjugate eye movement • Cerebellar dysfunction (without long tract signs) • Isolated contralateral homonymous hemianopia or cortical blindness	24	19
LACI	Maximum deficit from a single vascular event, *in the absence of*: visual field deficit, new higher cerebral dysfunction or impaired conscious level • PMS: unilateral motor weakness involving at least two out of three entire areas of face, arm and leg • PSS: unilateral sensory disturbance involving at least two out of three entire areas of face, arm and leg • SMS: unilateral motor weakness and sensory disturbance involving at least two out of three areas of face, arm and leg • AH: ipsilateral cerebellar dysfunction and motor weakness, with or without dysarthria	25	11

TACI = total anterior circulation infarction, PACI = partial anterior circulation infarction, POCI = posterior circulation infarction, LACI = lacunar infarction, PMS = pure motor stroke, PSS = pure sensory stroke, SMS = sensorimotor stroke, AH = ataxic hemiparesis.

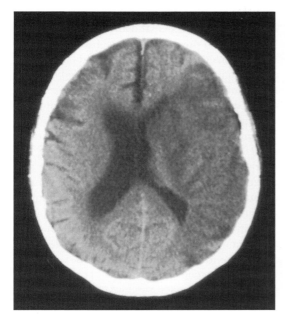

Figure 10.2 Computed tomography brain scan demonstrating left total anterior circulation infarction (TACI). There is extensive infarction throughout the entire territory of the left middle cerebral artery, with compression of the lateral ventricle. Note relative sparing of the left occipital cortex (supplied by the posterior cerebral artery) and anterior frontal lobe (supplied by the anterior cerebral artery). The patient presented with right hemiparesis, right facial nerve palsy, right homonymous hemianopia and right-sided hemi-neglect.

have a better chance of recovery but higher risk of early recurrent stroke.

The posterior circulation syndromes

This category encompasses infarcts in the verte-brobasilar territory – namely, the occipital lobes, medial/inferior temporal lobes, cerebellum, thala-mus and brainstem. The syndromes resulting from posterior circulation infarction (POCI) are perhaps the most heterogenous group, with diverse clinical presentations (see Table 10.1). In addition, a num-ber of classical syndromes resulting from POCI have been described, including lateral medullary syn-

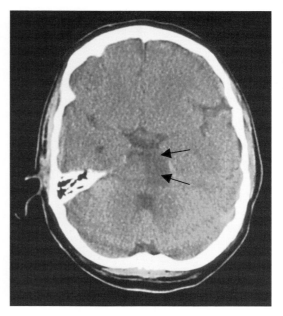

Figure 10.3 Computed tomography brain scan demonstrating posterior circulation infarction (POCI) in the left midbrain (arrowed). The patient presented with right hemiparesis and left third nerve palsy.

drome and various thalamic syndromes, but these rarely present in their complete form. The CT brain scan and clinical presentation of a patient presenting with POCI is shown in Figure 10.3. In hospital series, patients with POCI generally have a lower mortality than those with anterior circulation syndromes, but there is an appreciable risk of recurrent stroke.

The lacunar syndromes

'Lacunar infarction' (LACI) is a historical, pathologi-cal term to describe a small infarct in the territory of a single deep perforator. On CT or magnetic resonance imaging (MRI), LACIs are synonymous with small, deep infarcts less than 1.5 cm in diameter. The clin-ical presentation of a LACI depends on its anatomi-cal location. Many are asymptomatic, but lacunes in strategic sites may present with one of the classical lacunar syndromes (see Table 10.1), most frequently

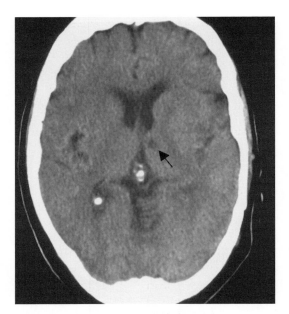

Figure 10.4 Computed tomography brain scan demonstrating lacunar infarction (LACI, arrowed) in the left thalamus (courtesy of Dr D. G. Hughes). The patient presented with sensorimotor stroke (SMS) affecting the right limbs and face.

pure motor stroke (PMS). Figure 10.4 illustrates the CT scan appearances of a patient with a lacunar infarct. Note that a lacunar syndrome is assigned in the absence of new higher cerebral dysfunction, visual field defect or altered level of consciousness. LACIs are commonly subcortical, occurring in the basal ganglia and internal capsule (anterior circulation), but they may also occur in the brainstem or thalamus (posterior circulation). It is therefore evident that classical lacunar syndromes may be due to infarcts in *either* the anterior or posterior circulation. As a clinical subgroup, LACIs have a lower case fatality and recurrence rate, with approximately 60% of patients independent at 12 months.

Aetiology of cerebral ischaemia

Brain cells are largely dependent on oxidative metabolism of glucose for production of energy and maintenance of electrochemical gradients. Cerebral blood flow (CBF) is maintained under varying conditions to meet this demand and depends on cerebral profusion pressure and cerebrovascular resistance. In healthy individuals, CBF is proportional to mean arterial pressure and is maintained by cerebral autoregulation. Brain cells are therefore sensitive to depletion of glucose and oxygen (reflecting reductions in CBF), with neurons being particularly vulnerable to ischaemic insult. A sudden, rapid reduction of CBF (hypoperfusion) in an arterial territory therefore leads to cellular energy failure and onset of cerebral ischaemia. The development and eventual extent of ischaemia depends on a number of factors, including the duration of reduced CBF, integrity of autoregulation, provision of collateral flow and reperfusion of the affected vascular territory. Cerebral ischaemia may therefore be temporary or permanent, depending on whether blood flow is restored to the affected vascular territory. Reperfusion may restore vital nutrients to ischaemic brain tissue but may also be detrimental by exacerbating ischaemic damage (reperfusion injury).

Pathophysiological mechanisms initiating cerebral ischaemia

Cerebral hypoperfusion and, therefore, cerebral ischaemia, is most frequently initiated by arterial occlusion. This is most often caused by proximal thromboembolism from large-artery atheroma (atherothromboembolism, approximately 50% of cases) or a cardiac source (cardioembolism, approximately 20% of cases). In situ occlusion in an artery is less common, usually occurring in small intracranial arteries (small vessel disease, 25% of cases).

Atherothromboembolism

Clinically relevant atheroma commonly occurs in the aortic arch, carotid bifurcation and BA (the aetiological factors involved in atherogenesis are discussed in Chapter 8). The severity of ICA stenosis is an important predictor of the risk of recurrent cerebral ischaemic events, but plaque instability and the tendency to atherothromboembolism are also important factors. Thromboembolism may also arise from large arteries, as occurs in carotid arterial dissection, without the presence of underlying atherosclerosis

Cardioembolism

The most frequent source of cardioembolism is the left atrium, associated with atrial fibrillation. Other important sources of thrombus are the mitral and aortic valves (mitral stenosis, valve prostheses, infective endocarditis) and left ventricle (recent acute myocardial infarction, aneurysm, dilated cardiomyopathy). There are many other recognised cardiac sources of cerebral thromboembolism, which are less commonly seen in clinical practice.

Small vessel disease

Small vessel disease affects the intracranial arteries, and encompasses several pathologies including lipohyalinosis and arteriosclerosis. Lacunar infarcts are believed to arise from occlusion within a single deep perforator, or hypoperfusion associated with disordered autoregulation, on a background of intrinsic small vessel disease. Occlusion is likely to be caused by in situ thrombosis, although the role of embolism in the aetiology of lacunar infarction is not well defined.

Haemodynamic infarction

Cerebral hypoperfusion can also be caused by a profound, rapid reduction in arterial blood pressure *without* arterial occlusion (low-flow or haemodynamic infarction) – for example, hypotension complicating acute ventricular tachycardia. This mechanism can also occur in the setting of a severely stenosed artery – for example, severe ICA stenosis. This type of infarction often affects boundary zones between distal beds of major cerebral arteries, so-called boundary zone or "watershed" infarction.

Risk factors for ischaemic stroke

Stroke is a multifactorial disorder; both environmental and genetic influences modifying the risk of ischaemic stroke have been described. In general, the major risk factors associated with ischaemic stroke are those associated with atherosclerosis and pro-thrombotic tendency. These include increasing age, male sex, hypertension, cigarette smoking, atrial fibrillation, diabetes mellitus, dyslipidaemia and coronary and peripheral vascular disease. In addition, many less common inflammatory and vascular conditions are associated with increased risk of stroke.

Acute ischaemia of the MCA territory: mechanisms of ischaemic injury

The pathophysiology of cerebral ischaemia has been studied most extensively in focal ischaemia of the MCA territory. This type of ischaemia is represented by reproducible preclinical models; it is a clinically common and relevant presentation of ischaemic stroke and TIA. For these reasons, we have chosen to focus on the pathophysiological mechanisms involved in acute ischaemia of the MCA territory.

Dynamic evolution of cerebral ischaemia: the ischaemic penumbra

Cerebral injury developing after the onset of focal ischaemia is a dynamic process, and infarct evolution may occur over hours (even beyond 24 h). After the onset of cerebral ischaemia, two ischaemic zones have been described, based on their extent of CBF compromise and altered metabolic parameters. When CBF falls below a critical threshold level, a central area of irreversibly damaged tissue, the *ischaemic core*, rapidly develops. Tissue surrounding this core, with less critically impaired CBF, is termed the *ischaemic penumbra*. This tissue maintains structural integrity, although ion homeostatic function is jeopardised. The ischaemic core and penumbra have been operationally defined in experimental cerebral ischaemia and in ischaemic stroke patients. Figure 10.5 illustrates the appearances, by MRI, of the ischaemic core and penumbra in a patient with acute infarction of the MCA territory. The penumbra is important clinically as it is potentially viable tissue; if intervention is available early enough, it may halt its progression to evolved infarction. *Reperfusion*

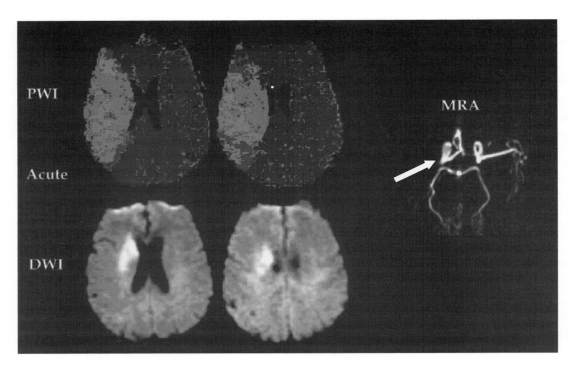

Figure 10.5 Magnetic resonance imaging (MRI) within 2 hours of a patient presenting with occlusion (arrow) of the right middle cerebral artery (MCA) on magnetic resonance angiography (MRA). Perfusion-weighted imaging (PWI) demonstrates a large area of moderate to severe hypoperfusion (represented here by light and medium grey areas) in the territory of the right MCA. On the diffusion-weighted imaging (DWI), the high signal (white) area represents an area of acute energy failure and cytotoxic oedema: the ischaemic core. The area of hypoperfusion not matched by the DWI lesion (the DWI-PWI mismatch) represents the at-risk ischaemic penumbra. (Parsons, M. W. *et al.* Diffusion- and perfusion-weighted MRI response to thrombolysis in stroke, *Annals of Neurology* (2002), **51**, 28–37. Reprinted with permission of John Wiley and Sons, Inc.)

therapy aims to limit the extent of the ischaemic lesion by restoring blood flow, whilst *neuroprotection* aims to rescue the ischaemic penumbra from irreversible damage. The period of time in which the ischaemic penumbra remains viable and potentially amenable to salvage largely determines the therapeutic time window of neuroprotection.

Overview of the ischaemic cascade

The onset of focal cerebral ischaemia initiates a series of pathophysiological events, termed the *ischaemic cascade*, resulting in cellular death in the ischaemic core, extension to the penumbra and infarct evolu-

tion. A diagrammatic overview of the main events of the ischaemic cascade is shown in Figure 10.6. An understanding of the mechanisms involved in this cascade is crucial for developing potential new therapies for the acute phase of ischaemic stroke. The components of the ischaemic cascade are discussed in more detail below.

Excitotoxicity

Within minutes of the onset of cerebral ischaemia, impaired CBF leads to neuronal energy failure with decreased production of mitochondrial adenosine triphosphate (ATP). Failure of ATP-dependent

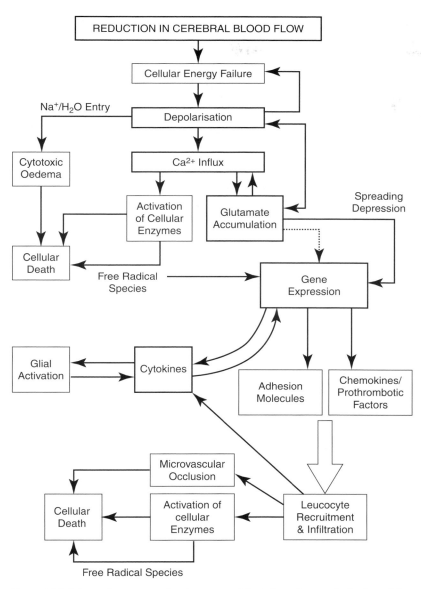

Figure 10.6 Schematic overview of major events of the ischaemic cascade. Excitotoxicity, gene expression, inflammation and cell death are described in more detail in the text.

membrane ion pumps causes changes in neuronal cell membrane permeability (depolarisation), further depleting ATP. These changes in ionic gradients, particularly calcium (Ca^{2+}), sodium (Na^+), chloride (Cl^-) and potassium (K^+) ions, are critical in the development of cytotoxic cell death (Figure 10.6). Excitotoxicity describes the cascade of events leading to neuronal injury secondary to excessive accumulation of excitatory amino acids. Potassium efflux and Ca^{2+} influx lead to excessive release of the excitatory neurotransmitter glutamate into the extracellular space. Glutamate binds to surface membrane receptors, including the N-methyl-D-aspartate (NMDA) and α-amino-3-hydroxy-5-methyl-4-isoxazole propionic acid (AMPA) receptors, facilitating influx of Na^+ and Cl^- ions while potentiating further Ca^{2+} influx. The Na^+ and Cl^- influx facilitates osmotic transport of water into the injured cells, causing swelling and the development of *cytotoxic oedema*. The sustained Ca^{2+} influx further promotes cell death via activation of various cellular enzymes, leading to the formation of free radicals, lipid–membrane peroxidation and degradation of structural proteins and nuclear components.

Excitotoxicity results in rapid cellular death in the ischaemic core, but prolonged excitotoxicity may contribute to more delayed neurodegeneration over several hours. Accumulating extracellular glutamate and K^+ ions potentiate irreversible anoxic depolarisations in the ischaemic core, extending into the penumbra (*spreading depression*). Cells in the penumbra have limited capacity to repolarise at the expense of ATP reserves, undergoing intermittent *peri-infarct depolarisations*, which contribute to the loss of penumbral viability. Furthermore, excitotoxic events, including spreading depression and free-radical generation, are believed to initiate the subsequent inflammatory response to cerebral ischaemia by inducing pro-inflammatory genes.

Inflammatory responses to cerebral ischaemia

There is considerable evidence that cerebral ischaemia initiates an inflammatory response contributing to ischaemic brain injury, mainly in the penumbral tissue. The extent of inflammatory injury may depend on whether the ischaemic insult is permanent or whether it is transient and followed by reperfusion. In addition, the inflammatory response within the brain may also modulate cerebral repair processes and regulate inflammation in the peripheral circulation.

The vascular endothelial/blood–brain barrier (BBB) interface is a major focus of inflammation in response to focal cerebral ischaemia. A number of cell types are involved, including resident glia, cerebrovascular endothelia and blood leucocytes. The interactions between these cells are mediated by a variety of inflammatory gene products, including the cytokines IL-1 and tumour necrosis factor -α (TNF-α). Key inflammatory events include activation of resident glial cells, expression of inflammatory mediators including cytokines and adhesion molecules, infiltration and activation of leucocytes, generation of oxidative stress, changes in vascular tone and disruption of the BBB. The humoral and cellular elements (Figure 10.6) of the inflammatory response to cerebral ischaemia are discussed in detail below.

Activation of glia

Microglia, resident tissue macrophages of monocytic lineage, are implicated in central nervous system (CNS) inflammation. Microglia and other glial cells are rapidly activated after the onset of cerebral ischaemia, undergoing morphological transformation and producing inflammatory mediators, such as IL-1, TNF-α and cytotoxic products. Activated microglia are likely to be the key cells mediating the inflammatory response to cerebral ischaemia, as they are activated prior to neutrophil and macrophage infiltration into the ischaemic lesion.

Inflammatory gene expression

Numerous genes expressed after the onset of focal cerebral ischaemia can modulate inflammation, cell death and, ultimately, repair processes. A schematic representation of the temporal "waves" of expression of inflammatory genes after the onset of cerebral ischaemia is shown in Figure 10.7. Several transcription factors, including c-fos and c-jun, are expressed within minutes (immediate-early genes or IEGs) and may play a role in mediating further inflammatory gene expression. Nuclear factor-κB (NF-κB), a transcription factor translocated to the nucleus when activated by free radicals or cytokines, may be important in regulating inflammatory gene expression

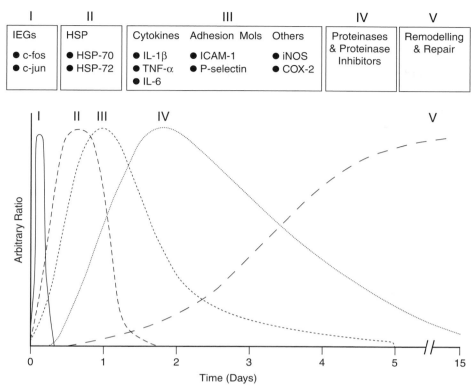

Figure 10.7 Time course of gene expression following experimental focal cerebral ischaemia, illustrating 'waves' of gene expression. *Wave I*, immediate early genes (IEGs). *Wave II*, heat-shock proteins (HSPs). *Wave III*, cytokines, adhesion molecules and prooxidant enzymes. *Wave IV*, proteinase and proteinase inhibitors. *Wave V*, delayed expression of genes involved in remodelling and repair. (Reproduced with kind permission from Barone, F. C., Feuerstein, G. Inflammatory mediators and stroke: new opportunities for novel therapeutics, *Journal of Cerebral Blood Flow and Metabolism* (1999), 19, 819–34. Published by Lippincott Williams & Wilkins, Inc.)

in response to focal cerebral ischaemia. NF-κB regulates expression of a number of inflammatory genes, including IL-1, TNF-α, IL-6, intercellular adhesion molecule-1 (ICAM-1), cyclooxygenase-2 (COX-2) and inducible nitric oxide synthase (iNOS).

Cytokines: IL-1, TNF-α and IL-6

IL-1 and TNF-α are the primary pro-inflammatory cytokines, up-regulating expression of each other, endothelial procoagulant factors, pro-inflammatory enzymes such as COX-2, leucocyte-endothelial adhesion molecules (e.g. ICAM-1) and activat-

ing neutrophils. By contrast, IL-6 has both pro-inflammatory and anti-inflammatory actions and is neurotrophic.

IL-1 is strongly implicated in cerebral ischaemic injury. The IL-1 family comprises several members, including the agonists IL-1β and IL-1α and the highly selective, competitive antagonist of IL-1, IL-1 receptor antagonist (IL-1ra). IL-1β is rapidly expressed in experimental cerebral ischaemia, and central administration of IL-1 at the onset of ischaemia markedly exacerbates brain oedema, volume of infarction and extent of neutrophil infiltration. By contrast, endogenous IL-1 blockade using IL-1ra is neuroprotective, dramatically attenuating the extent of experimental cerebral injury by more than 50%.

Whereas TNF-α and IL-6 are also rapidly expressed after experimental cerebral ischaemia, their roles are less clear. TNF-α appears to have both deleterious and neuroprotective roles in experimental cerebral ischaemia. IL-6 appears to be neuroprotective in some models of experimental ischaemia, reducing the extent of cerebral tissue injury. TNF-α and IL-6 have been detected in the cerebrospinal fluid (CSF) and peripheral circulation of patients with acute ischaemic stroke and correlate with cerebral infarct volume and poor outcome.

Nitric oxide synthase (NOS)

NOS catalyses conversion of L-arginine to nitric oxide (NO) and exists in three isoforms, endothelial NOS (eNOS), neuronal NOS (nNOS) and inducible NOS (iNOS). NO generated by eNOS and nNOS is mainly constitutive and Ca^{2+}-dependent, whereas iNOS is Ca^{2+}-independent. NO can be further oxidized to reactive nitrogen oxide species, including peroxynitrite.

eNOS and nNOS are expressed very rapidly after the onset of cerebral ischaemia, while iNOS expression occurs some hours later, producing excessive NO. NO has diverse biological effects and may have neuroprotective or deleterious effects in the ischaemic brain. For example, NO generation following eNOS expression has vasodilatory effects on cerebral vasculature, serving an early neuroprotective role in ischaemic brain tissue, particularly the penumbra (see below). Conversely, nNOS and iNOS exacerbate ischaemic injury. Several mechanisms have been proposed for NO-mediated ischaemic brain injury, including production of pro-oxidant species, inhibition of mitochondrial respiration, Ca^{2+}-dependent excitotoxic mechanisms and induction of apoptosis.

COX-2

Cyclooxygenase (COX) catalyses the conversion of arachidonic acid to prostaglandin H_2, the common precursor of inflammatory eicosanoids (prostaglandins, thromboxanes) – a process that also generates superoxide radicals. COX-2, an isoenzyme of COX, is markedly upregulated in inflammatory conditions. In response to cerebral ischaemia, COX-2 is rapidly expressed by glia, infiltrating leucocytes and endothelial cells and it exacerbates neuronal injury. Deleterious COX-2 products, particularly prostaglandin E_2, appear to mediate neuronal injury by contributing both to glutamate excitotoxicity and inflammatory injury.

Oxidative stress

Cerebral ischaemia/reperfusion induces *oxidative stress*, an excess of pro-oxidant over anti-oxidant species, leading to further brain injury. NO and superoxide are two key pro-oxidant products of excitotoxic and inflammatory pathways, which are substrates for the generation of other pro-oxidants such as hydrogen peroxide, peroxynitrite and hydroxyl radicals. Pro-oxidant species directly cause early neuronal death by lipid peroxidation, protein and DNA oxidation, but they may also act as signaling molecules via mitochondrial proteins, NF-κB and other transcription factors.

BBB permeability

The BBB is a complex structure comprising cerebral endothelial cells, extracellular matrix–containing basal lamina and astrocytes. Cerebral ischaemia results in loss of cerebral microvascular integrity in the ischaemic core. Disruption of BBB permeability is initiated by loosening of endothelial intercellular junctions and expression of matrix metalloproteinases, which degrade the basal lamina. These early changes in BBB permeability, along with effects mediated by bradykinin and thrombin, contribute to the development of cerebral oedema.

Changes in vascular tone

Cerebral endothelia regulate vascular smooth muscle tone by producing vasoactive mediators. Endothelin-1 (ET-1) and platelet-activating factor (PAF) are both potent vasoconstrictors implicated in cerebral ischaemic injury. In experimental animals, ET-1 causes MCA constriction and induction of focal cerebral ischaemia; it is also expressed in the ischaemic cortex following the onset of experimental ischaemia. Administration of antagonists to ET-1 or PAF confers neuroprotective effects in experimental cerebral ischaemia. ET-1 is also elevated in the CSF of patients within hours of ischaemic stroke and correlates with infarct volume. By contrast, production of other vasoactive mediators, including prostacyclin and NO derived from eNOS, may have neuroprotective properties by vasodilating cerebral vasculature.

Intravascular coagulation

The cerebral endothelial surface is usually maintained in an anticoagulant, antithrombotic state owing to the expression of molecules such as thrombomodulin, tissue factor pathway inhibitor, tissue plasminogen activator and prostacyclin. Experimental cerebral ischaemia induces expression of procoagulant and thrombotic factors, including tissue factor, PAF, thromboxane A_2 (TXA_2) and tissue plasminogen activator inhibitor, facilitating platelet aggregation and microvascular thrombotic occlusion.

Recruitment and infiltration of blood leucocytes

In response to cerebral ischaemia, cerebral endothelia express chemokines that mediate recruitment of blood leucocytes to the ischaemic tissue. Neutrophils and monocytes express surface integrins that interact with specific adhesion molecules expressed by cerebral endothelia – in particular intercellular adhesion molecules (ICAMs) and the selectins. Endothelial ICAM-1, E-selectin and P-selectin are rapidly up-regulated following the onset of cerebral ischaemia. Neutrophils occlude the microvasculature of the ischaemic cortex and infiltrate the ischaemic parenchyma after several hours. This is followed by occlusion of the cerebral microvasculature by platelets and later by microvascular accumulation and infiltration of monocytes.

Experimental studies of focal cerebral ischaemia suggest that neutrophils and adhesion molecules play an important role in the development of inflammatory reperfusion injury. In patients with cerebral infarction, neutrophils are detected in the CSF, and radiolabelled peripheral neutrophils accumulate in cerebral ischaemic lesions within hours.

Brain/body temperature

Fever, or pyrexia, is a regulated rise in core temperature due to alteration of the hypothalamic set point, whereas hyperthermia is due to heat production exceeding heat loss. Hyperthermia during or following the onset of experimental focal cerebral ischaemia worsens outcome. Conversely, intra-ischaemic or reperfusion hypothermia confers neuroprotection in experimental cerebral ischaemia. Hyperthermia may act through several mechanisms to exacerbate cerebral ischaemic injury, including enhanced excitotoxicity and spreading depression or by altering inflammatory gene expression.

Elevated body temperature is common in acute stroke patients, occurring in around 40% to 60% of patients, and is associated with severity of stroke and worse outcome. In acute stroke patients, elevated body temperature is generally assumed to be fever, although the underlying mechanisms are not well understood. The effects of antipyretics or hypothermia (induced by surface cooling or endovascular techniques) on body temperature in acute stroke have been evaluated in several small studies. However, whether antipyretics or induced hypothermia modify outcome after acute stroke is yet to be established in large, placebo-controlled intervention trials.

Hypothalamic-pituitary-adrenal (HPA) axis

Corticotropin-releasing factor and glucocorticoids have been implicated in experimental cerebral ischaemic injury. Increased serum adrenocorticotropic hormone, plasma and urinary free cortisol have been reported in patients after acute ischaemic stroke and are associated with stroke severity and worse outcome. Although several clinical trials have evaluated the use of corticosteroids as a treatment for acute stroke, systematic review of the trials administering intravenous or intramuscular corticosteroids within 48 h of acute stroke failed to demonstrate any treatment benefit compared to placebo.

Acute-phase proteins

Plasma fibrinogen and C-reactive protein (CRP) are elevated in patients after acute ischaemic stroke and predict recurrent vascular events and poor outcome. However, the role of these acute-phase proteins in adverse outcome remains unclear. Fibrinogen or CRP may contribute to ischaemic injury or recurrent atherothromboembolic events as a result of adverse rheological or pro-inflammatory effects, or these may simply be markers of CNS/peripheral inflammation. For example, CRP activates the classical complement pathway, also stimulating induction of tissue factor by macrophages and further induction of cytokines, including IL-1.

Cell death in cerebral ischaemia

The mode of cell death after ischaemic brain injury is complex and remains incompletely understood.

In acute neurodegeneration, features of *both* necrosis and apoptosis-like pathways are apparent in many ischaemic lesions. Ischaemic cells in the core of an infarct may die by necrosis as ATP levels drop below critical levels; cells further from the infarct core may initiate apoptosis after the ischaemic insult and then switch to necrosis when the ATP levels drop below a critical threshold. There may be cells in the ischaemic penumbra that die in a delayed fashion from the effects of apoptosis alone.

Regulation of cell death following cerebral ischaemia is not fully understood. Caspases are proteolytic enzymes that appear to be important in mediating apoptosis following experimental cerebral ischaemia. Oxidative stress may induce mitochondrial injury, which initiates a caspase cascade leading to apoptosis. The Bcl-2 gene family are key regulators of apoptotic cellular death (e.g. Bcl-2 itself is protective against cell death, whereas Bax promotes cell death). In experimental cerebral ischaemia, Bcl-2 is expressed in neurons, glia and endothelia, predominantly in the penumbra. Overexpression of Bcl-2 in transgenic models of cerebral ischaemia is neuroprotective, resulting in reduced infarct volumes.

Therapeutic strategies in acute ischaemic stroke

Stroke management is emerging from years of therapeutic nihilism, but there are still very few evidence-based treatment strategies available. Although stroke management incorporates both acute management and secondary prevention strategies, this section focuses only on the management of acute ischaemic stroke.

Brain imaging in acute stroke

In clinical practice, the role of brain imaging in acute stroke is to differentiate PICH from ischaemic stroke and to exclude certain pathologies mimicking stroke. In the UK, non-contrast CT is the first-line investigation in patients presenting with acute stroke and is recommended within 24 h of symptom onset. CT brain scanning is now rapid and widely available; it is both specific and highly sensitive in detecting PICH in acute stroke.

Stroke units

Management of patients on a stroke unit compared to a general ward is associated with lower rates of death, dependency or need for institutional care. Although the effective components of stroke unit care are not well defined, stroke units provide a setting for coordinated, multidisciplinary care directed at prophylaxis and treatment of common complications (e.g. infection, venous thromboembolism, hyperglycaemia, pressure area care), nutritional support, early rehabilitation and initiation of secondary prevention.

Pharmacological treatment

Aspirin is currently the mainstay of pharmacological treatment of acute ischaemic stroke. The beneficial effects of aspirin relate to its inhibitory effect on platelet TXA_2 synthesis via COX inhibition, thereby reducing platelet aggregation. When started within 48 h of ischaemic stroke, aspirin produces a small benefit (12 fewer patients per 1 000 dead or disabled) at 3 to 6 months.

Thrombolytic drugs have gained much interest in acute ischaemic stroke. Tissue plasminogen activator (t-PA) enhances conversion of plasminogen to plasmin, activating intravascular fibrinolysis and enabling reperfusion. Intravenous thrombolysis with recombinant t-PA administered within 3 h of symptom onset improves outcome in selected patients (140 fewer patients dead or dependent per 1 000 treated) at 3 months. Only a small proportion of all acute ischaemic stroke patients are eligible even in experienced centres (around 1% to 6%), and thrombolysis is associated with an excess of symptomatic intracranial haemorrhage (around 60 per 1 000 patients treated).

Neuroprotective strategies have so far been directed at modulating various deleterious steps in the ischaemic cascade, including excitotoxicity, free radical generation, inflammatory responses and apoptosis. However, despite showing promise in experimental models, numerous putative neuroprotectants have failed in clinical trials in patients with acute ischaemic stroke. There are a number of potential explanations for the failure of neuroprotective therapies in human stroke patients, with issues surrounding the limitations of preclinical models, optimum drug dose, delivery, dose-limiting side effects, therapeutic time window, appropriate patient selection, clinical trial design and assessment of outcome measures.

Future neuroprotective strategies may target specific genes involved in cerebral ischaemic injury. Combining reperfusion with neuroprotection is a logical approach to therapy in acute ischaemic stroke, as restoring blood flow may facilitate delivery of neuroprotective agents to ischaemic brain tissue. Advances in imaging techniques in the acute phase may aid more appropriate selection of patients with a viable penumbra for neuroprotective therapy.

Summary

Stroke is a major cause of mortality and morbidity. Cerebral ischaemia is the underlying cause of brain damage in several acute neurological disorders, including ischaemic and haemorrhagic stroke. The onset of cerebral ischaemia initiates an ischaemic cascade, resulting in immediate and delayed neurodegeneration in the ischaemic core and penumbra. Immediate cellular energy failure leads to loss of electrochemical gradients, calcium ion influx and excitotoxicity. Activation of an inflammatory response contributes to further ischaemic brain injury, mainly in the ischaemic penumbra. Key inflammatory events include activation of resident glial cells, expression of inflammatory mediators (including cytokines and adhesion molecules) and infiltration of blood leucocytes. The cytokine IL-1 is a major pro-inflammatory mediator and is strongly implicated in ischaemic brain injury. Despite advances in our understanding of the pathophysiology of cerebral ischaemia, pharmacological approaches to neuroprotection have been disappointing in clinical trials. Future research directed at the risk factors, pathophysiology and treatment of cerebral ischaemia may have an impact in reducing the burden of stroke.

Clinical scenarios

Scenario 1

A 68-year-old man developed sudden onset of isolated speech disturbance. His wife described his inability to 'get the right words out'. He was recovering from an acute anterior myocardial infarction that occurred 10 days previously, but had not been thrombolysed for this. Other past medical

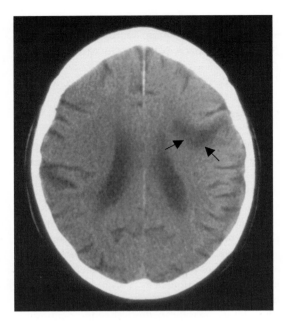

Figure 10.8 Computed tomography brain scan demonstrating cerebral infarction (arrowed), accompanying question 1.

history included hypercholestrolaemia, type 2 diabetes mellitus and hypertension; he was already taking aspirin. On examination, his blood pressure was 138/90; he appeared frustrated with faltering, non-fluent speech and impairment of word initiation. He had difficulty correctly naming objects but appeared to understand verbal commands and was not dysarthric. The remaining neurological examination was normal. Electrocardiography showed sinus rhythm and persistent ST-segment elevation in the anterior chest leads. His CT brain scan taken 3 days after the onset of symptoms is shown in Figure 10.8.

1. What is this disturbance of speech called?
2. Which OCSP subtype describes this presentation?
3. From the clinical presentation and CT brain scan, what is the most likely anatomical location and vascular territory of his infarction?
4. What further non-invasive cardiological investigation is required?
5. What is the most likely cause of this patient's ischaemic stroke, and how should it be treated?

Scenario 2

A 62-year-old woman presented with sudden, painless visual loss in the right eye that had occurred a week previously. On questioning, she described the sensation of a 'curtain descending' her right visual field from 'top to bottom'. The symptoms resolved completely within 5 min. She was a lifelong smoker, on treatment for hypertension. Fundoscopy was normal. She was in sinus rhythm and her blood pressure was 194/100. Fasting blood sugar was normal. Carotid duplex scanning revealed 80% stenosis of the right internal carotid artery.

1. What is the visual symptom this patient was describing?
2. What is the likely underlying mechanism?
3. Would she be a suitable candidate for consideration of carotid endarterectomy?

Scenario 3

A 72-year-old man was referred with a 2-year progressive history of poor memory. Further history from his wife revealed that he had difficulty finding his way around the house, difficulty with names, inability to recognise family members and unsteadiness when walking. He was also incontinent of urine. Past medical history included hypertension, angina pectoris and peripheral vascular disease. He was a lifelong smoker of 20 cigarettes per day. On examination, he had an expressionless face, difficulty initiating gait and impairment in multiple cognitive domains (language, praxis, visuospatial impairments and memory). Blood pressure was 190/110. Neurological examination revealed a left upper motor neuron facial weakness, mild left upper and lower limb weakness, brisk limb reflexes and extensor plantars.

1. What is the likely diagnosis of this patient's cognitive impairment?
2. What investigations would you perform?
3. What is your management plan?

Scenario 4

A 63-year-old woman presented to Casualty with a history of a sudden left-sided headache preceding right arm and leg weakness. She had a past

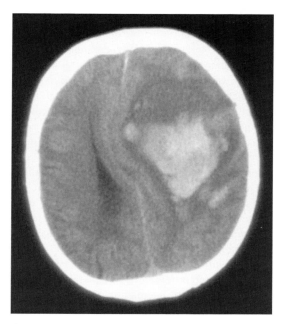

Figure 10.9 Computed tomography brain scan, accompanying scenario 4.

history of atrial fibrillation and was taking digoxin and warfarin; her international normalized ratio (INR) was 6.8. On arrival she was alert but had an expressive dysphasia, right homonymous hemianopia and right hemiparesis. While awaiting further assessment her level of consciousness deteriorated (eye opening to speech, making incomprehensible sounds and localising to painful stimuli with her left hand). An urgent CT brain scan (Fig. 10.9) was arranged. Her management was then discussed with the local neurosurgeons, who elected to take over her care.

1. On this patient's arrival in Casualty, what was the differential diagnosis?
2. What is her immediate management and what are the available management options in primary intracerebral haemorrhage (PICH)?

Answers

Scenario 1

1. Expressive dysphasia. In this particular case there is no receptive difficulty.

2. PACI (isolated higher cerebral dysfunction; i.e dysphasia)
3. The classical cortical representation is Broca's area in the inferior frontal area of the dominant hemisphere. Computed tomography of the brain in this case confirms restricted cortical infarction in the left fronto-parietal region, within the territory of the left middle cerebral artery.
4. Trans-thoracic echocardiogram.
5. The history of recent anterior myocardial infarction suggests associated left ventricular thrombus and cardioembolic cerebral infarction. The echocardiogram revealed evidence of a hypokinetic anterior wall with overlying mural thrombus. Management would be to temporarily discontinue aspirin and commence oral anticoagulation for 12 to 24 weeks provided that there was no contraindication.

Scenario 2

1. This woman is presenting with an ocular transient ischemic attack (TIA) in the territory of the right carotid circulation. Her description of transient monocular blindness is fairly typical of amaurosis fugax.
2. Atherothromboebolism from the right internal carotid artery (ICA) to the right central retinal artery.
3. Yes. Criteria for consideration of carotid endarterectomy are definite symptoms in the territory of the anterior circulation (TIA or ischaemic stroke with good recovery), preferably within 3 months, with significant stenosis (70% to 99%) in the ipsilateral ICA.

Scenario 3

1. The differential diagnosis of progressive cognitive impairment with abnormalities in multiple cortical areas is between a vascular dementia ('multi-infarct dementia') and a neurodegenerative disease such as Alzheimer's disease. There is considerable overlap between the two, but in this case evidence of vascular disease outside the brain, with vascular risk factors (hypertension, cigarette

smoking) suggests a vascular cause. This is supported by the patient's asymmetrical neurological signs, which suggest previous stroke. Multiple infarcts especially in the midline frontal lobes can mimic idiopathic Parkinson's disease (gait apraxia; 'pseudo-Parkinson's').

2. Useful investigations include the assessment of vascular risk factors (e.g. fasting blood sugar and lipids, electrocardiogram to assess rhythm and left ventricular hypertrophy) and a CT brain scan to demonstrate multiple cortical infarctions (a degenerative dementia tends to be associated with a CT scan that may be normal or reveal generalised atrophy).

3. The management plan will include secondary prevention management of vascular risk factors (optimum blood pressure control, treatment with an anti-platelet agent, smoking cessation) but more importantly support for the patient and carer to allow him to continue living at home for as long as possible. Such support would include social work and community psychiatric input.

Scenario 4

1. Anticoagulation in chronic atrial fibrillation (INR target 2.0 to 3.0), reduces the relative risk of ischaemic stroke by around 60%, so there is still a risk of ischaemic stroke. The differential diagnosis at presentation includes infarction in the territory of the left middle cerebral artery (total anterior circulation infarction or TACI) and primary intracerebral haemorrhage (PICH) of the left hemisphere associated with over-anticoagulation. Within hours of onset, CT brain scan is required to exclude or confirm the presence of haemorrhage, and in this case shows extensive deep PICH in the left hemisphere. The majority (around 90%) of PICHs occur in the supratentorial compartment, and most of these are deep in the hemisphere. Classically patients present with a focal deficit of smooth, progressive onset over minutes to hours and may have a diminished level of consciousness. Headache is not a distinguishing feature of PICH and occurs in around 20% of patients with cerebral infarction.

2. Immediate management would be assessment of airway, breathing and circulation. Further management options for supratentorial PICH include supportive care (correction of coagulopathies, including over-anticoagulation, treatment of hypertension and prophylaxis for deep venous thrombosis) or consideration of surgical intervention and haematoma evacuation. The International Surgical Trial in Intracerebral Haemorrhage (STICH) has recently reported no overall benefit from early surgical evacuation compared to initial conservative management in spontaneous supratentorial PICH. There is more evidence favouring surgical intervention in patients with infratentorial haematomas, particularly those with haematomas larger than 3cm in diameter or impaired consciousness level and smaller haematomas.

Abbreviations

ACA: anterior cerebral artery
ACoA: anterior communicating artery
AH: ataxic hemiparesis
AMPA: α-amino-3-hydroxy-5-methyl-4-isoxazole propionic acid
ATP: adenosine triphosphate
BA: basilar artery
BBB: blood-brain barrier
Ca^{2+}: calcium ions
CBF: cerebral blood flow
Cl^-: chloride ions
CNS: central nervous system
COX: cyclooxygenase
COX-2: cyclooxygenase-2
CRP: C-reactive protein
CSF: cerebrospinal fluid
CT: computed tomography
ET-1: endothelin-1
eNOS: endothelial nitric oxide synthase
HPA: hypothalamic-pituitary-adrenal

HSP: heat-shock protein
ICA: internal carotid artery
ICAM-1: intercellular adhesion molecule-1
ICP: intracranial pressure
IEG: immediate-early gene
IL-1: interleukin-1
IL-6: interleukin-6
IL-1ra: interleukin-1 receptor antagonist
iNOS: inducible nitric oxide synthase
INR: international normalized ratio
K$^+$: potassium ions
LACI: lacunar infarction
MCA: middle cerebral artery
MRI: magnetic resonance imaging
Na$^+$: sodium ions
NF-κB: nuclear factor-κB
NMDA: N-methyl-D-aspartate
nNOS: neuronal nitric oxide synthase
NO: nitric oxide
NOS: nitric oxide synthase
OCSP: Oxfordshire Community Stroke Project
PACI: partial anterior circulation infarction
PAF: platelet activating factor
PCA: posterior cerebral artery
PCoA: posterior communicating artery
PICH: primary intracerebral haemorrhage
PMS: pure motor stroke
PSS: pure sensory stroke
POCI: posterior circulation infarction
SAH: subarachnoid haemorrhage
SMS: sensorimotor stroke
TACI: total anterior circulation infarction
TXA$_2$: thromboxane A$_2$
TIA: transient ischaemic attack
TNF-α: tumour necrosis factor alpha
tPA: tissue plasminogen activator
VA: vertebral artery

FURTHER READING

General introduction to stroke and useful links

The Internet Stroke Center at Washington University. http://www.strokecenter.org/

Pathophysiology of cerebral ischaemia and neuroprotection

Arundine, M., Tymianski, M. (2004). Molecular mechanisms of glutamate-dependent neurodegeneration in ischemia and traumatic brain injury. *Cellular and Molecular Life Sciences* **61**, 657–68.

Muir, K. W., Tyrrell, P., Sattar, N., Warburton, E. (2007). Inflammation and ischaemic stroke. *Current Opinion in Neurology* **20**, 334–42.

Lucas, S. M., Rothwell, N. J., Gibson, R. M. (2006). The role of inflammation in CNS injury and disease. *British Journal of Pharmacology* **147** (Suppl 1), S232–40.

Ginsberg, M. D. (2003). Adventures in the pathophysiology of brain ischemia: penumbra, gene expression, neuroprotection. *Stroke* **34**, 214–23.

Iadecola, C., Gorelick, P. B. (2005). The janus face of cyclooxygenase-2 in ischemic stroke: shifting toward downstream targets. *Stroke* **36**, 182–5.

Keynes, R. G., Garthwaite, J. (2004). Nitric oxide and its role in ischaemic brain injury. *Current Molecular Medicine* **4**, 179–91.

Liu, L., Yenari, M. A. (2007). Therapeutic hypothermia: neuroprotective mechanisms. *Frontiers in Bioscience* **12**, 816–25.

Warner, D. S., Sheng, H., Batinic-Haberle, I. (2004). Oxidants, antioxidants and the ischemic brain. *Journal of Experimental Biology* **207**, 3221–31.

Clinical stroke

Intercollegiate Working Party for Stroke. (2004). National Clinical Guidelines for Stroke, 2nd ed. London: Royal College of Physicians. http://www.rcplondon.ac.uk/pubs/books/stroke/index.htm

Davalos, A. (2005). Thrombolysis in acute ischemic stroke: successes, failures, and new hopes. *Cerebrovascular Diseases* **20** (**Suppl 2**), 135–9.

Van der Worp, H. B., van Gijn, J. (2007). Clinical practice. Acute ischemic stroke. *New England Journal of Medicine* **357**, 572–9.

Muir, K. W., Buchan, A., von Kummer, R., Rother, J., Baron, J. C. (2006). Imaging of acute stroke. *Lancet Neurology* **5**, 755–68.

Warlow, C. P., Dennis, M. S., van Gijn, J. *et al.* (2001). Stroke: a practical guide to management, 2nd ed. Oxford, UK: Blackwell Science.

Warlow, C., Sudlow, C., Dennis, M. *et al.* (2003). Stroke. *Lancet* **362**, 1211–24.

11

Diabetic neuropathy

Adam Greenstein, Moaz Mojaddidi, Andrew J. M. Boulton and Rayaz A. Malik

Introduction

Of all the long-term complications of diabetes, none affects as many organs or systems of the human body as the group of conditions included under the term 'diabetic neuropathies'.

Definitions and classification

A simple definition as to what constitutes diabetic neuropathy is 'the presence of symptoms and signs of peripheral nerve dysfunction in people with diabetes after the exclusion of other causes'.

To quantify neuropathy, the following assessments are required:

1. Neuropathic symptoms (neuropathy symptom score, or NSS)
2. Neuropathic deficits (neuropathy impairment score, or NIS)
3. Motor/sensory nerve conduction velocity (MS NCV)
4. Quantitative sensory testing (QST)
5. Autonomic function testing (AFT)

The minimum criteria for a diagnosis of neuropathy require at least two abnormalities among the listed criteria, with at least one being number 3 or 5.

Staging is as follows:

N0 = No neuropathy (minimum criteria unfulfilled)

N1 = asymptomatic neuropathy (NSS = 0)

N2 = symptomatic neuropathy

N3 = disabling neuropathy

Epidemiology

The prevalence of symptomatic neuropathy varies from 22.5% to 28.5%; It is thought to be present in 5% to 10% of patients at diagnosis of type 2 diabetes and, depending on the tests used to define neuropathy, may affect 60% to 90% of diabetic patients.

Clinical features of diabetic neuropathies

Focal/multifocal

Focal/multifocal neuropathies account for no more than 10% of all diabetic neuropathies. Most tend to occur in older type 2 patients with a rapid onset of focal pain and sensori-motor deficit, which resolves partially or completely.

Cranial mononeuropathies

The nerves supplying the extra-ocular muscles are most commonly affected. Diabetic ophthalmoplegia (third nerve palsy) is relatively rapid in onset and presents with pain in the orbit, diplopia and ptosis. The exclusion of other causes, particularly rupture of a posterior communicating aneurysm, is essential. Investigation should include high-resolution computed tomography (CT) or magnetic resonance imaging (MRI) of the brain, in particular the posterior fossa, to exclude a tumour. Although these neuropathies were traditionally believed to be due to acute ischemia within the nerve, there is now evidence for micro-infarcts within the third nerve nucleus.

Isolated and multiple mononeuropathies

A number of nerves are prone to damage in diabetes: by far the commonest is the median nerve as it passes under the flexor retinaculum. Up to 10% of diabetic patients may be affected by characteristic symptoms, including pain and paraesthesiae in the distribution of the median nerve radiating to the forearm and sometimes the arm. However, 30% of patients may show electrophysiological evidence of median nerve compression. Other entrapment neuropathies are less frequently seen and may involve the ulnar nerve, the lateral cutaneous nerve of the thigh (meralgia paraesthetica), the radial nerve (wrist drop) and the peroneal nerve (foot drop). 'Mononeuritis multiplex' simply describes the occurrence of more than one isolated mononeuropathy in an individual patient.

Truncal neuropathies

Truncal neuropathy typically presents with sensory (dull, aching, boring pain together with burning discomfort or allodynia occurring in a band distribution around the chest or abdomen in a dermatomal distribution) but very occasionally motor (unilateral bulging of abdominal muscles) manifestations. Electrophysiological investigation, including needle electromyographic examination, is diagnostic and should be performed in any patient suspected of this diagnosis. The natural history for symptoms and signs is good, with recovery the rule.

Proximal motor neuropathy (amyotrophy)

Typically affecting older, male, type 2 diabetic patients, this condition presents with pain, wasting and weakness in the proximal muscles of the lower limbs, either unilaterally or with asymmetrical bilateral involvement together with a distal symmetrical sensory neuropathy. Weight loss, as much as 40% of pre-morbid body mass, may occur. Stable glycaemic control together with physiotherapy is cur-

rently recommended. In most cases, recovery is gradual but may take years rather than months. Recent neuropathological studies have suggested that a significant proportion of patients have a vasculitis that responds dramatically to immunosuppression. Thus both high-dose corticosteroids and intravenous immunoglobulin therapy have been advocated and large multicentre trials are currently under way to assess their benefit.

Symmetrical neuropathies

Distal sensory neuropathy

This is a diffuse symmetrical disorder, mainly affecting the feet and lower legs in a stocking distribution but rarely also involving the hands in a glove distribution. The clinical presentation is extremely variable, ranging from the severely painful (positive) symptoms at one extreme to the completely painless variety, which may present with an insensitive foot ulcer. The neuropathic symptoms may be difficult for the patient to describe but typically fall into a recognisable pattern, ranging from the severely painful 'positive symptoms' at one extreme, with burning pain, stabbing and shooting sensations, uncomfortable temperature sensations, paraesthesiae, hyperaesthesia and allodynia, to mild or 'negative symptoms' such as decreased pain sensation, deadness and numbness. Symptoms fluctuate with time but tend to be extremely uncomfortable and distressing and also prone to nocturnal exacerbation with bedclothes hyperaesthesia. As the disease progresses, there is usually also some motor dysfunction (including small muscle wasting: sensorimotor neuropathy).

Painful neuropathies

Hyperglycaemic neuropathy may occur in newly diagnosed patients and is characterized by transient positive symptoms associated with rapidly reversible abnormalities of nerve function. An acute sensory neuropathy is recognized, with rapid onset of severe painful symptoms, which often follows a period of severe metabolic instability or may be precipitated by a sudden improvement of control ('insulin neuritis'). A specific small-fibre neuropathy with neuropathic pain and autonomic dysfunction but few signs also exists. This shares many similarities with the acute sensory neuropathy, but symptoms tend to be more persistent.

Autonomic neuropathy

This is a common and under-diagnosed manifestation of the neuropathies that affects principally cardiovascular, urogenital, gastrointestinal, thermoregulatory and sudomotor function.

Cardiac neuropathy

Cardiac autonomic neuropathy manifests initially as an increase in heart rate secondary to vagal denervation followed by a decrease due to sympathetic denervation. Finally, a fixed heart rate supervenes, which responds only minimally to physiological stimuli; it is suggestive of almost complete denervation and bears similarities to the transplanted heart. In type 1 diabetes, 25% of children display some degree of cardiac autonomic dysfunction at diagnosis. In type 2 diabetic patients, parasympathetic dysfunction is present in 65%, with combined parasympathetic/sympathetic neuropathy in 15.2% at 10 years after diagnosis. Postural hypotension, defined as a drop in the systolic and diastolic blood pressures of 20 and 10 mm Hg respectively, occurs as a consequence of impaired vasoconstriction in the splanchnic and cutaneous vascular beds due to efferent sympathetic denervation.

Gastrointestinal neuropathy

Gastrointestinal neuropathy manifests as an abnormality in motility, secretion and absorption through derangement of both extrinsic parasympathetic (vagus and spinal S2-S4) and sympathetic as well as intrinsic enteric innervation provided by Auer-

bach's plexus. Clinically, patients present with two major problems: diabetic gastroparesis – manifest by nausea, postprandial vomiting and loss of appetite – and alternating nocturnal diarrhoea and constipation. Gastroparesis can result in poorly controlled diabetes because of delayed gastric emptying and vomiting. Both of these may cause variability in glucose absorption and thus mismatched insulin action and glucose peaks resulting in hyperglycaemia as well as hypoglycaemia.

Erectile dysfunction

Erectile dysfunction in diabetes is usually of multifactorial aetiology; in most series, autonomic neuropathy is a major contributory factor in up to 40%. Cholinergic and non-cholinergic noradrenergic neurotransmitters mediate erectile function by relaxing smooth muscle in the corpus cavernosum. Other features include occasional retrograde ejaculation, although some ejaculation and orgasm are maintained. Consideration of other potential causes – including vascular disease, medications, local problems such as Peyronie's disease and psychological factors – are essential before considering therapeutic approaches.

Bladder dysfunction is also well recognized as a consequence of autonomic neuropathy in some patients: this 'cystopathy' is usually the result of neurogenic detrusor muscle abnormality. In extreme cases, gross bladder distension with abdominal distension and overflow incontinence may occur.

Sweating abnormalities

Abnormalities of sweating are common but often neglected symptoms of autonomic neuropathies. The sweat gland has a complex peptidergic as well as cholinergic innervation, and neuropeptide immunoreactivity (especially for vasoactive intestinal peptide or VIP) is low in the sudomotor nerves of diabetic patients. The most common presentation is reduced sweating in the extremities, particularly the feet, which is a manifestation of sympathetic dysfunction. In contrast, some patients may complain of a paradoxical compensatory drenching with truncal sweating, particularly at night. Gustatory sweating, which is profuse sweating over the head and neck region on eating certain foods, is a highly characteristic symptom of diabetic autonomic neuropathy.

Measures of neuropathy

Clinical symptoms

A number of instruments have been developed to quantify neuropathic symptoms that might aid in diagnosis and in longitudinal studies:

- The McGill pain questionnaire, consisting of a number of descriptors of symptoms from which patients select those that best describe their experience
- The neuropathy symptom score (NSS), a standardized list of questions and neuropathic symptoms applied by a trained individual in a standardized manner
- The symptom profile or change scores (NSP and NSC derived from the NSS

Quantitative sensory tests (QST)

This test assesses the patient's ability to detect a number of sensory stimuli at the most vulnerable site – the foot. However, these are complex psycho-physiological tests that rely on a patient's co-operation and concentration; abnormal findings do not necessarily confirm that the abnormality lies in the peripheral nerve, as it might lie anywhere in the afferent pathway. Some of the more commonly used techniques are listed below.

Semmes–Weinstein monofilaments
These comprise sets of nylon filaments of variable diameter that buckle at a pre-defined force when applied to the testing site. Inability to perceive pressure of a 10-g Semmes-Weinstein 5.07 monofilament identifies subjects at risk of neuropathic foot ulceration.

Vibration perception
A number of devices (e.g. the Biothesiometer) quantify vibration perception thresholds (VPT) and assess viability of the large myelinated fibres. A reading of greater than 25 V is associated with a high risk of foot ulceration.

Thermal/cooling thresholds
Warm and cold sensation is transmitted via small myelinated and unmyelinated fibres and can be assessed using a number of devices. Those employing a forced-choice technique with the method of limits are the most reproducible.

Autonomic function testing

Cardiovascular autonomic dysfunction is evaluated using a battery of five tests:

- The average inspiratory-expiratory heart-rate difference/6 deep breaths
- The Valsalva ratio
- The 30:15 ratio
- The diastolic blood pressure response to isometric exercise
- The systolic blood-pressure fall to standing

Spectral analysis allows an assessment of the modulation in sinus node activity and, depending on which frequency one assesses, may allow dissection of the component contribution of both autonomic input and circulating neurohumoral factors.

Gastroparesis may be investigated with barium meals and manometry to determine delayed gastric emptying and possible reflux.

Electrophysiology

Electrophysiological (EP) testing is currently the most reliable and reproducible methodology (coefficients of variability of 3% to 4% for motor and sensory nerve conduction velocities). For these reasons, EP variables such as nerve conduction velocities and amplitudes are frequently used as surrogate end points in clinical trials and for differentiating axonal degeneration from demyelination, thus aiding accurate diagnosis.

Pathology

Pathological changes in peripheral neuropathy are evaluated by biopsy of a sensory nerve, most commonly the sural nerve. Nerve biopsy is indicated only if, after performing neurophysiological and relevant diagnostic tests to evaluate a peripheral neuropathy, the diagnosis is not clear. The procedure itself is performed by a neurosurgeon under local anaesthesia, and fascicular rather than whole nerve biopsy is preferred. It may leave mild mechanically elicited sensory symptoms for approximately a year, but recovery via collateral sprouting appears to be good and no different from that in patients without diabetes. Other alternatives include skin biopsy, which allows an assessment of epidermal nerve fibre morphology. Neuropathological studies are extremely sensitive, as they can show a significant abnormality in the presence of entirely normal clinical and neurophysiological tests of neuropathy. Abnormalities may be observed in the myelinated or unmyelinated nerve fibres. Several stages of pathological change may be defined from the type and severity of damage.

Myelinated fibres

Studies in diabetic patients without evidence of neuropathy demonstrate demyelination without axonal loss or atrophy of the myelinated nerve fibres, suggesting that demyelination and hence involvement of the Schwann cell is primary. Patients with mild to moderate neuropathy demonstrate progressive demyelination, but with additional axonal degeneration and regeneration. Patients with established neuropathy demonstrate a mixture of both demyelination and axonal degeneration consistent with the observed reduction in nerve conduction velocity and amplitude.

A range of ultrastructural abnormalities of the Schwann cell have been described and include those that are:

- Reactive (accumulation of lipid droplets, pi, Reich and glycogen granules)
- Degenerative (mitochondrial enlargement, effacement of cristae, degeneration of abaxonal and adaxonal cytosol and organelles)
- Axonal atrophy, presumed secondary to ineffective axonal transport (This was considered to be a key feature of diabetic neuropathy, but recent studies have failed to confirm this abnormality.)

Loss of myelinated fibres correlating with reduced nerve conduction velocity and altered quantitative sensory testing

Unmyelinated fibres

Axonal degeneration with active regeneration occurs early in the evolution of neuropathy. Importantly, however, their regenerative capacity is maintained long after the myelinated fibres have lost their capacity to regenerate in severe neuropathy. Thermal thresholds have been related to the median unmyelinated axon diameter.

Pathological studies of autonomic tissue are limited and have not been adequately quantified. However, qualitative changes include chromatolysis, cytoplasmic vacuolization and pyknotic changes. Axonal degeneration and demyelination have been reported in a variety of biopsied tissues including preganglionic white rami communicantes, sympathetic chain, paravertebral and prevertebral autonomic ganglia, dorsal root ganglia, as well as more distal autonomic nerves such as the splanchnic, vagus and intramural nerves to the bladder and corpora cavernosa.

Pathogenesis

Risk factors for the development of neuropathy include:
- Diabetes duration, poor glycaemic control
- Deranged lipid profile and hypertension
- Height, age and smoking
- Haemorheological abnormalities (platelet activation, levels of fibrinogen)

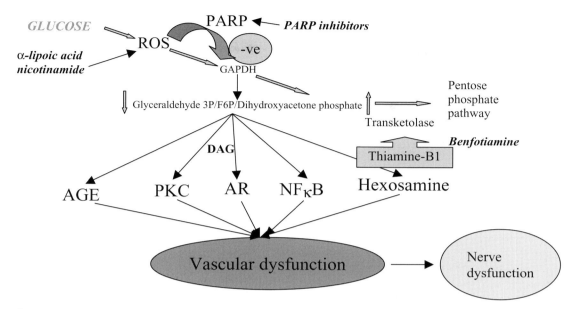

Figure 11.1 Possible mechanisms involved in the diversion of substrate (glucose) flux leading to diabetic neuropathy. Abbreviations: ROS: reactive oxygen species; PARP: poly(ADP-ribose) polymerase; DAG: diacylglycerol; AGE: advanced glycation end-product; PKC: protein kinase C; AR: aldose reductase; NF$\kappa\beta$; GADPH: glyceraldehyde-3-phosphate dehydrogenase. (See colour plate section.)

- Enhanced endothelial cell activation (von Willebrand factor, P-selectin, E-selectin and ICAM-1)

Studies in animal models and cultured cells provide a conceptual framework for the cause and treatment of diabetic neuropathy. It has been suggested that overproduction of superoxide by the mitochondrial electron transport chain partially inhibits glyceraldehyde-3-phosphate dehydrogenase, which diverts substrate flux from glycolysis to pathways of glucose over-utilization (Fig. 11.1). These latter pathways include increased polyol pathway flux, increased formation of advanced glycation end products (AGEs), activation of protein kinase C (PKC) and increased hexosamine pathway flux. Although preliminary experimental evidence *in vivo* suggests that this new paradigm provides a novel basis for research and drug development, limited translational work in diabetic patients continues to generate much debate and controversy over the relevance to human diabetic neuropathy.

Hyperglycaemia

In patients with impaired glucose tolerance (IGT), sural nerve amplitude and myelinated fibre density do not differ significantly from those found in individuals with normal glucose tolerance, suggesting a glycaemic threshold. However, 25% of patients with painful neuropathy and electrodiagnostic evidence of axonal injury and epidermal nerve fibre abnormalities have impaired glucose tolerance. In patients with established diabetes, longitudinal data have suggested that the duration and severity of exposure to hyperglycaemia are related to the severity of neuropathy. Improvement of glycaemic control improves neuropathy in type 1 but perhaps not type 2 diabetes.

Important downstream transducers of hyperglycaemia that may act as useful therapeutic targets to prevent nerve damage include:

- The polyol pathway

- Advanced glycation
- Cellular redox state and oxidative stress
- Intracellular diacylglycerol levels and enhanced protein kinase Cß activity
- Stress-activated protein kinases [ERK (extracellular signal-regulated kinase], JNK (c-Jun N-terminal kinase) and p38

Polyol pathway

Animal models consistently demonstrate an association between increased polyol pathway flux and a reduction in nerve conduction velocity (NCV), which can be ameliorated with aldose reductase inhibitors (ARIs).

$$D\text{-glucose} + NADPH + H^+ \xrightarrow{\text{aldose reductase}} Sorbitol + NADP^+$$

$$Sorbitol + NAD^+ \xrightarrow{\text{polyol dehydrogenase}} D\text{-fructose} + NADH + H^+$$

The potential role of the polyol pathway has been perhaps oversimplified and oversold. Certainly in diabetic patients, considerable heterogeneity has been observed in the level of polyol pathway metabolites. Type 2 diabetic patients, but not those with IGT, demonstrate an elevation in nerve sorbitol, suggestive of a glycaemic threshold for activation of this pathway. It would also appear that those at greatest risk of developing the complications are those with a higher set point for AR activity. This may be further modulated by the interaction with sorbitol dehydrogenase (SDH) expression. A meta-analysis of 19 randomised controlled trials of ARIs demonstrated a small but statistically significant reduction in decline of median and peroneal motor nerve conduction velocity without benefit in sensory nerves. Several other interventional studies suggest there may be a dose–response relationship between the degree of AR inhibition and nerve regeneration.

Glycation

The ubiquitous process of glycation occurs in nerve, retina, kidney and plasma protein of diabetic animals and induces a range of cellular and sub-cellular alterations that have far-reaching effects on tissue biology. Glycation may affect matrix metalloproteinases (MMPs), and tissue inhibitors of MMPs (TIMP-1 and -2) as well as transforming growth factor-β (TGF-ß). These have been shown to prevent epidermal growth factor–induced auto-phosphorylation and activation of extra-cellular signal-regulated kinases (ERKs). Sural nerves obtained from diabetic patients at amputation demonstrate significantly elevated pentosidine levels in both cytoskeletal and myelin protein. Pyrraline, an advanced glycation end product, is also increased in post-mortem samples of optic nerve from diabetic patients. The formation of AGEs can be limited by inhibitors, such as the nucleophilic compounds pyridoxamine, tenilsetam, 2,3-diaminophenazone and aminoguanidine. Additionally, recombinant RAGE may hinder the AGE–RAGE interaction.

Oxidative stress

An increasing body of data supports the role of oxidative stress in the pathogenesis of diabetic neuropathy in animal models. Whereas the evidence in patients is not so compelling, alpha-lipoic acid (LA), a powerful antioxidant that scavenges hydroxyl, superoxide and peroxyl radicals and regenerates glutathione has been shown to be beneficial.

Vascular factors

A large body of data implicates vascular disease in the pathogenesis of diabetic neuropathy. Large vessel revascularization improves both microvascular perfusion and nerve conduction velocity.

Pharmacological intervention with the ACE inhibitor trandalopril demonstrates an improvement in peroneal motor nerve conduction velocity, M-wave amplitude, F-wave latency and sural nerve amplitude.

Activation of PKCß induced by 1, 2-diacylglycerol (DAG) has been proposed to play a major role in diabetic neuropathy. Although a fall in DAG levels and a consistent pattern of change in PKC activity have not been observed in diabetic animal models, inhibition of PKCß in diabetic rats appears to correct reduced nerve blood flow and nerve conduction velocity. Phase II clinical trial data have demonstrated some benefit in diabetic neuropathy; multi-centre, randomized, double-blind, placebo-controlled trials to conclusively assess efficacy are currently underway.

An increasing body of evidence suggests that conventional risk factors for macrovascular disease, such as deranged lipids, are also important in the pathogenesis and progression of human diabetic neuropathy. Conventional wisdom suggests that HMG-CoA reductase inhibitors are beneficial principally by reducing levels of low-density-lipoprotein cholesterol. However, recent studies show that this class of compounds may have multiple benefits that are particularly relevant to diabetes-related complications; they can completely prevent AGE- and NF-$\kappa\beta$ induced protein-1 activation and up-regulation of VEGF mRNA in microvascular endothelial cells. Moreover, simvastatin has shown a trend towards slower progression of vibration perception threshold without a change in the status of clinical neuropathy.

Growth factors

Factors that may aid repair include:

- Nerve growth factor (NGF)
- Ciliary neurotrophic factor (CNTF)
- Neurotrophin-3 (NT-3)
- Brain-derived neurotrophic factor (BDNF)
- Insulin-like growth factor (IGF)
- C-Peptide
- Vascular endothelial growth factor
- Hedgehog proteins

Neurotrophins promote neuronal survival by inducing morphological differentiation, enhancing nerve regeneration and stimulating neurotransmitter expression. Although data implicating deranged neurotrophic support is compelling in animal models, data in diabetic patients are somewhat contradictory. Thus, whereas dermal NGF protein levels are reduced in diabetic patients with sensory fibre dysfunction, skin mRNA NGF and NT-3 are increased and sciatic nerve ciliary neurotrophic factor (CNTF) levels remain unchanged. Furthermore, *in situ* hybridization studies demonstrate increased expression of TrkA (NGF-receptor) and TrkC (NT-3 receptor) in the skin of diabetic patients. However, whilst a phase II clinical trial of recombinant human nerve growth factor demonstrated a significant improvement in neuropathy, a phase III trial failed to demonstrate a significant benefit. More recently brain-derived neurotrophic factor (rhBDNF) has demonstrated no significant improvement in nerve conduction, quantitative sensory and autonomic function tests, including the cutaneous axon reflex.

Insulin-like growth factors (IGFs)

In cultured Schwann cells and the STZ-diabetic rat, IGF-1 demonstrates a protective effect via PI 3-kinase in preventing glucose-mediated apoptosis. Both the STZ-diabetic and BB/W rat develop severe hyperglycaemia, a deficiency in circulating IGF-I levels and neuroaxonal dystrophy (NAD) in nerve terminals of the prevertebral sympathetic ganglia and the distal portions of noradrenergic ileal mesenteric nerves. In contrast, the Zucker diabetic fatty (ZDF) rat, an animal model of type 2 diabetes also develops severe hyperglycaemia comparable to that in the STZ- and BB/W diabetic rats. However, the ZDF rat maintains normal levels of plasma IGF-I and fails to demonstrate NAD in sympathetic ganglia and ileal mesenteric nerves as assessed by quantitative ultra-structural techniques. Furthermore, IGF I and IGF-I receptor mRNA levels are unaltered in the sural nerve of diabetic patients compared with control subjects.

C-Peptide

Impaired insulin/C-peptide action has emerged as a prominent pathogenetic factor. Pre-clinical studies have demonstrated a range of actions that include effects on Na(+)/K(+)-ATPase activity, endothelial nitric oxide synthase, expression of neurotrophic factors, regulation of molecular species underlying the degeneration of the nodal apparatus in type 1 diabetic nerves, as well as DNA binding of transcription factors and modulation of apoptotic phenomena. These findings have recently been effectively translated into benefits in patients with type 1 diabetes, with the demonstration of a significant improvement in sural sensory nerve conduction velocity and vibration perception but without a benefit in either cold or heat perception after 12 weeks of daily subcutaneous C-peptide treatment.

Vascular endothelial growth factor (VEGF)

VEGF was originally discovered as an endothelial-specific growth factor with a predominant role in angiogenesis. However, recent observations indicate that VEGF also has direct effects on neurons and glial cells stimulating their growth, survival and axonal outgrowth. Thus with its potential for a dual impact on both the vasculature and neurons, VEGF could represent an important therapeutic intervention in diabetic neuropathy. Both the STZ diabetic rat and the alloxan-induced diabetic rabbit have demonstrated restoration of nerve vascularity, blood flow and both large and small fibre dysfunction 4 weeks after intramuscular gene transfer of plasmid DNA encoding VEGF-1 or VEGF-2, with confirmed constitutive over-expression of both transgenes in tissue. In contrast, immunohistochemistry of sciatic nerves and dorsal root ganglia from STZ diabetic rats demonstrates intense VEGF staining in cell bodies and nerve fibres, whereas controls express no or very little VEGF and animals treated with insulin or NGF show significantly lower immunostaining for VEGF. Thus there is an intrinsic capacity to up-regulate VEGF, but this appears insufficient and may require exogenous delivery, possibly via gene ther-

apy. A phase I/II single-site dose escalating double-blind placebo-controlled study to evaluate the safety and impact of phVEGF165 gene transfer on sensory neuropathy in diabetic patients with or without macrovascular disease involving the lower extremities is currently under way and will involve 192 patients over a period of 4 years.

Hedgehog proteins

The hedgehog (sonic, desert and Indian) proteins were originally thought to principally modulate the development of the central and peripheral embryonic nervous system. However, it is now apparent that this family of proteins constitutes a major regulatory pathway for the maintenance, repair and regeneration of a number of tissues including nerve. mRNAs for desert hedgehog (dHh) and its receptor patched (ptc) are expressed in Schwann cells and perineurial mesenchyme, respectively. In dHh-/-mice, epineurial collagen is reduced, the perineurium is thin and disorganized with patchy basal lamina and perineurial tight junctions are abnormal. Recently, desert hedgehog mRNA was found to be significantly reduced in the nerve of STZ diabetic rats. Treatment with a sonic hedgehog–IgG fusion protein fully restored motor- and sensory-nerve conduction velocities and thermal hypoalgesia. This was associated with maintenance of axonal calibre of large myelinated fibres and a restoration of sciatic nerve growth factor, calcitonin gene–related product and neuropeptide Y.

Immune mechanisms

Studies suggest that sera from type 2 diabetic patients with neuropathy contain an autoimmune immunoglobulin that induces complement-independent, calcium-dependent apoptosis in neuronal cells. The expression of these cytotoxic factors has been related to the severity of neuropathy and the type of neuronal cell killed. Thus it has been suggested that such toxic factors may contribute to diabetic neuropathy by acting in concert with hyperglycaemia to damage sensory/autonomic neurons.

Painful neuropathy

Neuropathic pain is characterized by neuronal hyper-excitability in areas of neuronal damage that may be present in the peripheral nociceptor, dorsal root ganglia, ascending spinothalamic pathways and brain. A variety of intracellular and cell receptor changes occur and include abnormal expression of sodium channels, altered cellular influx of calcium, altered glutamate receptor expression and gamma-aminobutyric acid (GABA-ergic) inhibition, as well as N-methyl-D-aspartate (NMDA) receptor hypofunction (NRHypo). Additionally, peripheral nerve endings may exhibit abnormal spontaneous and increased evoked activity and central neuronal hyper-excitability, leading to spontaneous pain and allodynia. However, there is limited evidence that the spontaneous activity of A- and C-fibres is increased in diabetic neuropathy; in fact, the converse is true, as sensory input to the spinal cord is decreased. Spinal or supra-spinal modulation of sensory processing may be of prime importance, especially with the demonstration of spinal cord atrophy in diabetic neuropathy. Haemodynamic factors may also play an important role in the pathogenesis of neuropathic pain, as sural nerve epineurial blood flow has been found to be increased in those with painful neuropathy.

The effective treatment of patients with painful diabetic neuropathy represents a formidable therapeutic challenge to clinicians. Few of the currently prescribed treatments have a sound scientific basis and even fewer have been rigorously assessed in large studies to justify use in this era of evidence-based medicine.

Tricyclic drugs

Until new therapies are proven to relieve symptoms in appropriately designed trials, the tricyclic drugs, such as amitryptyline and imipramine, will remain the first-line agents for painful neuropathy. Their efficacy has been confirmed in several randomized, placebo-controlled trials. There is a clear dose-response relationship, but sedative and anticholinergic side effects are also dose-related and troublesome, often restricting the use of these drugs.

Anticonvulsants

Carbamazepine is widely used in the management of neuropathic pain. Its use is supported by some clinical trial data, although side effects limit its use in a proportion of patients. More recently, the new anticonvulsant gabapentin has been shown to be efficacious in the treatment of painful neuropathy, with adverse effects less pronounced than those associated with tricyclic therapy. Newer compounds such as pregabelin and topiramate have not proven to be as efficacious, with side effects limiting efficacy.

Other agents

A number of other drug therapies – including phenytoin, mexilitene, lidocaine and transdermal clonidine – have been reported to be useful in the management of painful or paraesthetic symptoms. Topical therapy with capsaicin relieves pain but does so by causing dermal nerve fibre degeneration and therefore is not recommended. Tramadol is a centrally acting analgesic, whose efficacy in painful neuropathy has been confirmed in a randomized controlled trial. Finally, traditional therapies such as acupuncture have also been employed in symptomatic neuropathy, with good results.

Autonomic neuropathy

Diabetic gastroparesis

This condition can be extremely difficult to treat and manage. The main treatment goal for gastroparesis related to diabetes is to regain control of blood glucose levels. Treatment may include insulin; oral medications to increase gastric motility, such as erythromycin and metoclopramide; changes in what and when the patient eats; and, in severe cases, tube or parenteral feeding.

It is important to note that in most cases treatment does not cure gastroparesis, as it is usually a chronic condition. Treatment is aimed at managing the symptoms.

Erectile dysfunction

Psychosexual counselling and altering drug therapy, to remove those associated with ED, is beneficial in many cases. The orally active phosphodiesterase (PDE) inhibitor sildenafil is efficacious for erectile dysfunction in diabetic males, with a response rate (defined as at least one successful attempt at sexual intercourse) of 61% in sildenafil-treated subjects versus 22% on placebo. More recently two newer agents, vardenafil and tadalafil, have become available. Both agents are more selective for PDE 5, the subtype found in greatest concentration in the smooth muscle of the corpus cavernosum; they have little or no impact on PDE 6, inhibition of which is responsible for the visual side effects associated with sildenafil. Most diabetic patients require the higher doses of these agents. Care must be taken if there is any history of ischaemic heart disease, and these agents must never be given to any patients on nitrate therapy. Older therapies include intracavernosal injections, alprostadil and vacuum devices.

Sweating disorders

The first specific treatment for gustatory sweating has been reported: Glycopyrrolate is an antimuscarinic compound that, when applied topically to the affected area, results in a marked reduction of sweating while the subject is eating "trigger" foods.

Late sequelae

Foot ulceration

Distal sensory and sympathetic neuropathies are the most important component causes leading to foot ulceration, being present in 78% of cases.

However, the neuropathic foot does not spontaneously ulcerate: it is the combination of neuropathy with other risk factors, such as deformity and unperceived trauma, that results in ulceration (Fig. 11.2). Clinical management of neuropathy emphasizes the importance of regular foot examination and education in self foot care.

Charcot neuroarthropathy

Charcot neuroarthropathy is a relatively rare but clinically important and potentially devastating disorder (Fig. 11.2). Permissive features for the development of a Charcot joint include:
- Sensorimotor neuropathy
- Sympathetic denervation in the foot
- Intact peripheral circulation
- Minor, often unperceived trauma

Thus, repetitive minor trauma causes bone fracture, which in turn induces osteoblastic activity stimulating the remodelling of bone. Treatment involves damage limitation with complete off-loading using an air-cast boot along with oral or intravaenous bisphosphonate therapy.

Summary

Diabetic neuropathy is the commonest and most costly long-term complication of diabetes. Focal/multifocal neuropathies occur in approximately 10% of all diabetic neuropathies; the remaining clinical presentation is that of a symmetrical sensory polyneuropathy that affects both somatic and autonomic systems. Autonomic neuropathy affects the cardiovascular, urogenital, gastrointestinal, thermoregulatory and sudomotor systems. Somatic abnormalities are associated with pain (~30%) and sensory loss, with foot ulceration (~5%) and amputation. The cause of diabetic neuropathy is not clearly understood, although multiple metabolic and vascular abnormalities mediated via hyperglycaemia have been proposed. At present there are no treatments to prevent or reverse nerve damage. Symptomatic treatment is available for painful

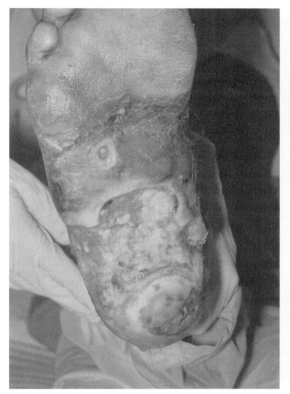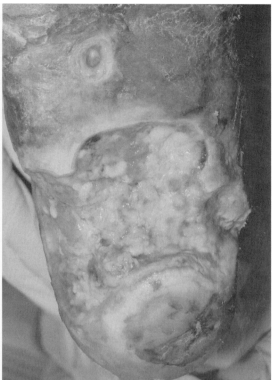

Figure 11.2 Plantar ulceration with necrosis. (See colour plate section.)

symptoms but is limited by side effects of the drugs used.

Clinical scenarios

Scenario 1

A 50-year-old man with type 1 diabetes and acute onset pain and swelling in the right calf is admitted to a university teaching hospital following a referral from his general practitioner.

Examination of his lower limbs demonstrates a tender (10 by 15 cm) swelling over the postero-medial aspect of the right calf (circumference, 53 cm; left calf, 40 cm).

Other results are as follows: sodium, 140 mmol/l (132 to 144); potassium, 4.8 mmol/l (3.5 to 5.5); urea, 15.1 mmol/l (3.5 to 7.4); creatinine, 210 μmol/l (0 to 110); ESR, 58 (0 to 5); CRP < 3; creatine kinase, 1080 U/l (0 to 190).

MRI (Fig. 11.3) demonstrates an extensive high signal abnormality on the T2 weighted sequence throughout the medial head of the gastrocnemius muscle and surrounding adjacent tissue planes. The appearance was that of a gross myositis with oedema and haemorrhage in and around the muscle. No abscess was identified, but there were areas of heterogeneity that may have represented muscle necrosis or focal haemorrhage.

The biopsy (Fig. 11.4) contained inflamed skeletal muscle with a severe active chronic inflammatory

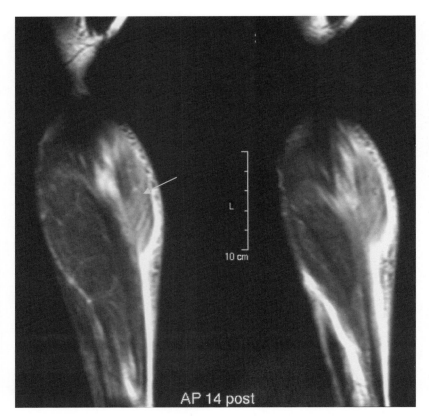

Figure 11.3 MR axial fat-suppressed T2-weighted turbo spin-echo sagittal sequences performed through the right calf demonstrating an extensive high signal abnormality throughout the medial head of the gastrocnemius muscle (→) and adjacent tissue with normal lateral head. (See colour plate section.)

cell infiltrate present between individual myocytes showing varying degrees of necrosis, characterized by loss of cross striations and nuclei together with fragmentation. Cellular debris, including nuclear dust, was associated with the infiltrate. No granulomas or micro-organisms were identified.

Questions

1. What is the differential diagnosis for the calf swelling?

2. Give an explanation for each of the results in bold.
3. What investigations would you perform?
4. What is the diagnosis and management?

Answers

1. The differential diagnosis of a swelling in the calf with inflammatory features includes neoplasia, infection, ischemia, trauma and vasculitis. Specifically one must consider deep venous thrombosis, ruptured Baker's cyst, acute exertional

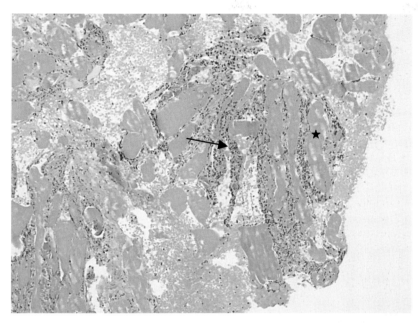

Figure 11.4 Inflamed skeletal muscle with a severe active chronic inflammatory cell infiltrate (→) between individual myocytes showing varying degrees of necrosis (·) characterized by loss of cross striations and nuclei together with fragmentation (H&E, ×100). (See colour plate section.)

compartment syndrome, muscle rupture, soft tissue abscess, haematoma, sarcoma, inflammatory or calcifying myositis and pyomyositis.

2. Raised urea/creatinine indicates impaired renal function (diabetic nephropathy/partial rhabdomyolysis/necrosis). Raised ESR indicates inflammation, myositis. Raised CK indicates myositis, skeletal muscle infarction, silent myocardial infarction.
3. Ultrasound calf, ECG, MRI, CT-guided biopsy for histology.
4. See below.

Treatment

The treatment of diabetic muscle infarction is supportive and usually includes the administration of analgesics and short-term immobilization of the involved leg. The short-term prognosis is excellent because the symptoms resolve spontaneously over weeks to months. However, contra-lateral or recurrent lesions may develop in almost half of such patients. Classically rhabdomyolysis accounts for 5% to 15% of cases with acute renal failure (acute tubular necrosis), the mechanism being myoglobin overload, hypovolemia and acidosis associated with creatinine kinase >16 000 U/l. In this case with the occurrence of skeletal muscle necrosis, one must consider a minor contributory role of this mechanism leading to decreased afferent renal blood flow and partial renal tubular obstruction.

Scenario 2

A 54-year-old man with type 2 diabetes is admitted to the renal unit with a 3-day history of nausea/

vomiting and deterioration in renal function. At presentation, the patient appears to be alert but slightly dehydrated. Physical examination reveals the following: weight, 94 kg; blood pressure,118/62 mm Hg supine and 96/50 standing; heart rate, 55 beats per minute and regular.

Other results are as follows: sodium, 140 mmol/l (132 to 144); potassium, 5.3 mmol/l (3.5 to 5.5); urea, 34.5 mmol/l (3.5 to 7.4); creatinine, 477 μmol/l (0 to 110); urine protein, 4.17 g/24 h; Hb, 10.9 g/dl (13 to 18); MCV, 88 fl (80 to 97); WBC, 7.9 x 10^9/l (4 to 11); platelets 170 x 10^9/l; C3, 0.98 g/l (0.62 to 1.6); C4, 0.21 g/l (0.14 to 0.39); IgG, 12.2 g/l (5.9 to 15.6); IgA, 3.9 g/l (0.6 to 5.0); IgM, 2.0 g/l (0.4 to 2.3); electrophoresis normal; ANCA negative; antibody to GBM, 1 U (<30); rheumatoid factor, <8 IU (<8); ANA, ve.

Questions

1. What is the differential for the nausea and vomiting?
2. What is the reason for the raised creatinine and 24-h urine protein?
3. Why were the immunology tests performed and what is their significance?
4. Give a differential for the low Hb.

Answers

1. Gastritis, gastroparesis diabeticorum, gastric/duodenal ulceration.
2. The deterioration in renal function was attributed to the prolonged episode of nausea and vomiting, with resultant hypotension evidenced by the significant postural hypotension on admission. This led to pre-renal decompensation of established renal impairment secondary to diabetic nephropathy.
3. To exclude other causes of renal impairment, consider pre-renal hypovolemia, hypotension secondary to constant vomiting, renal-diabetic nephropathy, glomerulonephritis, myeloma, post-renal renal stones, diabetic cystopathy.

4. Iron deficiency, B12 deficiency, folate deficiency or combination secondary to CRF, upper/lower GI bleed.

Questions

1. Diabetic neuropathy is associated with
   a. Smoking
   b. High LDL
   c. Hypertension
   d. Height
   e. Hypoglycaemia
2. Diabetic amyotrophy is
   a. A myopathy
   b. Responds to improvement in glycaemic control
   c. Responds to high-dose steroids
   d. Is due to a vasculitis
   e. Occurs primarily in type 2 diabetes
3. Painful neuropathy
   a. Responds to acupuncture
   b. Responds to gabapentin
   c. Is a good marker of neuropathic severity
   d. Responds to reduction in flux of glucose levels
   e. Occurs in 20% to 30% of diabetic patients
4. Of the mononeuropathies
   a. Median nerve compression occurs in 30% of diabetic patients
   b. Abducens nerve palsy is the commonest ocular palsy
   c. Ulnar nerve compression responds to transposition
   d. They improve with an improvement in glycaemic control
   e. They are associated with retinopathy
5. The neuropathological features of human diabetic neuropathy include
   a. Axonal atrophy
   b. Demyelination
   c. Axo-glial dysjunction
   d. Apoptosis
   e. Basement membrane thickening

Answers

1: a, T; b, T; c, T; d, F; e, T
2: a, F; b, F; c, T; d, T; e, T
3: a, T; b, T; c, F; d, T; e, T
4: a, T; b, F; c, T; d, F; e, F
5: a, F; b, T; c, F; d, T; e, T

REFERENCES AND FURTHER READING

UKPDS (1990). Intensive blood glucose control with sulpho-nylureas or insulin compared with conventional treat-ment and risk of complications in patients with Type 2 diabetes. *Lancet* **352,** 837–53

Diabetes Control and Complications Trial. (1995). Effect of intensive therapy on the development and progression of diabetic nephropathy in the Diabetes Control and Complications Trial. *Kidney Int* **47,** 1703–20.

Websites

Diabetes UK: www.diabetes.org.uk.
American Diabetes association: www.diabetes.org.

12

Renal cell carcinoma

Wasat Mansoor

Introduction

Overall, approximately 1.5% of males and 2.5% of females in the UK population are living with a diagnosis of cancer. These proportions increase steeply with age, with approximately 7.5% of people 65 years of age or above living with a diagnosis of cancer. Of the individual cancers, by far the highest prevalence (almost 1%) is seen for breast cancer in females and lung cancer in males (Forman *et al.*, 2003).

The mainstay of oncology treatment has remained unchanged for many tumour types over the last half century. Surgery continues to be the first line of therapy and often the only chance of cure for most patients. Radiotherapy and chemotherapy are generally palliative and mostly used as second-line modalities when surgery is not an option. Although the range and benefit of chemotherapeutic agents has increased over the last 50 years, they have continued, in general, to remain cytotoxic not only to tumour cells but also healthy cells, which leads to significant morbidity and mortality. Ultimately, this has limited the dose intensity and frequency of chemotherapy and hence the efficacy of cancer therapy. Traditionally, responses have been partial, often disappointingly brief and unpredictable, which has led to a growing body of interest in novel strategies to treat cancer.

The immunogenic nature of leukaemia and lymphoma is now accepted; hence immune therapies have become accepted therapies over the last decade. The establishment of similar treatment modalities for solid malignancies has, however, proven to be more difficult. The initial observation of the potential anti-cancer activity of the immune system against solid malignancies was made by William Coley in the 1890s, when he injected streptococcal toxin in the locality of a tumour and successfully observed clinical responses by stimulating local inflammation (Coley, 1893). Since these early days, our knowledge of the immune system and how to manipulate it has increased greatly, so that some 'immune therapies' have now firmly established themselves as standard cancer treatments while others are being developed as promising future therapies. This understanding has been complemented by a growing knowledge in other fields, such as molecular biology and gene transfer technology (see Chapter 1).

Renal cancer provides an exemplar of a cancer that had proven difficult to treat in the past, as standard cytotoxic therapies were found to be ineffective. However, with the realisation that renal cancer alters the immune system, the focus of treatment has changed to harnessing the immune system to effectively treat this particular tumour.

Renal cell cancer

Incidence

The incidence of renal cancer accounts for 2% of all cancers in the UK. There are approximately 5000 new cases annually, with a slight male preponderance, and the peak incidence is in the sixth and seventh decades.

Aetiology

Renal cancer is associated with smoking, chronic renal dialysis and obesity. Although only a small proportion of patients have affected family members, the risk is increased four-fold in first-degree relatives of patients. It is also commonly associated with Von Hippel–Lindau syndrome (characterised by cerebellar or retinal haemangioblastomas and an association with phaeochromocytoma). Recent research has shown that the von Hippel–Lindau gene (on chromosome 3q) is a classical tumour-suppressor gene whose inactivation leads to tumour development.

Clinical presentation

Renal cell carcinoma (RCC) commonly remains clinically occult; the classical triad of haematuria with flank pain and mass is uncommon (10%) and indicative of advanced disease. Approximately 25% to 30% of patients are asymptomatic, and their RCCs are found on incidental radiologic study.

The most common presentations are:
- Haematuria (50%)
- Flank pain (35%)
- A palpable mass in the flank or abdomen (25%)
    Other signs and symptoms include:
- Weight loss (33%)
- Fever (20%)
- Hypertension (20%)
- Hypocalcaemia (5%)
- Night sweats
- Malaise
- Varicocele, usually left-sided, due to obstruction of the testicular vein (2% of males)

Renal cell carcinoma is a unique and challenging tumour because of the frequent occurrence of paraneoplastic syndromes, including hypercalcaemia, erythrocytosis and non-metastatic hepatic dysfunction (i.e. Stauffer syndrome). Polyneuromyopathy, amyloidosis, anaemia, fever, cachexia, weight loss, dermatomyositis, increased erythrocyte sedimentation rate and hypertension may also be associated with RCC. These symptoms are believed to have an immune basis, where cytokine release by the tumour (e.g. IL-6, erythropoietin, nitric oxide) causes these paraneoplastic conditions. Resolution of symptoms or biochemical abnormalities frequently follows successful treatment of the primary tumour or metastatic foci.

Physical examination

This may reveal:
- Gross haematuria
- Look for hypertension, supraclavicular adenopathy and flank or abdominal mass with bruit.
- Approximately 30% of patients with renal carcinoma present with metastatic disease. Physical examination should include thorough evaluation for metastatic disease. Organs involved include:
    - Lung (75%)
    - Soft tissues (36%)
    - Bone (20%)
    - Liver (18%)
    - Cutaneous sites (8%)
    - Central nervous system (8%)

Histopathology

Renal cell carcinoma has five histological subtypes: clear cell (75%), chromophilic (15%), chromophobic (5%), oncocytoma (3%) and collecting duct (2%).
- Unusually, clear cells with a cytoplasm rich in lipids and glycogen characterize clear cell carcinoma, which is most likely to show 3p deletion (von Hippel–Lindau mutation).
- Chromophilic tumours tend to be bilateral and multifocal and may have trisomy 7 and/or trisomy 17.
- Large polygonal cells with pale reticular cytoplasm characterize chromophobic carcinoma, which does not exhibit 3p deletion.
- Renal oncocytoma consists predominantly of eosinophilic cells in a characteristic nested or

organoid pattern; it rarely metastasises and does not exhibit 3p deletion or trisomy 7 or 17.

- Collecting duct carcinoma is characterised by a very aggressive clinical course. This may present with local or widespread advanced disease. These cells can have three different types of growth patterns: (1) acinar, (2) sarcomatoid and (3) tubulopapillary. The sarcomatoid variant, which can occur with any histologic cell type, is associated with a significantly poorer prognosis.

Treatment

The treatment options for renal cell cancer are surgery, radiation therapy, chemotherapy, hormonal therapy, immunotherapy or combinations of these.

Surgery

Surgical resection remains the only known effective treatment for localized RCC, and it is also used for palliation in metastatic disease.

Radical nephrectomy remains the most commonly performed standard surgical procedure for treatment of localized renal carcinoma. It involves complete removal of the Gerota fascia and its contents, including resection of the kidney, perirenal fat and ipsilateral adrenal gland, with or without ipsilateral lymph node dissection. Radical nephrectomy provides a better surgical margin than simple removal of the kidney because perinephric fat may be involved in some patients. About 20% to 30% of patients with clinically localized disease develop metastatic disease after nephrectomy. Some surgeons believe that the adrenal gland should not be removed because of the low probability of ipsilateral adrenal metastasis and the morbidity associated with adrenalectomy. In the absence of distant metastatic disease with locally extensive and invasive tumours, adjacent structures such as bowel, spleen or psoas muscle may be excised en bloc during radical nephrectomy. Lymph nodes may be involved in 10% to 25% of patients. The 5-year survival rate in patients with regional node involvement is substantially lower than that in patients

with stage I or II disease. Regional lymphadenectomy adds little in terms of operative time or risk and should be included in conjunction with radical nephrectomy.

Approximately 5% of patients with RCC have inferior vena caval involvement. Tumour invasion of the renal vein and inferior vena cava usually occurs as a well-vascularized thrombus covered with its own intimal surface. In patients with renal vein involvement without metastases, radical nephrectomy is performed with early ligation of the renal artery but no manipulation of the renal vein. If the inferior vena cava is involved, then vascular control of the inferior vena cava is obtained both above and below the tumour thrombus and the thrombus is resected intact, with subsequent closure of the vena cava. Patients with actual invasion of the inferior vena caval wall have a poor prognosis despite aggressive surgical approaches.

At least three common approaches exist for the removal of kidney cancer: (1) the transperitoneal approach, (2) the flank approach and (3) the thoracoabdominal approach. The approach depends on tumour location and size and the body habitus of the patient. The thoracoabdominal approach offers the advantage of palpation of the ipsilateral lung cavity and mediastinum as well as the ability to resect solitary pulmonary metastases.

Laparoscopic nephrectomy is a less invasive procedure, incurs less morbidity and is associated with shorter recovery time and less blood loss. The need for pain medications is reduced, but operating room time and costs are higher. Disadvantages include concerns about spillage and technical difficulties in defining surgical margins. Laparoscopic partial nephrectomy can be considered at centres with experience in this procedure for early-stage renal cell cancer.

About 25% to 30% of patients have metastatic disease at diagnosis; fewer than 5% have solitary metastasis. Surgical resection is recommended in selected patients with metastatic renal carcinoma. This procedure may not be curative in all patients but may produce some long-term survivors. The possibility of disease-free survival increases after resection of the primary tumour and isolated excision of metastasis.

Chemotherapy

Options for chemotherapy and endocrine-based approaches are limited, and no hormonal or chemotherapeutic regimen is accepted as a standard of care. Objective response rates, either for single or combination chemotherapy, are usually lower than 15%.

Floxuridine [5-fluoro 2′-deoxyuridine 9FUDR)], 5-fluorouracil (5-FU) and vinblastine, paclitaxel (Taxol), carboplatin, ifosfamide, gemcitabine and anthracycline (doxorubicin) have been used. Floxuridine infusion has a mean response rate of 12%, while vinblastine infusion yields an overall response rate of 7%. 5-FU alone has a response rate of 10%, but when used in combination with interferon has shown a 19% response rate in some studies.

Renal cell carcinoma is refractory to most chemotherapeutic agents because of multi-drug resistance mediated by P-glycoprotein. Normal renal proximal tubules and RCC both express high levels of P-glycoprotein. Calcium channel blockers or other drugs that interfere with the function of P-glycoprotein can diminish resistance to vinblastine and anthracycline in human RCC cell lines.

Endocrine treatments have evolved from multiple studies using megestrol (Megace) in the treatment of RCC. No benefit has been shown except for appetite stimulation; therefore, megestrol currently is not recommended. Anti-estrogens such as tamoxifen (100 mg/m^2 per day or more) and toremifene (300 mg/day) have also been tried, with a response rate as low as that of most other chemotherapeutic agents.

Radiation

Radiation therapy may be considered as the primary therapy for palliation in patients whose clinical condition precludes surgery, either because of extensive disease or poor overall condition. However, it is now accepted that preoperative radiation therapy yields no survival advantage. Furthermore, controversies also exist concerning postoperative radiation therapy, but it may be considered in patients with perinephric fat extension, adrenal invasion or involved margins. A dose of 4 500 cGy is delivered, with consideration of a boost. Palliative radiation therapy is often used for local or symptomatic metastatic disease, such as painful osseous lesions or brain metastases, to halt potential neurological progression. Surgery should also be considered for solitary brain or spine lesions, followed by postoperative radiotherapy. About 11% of patients develop brain metastasis during the course of illness. Although RCC is a radioresistant tumour, radiation treatment of brain metastasis has been show to improve quality of life, local control and overall survival duration. Patients with untreated brain metastasis have a median survival time of 1 month, which can be improved with glucocorticoid therapy and brain irradiation. Stereotactic radiosurgery is more effective than surgical extirpation for local disease.

Immune therapies

Renal cell carcinoma is an immunogenic tumour, and spontaneous regressions believed to be immune-regulated have been documented. An increased understanding of the immune system and improved methodology in isolating and utilising immune agents has opened up some very promising avenues in the treatment of renal cell cancer and many other cancers. Many immune modulators have been tried, such as the following:

- Interferon
- IL-2 [aldesleukin (Proleukin)]
- Bacille Calmette–Guérin (BCG) vaccination
- Lymphokine-activated killer (LAK) cells plus IL-2
- Tumour-infiltrating lymphocytes
- Nonmyeloablative allogeneic peripheral blood stem-cell transplantation

The rationale for trying such therapies is better understood by first understanding certain basic principles of immunology.

The immune system–cancer interface: the basics of immunology

Initiation of a specific immune response

The immune system can be grossly divided into the innate and adaptive immune systems. In brief, the innate immune system is regarded as non-specific and forms a primary mechanism of protection against many pathogens (Medzhitov and Janeway, 2000). This includes the following:

- Anatomic barriers such as skin and mucous membranes
- Physiological barriers – e.g. acidic pH of stomach or chemical mediators such as lysozyme, which is cleaved from cells to cleave bacterial walls
- Phagocytic barriers – e.g. various cells (neutrophils, macrophages) that can internalise (phagacytose) whole micro-organisms
- Inflammatory barriers, where tissue damage induces leakage of fluid with anti-bacterial activity (Medzhitov & Janeway, 2000)

For the purposes of this chapter, the acquired immune system is of major interest, as it is believed to play an important role in the eradication of cancer. The acquired immune system specifically recognises, memorises and selectively eliminates foreign antigens. The generation of an effective immune response relies on two major groups of cells: lymphocytes and antigen-presenting cells (APCs). The two main populations of lymphocytes are B lymphocytes (B cells) and T lymphocytes (T cells). The acquired immune response can be divided into 'humoral' and 'cell-mediated' responses. The humoral response involves interaction of B cells with antigen and their subsequent proliferation and differentiation into antibody-secreting plasma cells. Cell-mediated immunity involves the activation of T cells. Although the humoral immune system may play a role in the generation of an anti-tumour immune response, several studies have demonstrated that T cells have a critical role in achieving tumour rejection (Golumbek *et al.*, 1991; Dranoff *et al.*, 1993). For this reason, much research regarding cancer immune therapies has focused on the manipulation of T cells.

T lymphocytes

Haematopoietic stem cells differentiate to become lymphoid stem cells, which then differentiate into T and B cells. However, unlike B cells, which mature in the bone marrow, immigrant stem cells migrate to the thymus gland to mature into T cells. There are two well-defined sub-populations of T cells: T-helper cells (Th cells) and cytotoxic T cells (CTLs). These T cells can be distinguished from one another by the presence of the membrane glycoproteins CD4 and CD8 (Fig. 12.1). Th cells generally display CD4 and are therefore often referred to as CD4+ T cells. Likewise, CTLs generally display surface CD8 and are therefore referred to as CD8+ cells.

The T-cell receptor

All T cells express the T-cell receptor (TCR) on their surface, which is a membrane-bound molecule composed of two disulfide-linked proteins referred to as α and β chains (Fig. 12.2). The function of the TCR is to recognise antigen presented to it on a platform referred to as the major histocompatibility complex (MHC). Where the peptide originates from a 'non-self' antigen, it will signal the T cell to eradicate any cells expressing this antigen. If the antigen is recognised as 'self', as might be the case with cancers, the T cell will go in to a state of reversible unresponsiveness referred to as anergy (Schultze *et al.*, 1996). The signalling is done through an integral part of the TCR called the CD3 complex (see Fig. 12.1). This is an associated complex of transmembrane polypeptides found mainly on the interior surface of the plasma membrane. The TCR (α and β chains) is non-covalently linked to the CD3 complex (see Fig. 12.1).

MHC restriction and the T-cell receptor

For a T cell to respond to a particular antigen, the antigen must be broken down and presented to the TCR in the form of a peptide presented in association with a major histocompatibility complex (MHC)

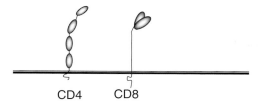

Figure 12.1 CD4 and CD8 structures. CD4 is a 428 amino acid protein. These are distributed into segments: 372 amino acid extra-cellular segment, 23 amino acid transmembrane segment and a 33 amino acid cytoplasmic segment. The extracellular region of the CD4 protein is a single-chain molecule that is made up of four tandemly arranged immunoglobin-like domains (D1 to D4). The D1 domain binds to MHC class II molecules. The CD8 structure comprises an α and β subunit. Both consists of an NH2 terminal domain homologous to Ig variable domains and a short 'hinge' region connecting the Ig-like domain to a membrane spanning region.

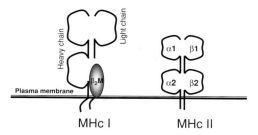

Figure 12.3 MHC class I and II. MHC class I molecules consist of three non-covalently associated components: a 45kDa heavy chain (HC), a 12-kDa light chain and a β2-microglobulin (β2-M) and a shor peptide antigen. The HC presents processed antigen peptide of 8 to 12 amino acids along to the TCR and has a binding site for the CD8 molecule (found on the T-cell surface). β2-M plays an important role in keeping the conformational shape of the extra cellular regions of the HC. The MHC class II molecule is comprised of an α and β chain which are associated with a third protein referred to as the invariant chain which stabilises the structure.

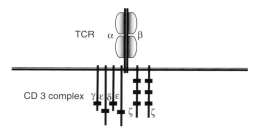

Figure 12.2 The T-cell receptor. The T-cell receptor is a membrane bound molecule composed of two disulfide-linked proteins referred to as α and β chains, which make contact with specific peptide-MHC ligands. The TCR (α and β chains) is non-covalently linked to the CD3 molecule, which consists of one molecule of invariant CD3 polypeptide chains γ and δ, two molecules of CD3ε and the disolplude linked ζ-ζ dimer. The intracellular potions of the CD3 γ, δ, ε and ζ subunits contain copies of immunoreceptor tyrosinc-based activation motifs (ITAMs). These serve as protein tyrosine kinase(PTK) subunits and are involved in initiating the TCR signalling. Each of the CD3 chains, except ζ, contain one ITAM, whereas each CD3-ζ contains three.

molecule. MHC molecules can be broadly divided into two classes, which are numbered I and II (Fig. 12.3). Both MHC classes are involved in antigen presentation. MHC class I molecules are generally expressed by the vast majority of nucleated cells and would therefore be expected to be found on cancers. MHC class I molecules allow circulating CD8[+] T cells to survey them for possible infection or improper protein expression, such as may be seen during tumour genesis. MHC class I molecules tend to present peptide antigens derived from endogenously synthesised proteins (Reits *et al.*, 2000). There is good evidence that cancers down-regulate their MHC or express faulty MHC that cannot present antigen properly, effectively making the T cells blind to the presence of cancer. MHC class II molecules are found mainly on the surface of APCs such as dendritic cells, monocytes, B cells and macrophages. These molecules tend to present exogenous peptide antigens to CD4[+] T cells (Cresswell *et al.*, 2005). The structure of MHC class I and II molecules are shown (see Fig. 12.3).

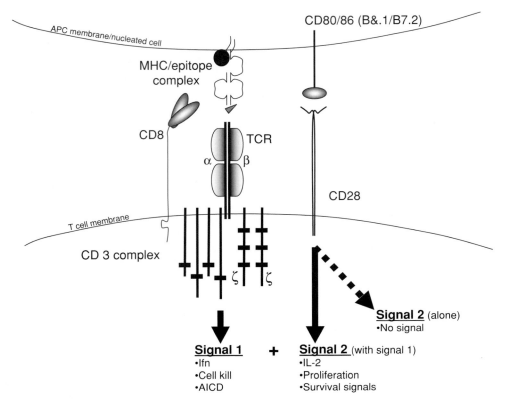

Figure 12.4 T-cell signalling. The T-cell receptor (TCR) comprising the α and β chains communicates with the MIC-eptitope complex of the antigen presenting cell. Presentation of a foreign ('non-self') epitope causes a conformational change in the TCR which activates the CD3 complex to initiate the primary activation signal referred to as signal 1; at the same time, interaction between the CD28 co-stimulatory molecule and its natural ligand CD80 or CD86 leads to co-stimulation (also referred to as signal 2). This leads to optimal activation of the T cell. In the absence of signal 1 (TCR and MIIC-epitope interaction), the CD80/CD86 and CD28 interaction does not lend to any signalling CD4 or CD8 (as shown) and enhance the TCR interaction with the MHC-epitope complex.

T-cell activation and co-stimulation

The activation of a T lymphocyte is initiated by a sig-nalling pathway originating from the TCR (see Fig. 12.4). This initial signal is referred to as the primary activation signal (signal 1e) (see Fig. 12.4). Confor-mational changes in the TCR and its associated CD3 molecule result in the activation of transcription fac-tors that control entry in the cell cycle from G0, reg-ulating expression of many cytokines that allow the cell to carry out its effector function. Two important effector functions include

1. The production of interferon γ
   • Upregulates MHC (makes cancer more visible)
   • Helps to co-ordinate an effective immune response
2. Target-cell kill (The target may be an invading organism or cancer.)

Importantly, activation when preceded by a strong TCR signal also results in the up-regulation of survival proteins that maintain the integrity and improve the survival of the cell, allowing it to carry out its function for a longer period. However, TCR occupancy in the absence of a strong MHC-peptide signal fails to generate an optimal T-cell response and may result in the induction of anergy, followed by premature cell death by up-regulation of pro-apoptotic proteins (Harding *et al.*, 1992). This process is also referred to as activation-induced cell death (AICD); it plays an important role in the evasion by tumours from the immune system and is discussed further on.

Optimal T-cell activation requires not only the primary activation signal but also the co-stimulatory signal, which is sometimes also referred to as signal 2 (see Fig. 12.4) (Boise *et al.*, 1995; Wulfing & Davis, 1998; Boonen *et al.*, 1999; Viola *et al.*, 1999). Co-stimulation is provided through surface receptors on the T cell referred to as co-stimulatory molecules. The most-documented and best-characterised of these molecules is the CD28 molecule, which is expressed by naïve and primed T cells (see Fig. 12.4). It is a 44-kDa glycoprotein, and its natural ligands are found on APCs. It binds with high affinity to B7–1 (CD80) and B7–2 (CD86), both of which are expressed on APCs only following appropriate stimulation (see Fig. 12.4). CD28 signalling in conjunction with the TCR binding to the MHC–epitope complex (signal 1) has been shown to:

- Increase IL-2 production by T cells. This is an important cytokine involved in T-cell survival, growth and proliferation. All these features can be suppressed by cancer.
- Induce up-regulation of anti-apoptotic proteins in the T cells to allow them to live longer in a suppressive cancer environment.
- Enhance T-cell proliferation.

Activation-induced cell death (AICD)

'Activation-induced cell death' (AICD) is the phrase used to describe the death of a T cell following activation through the TCR. It is an in vitro observation, which may play an important role in vivo as a mechanism to reduce the number of effector T cells in the periphery at the end of an immune response. If this mechanism were not set in place, unchecked proliferation of T cells can lead to malignant transformation or auto-immunity. In contrast, premature AICD can lead to ineffectual immunity.

It is now known that AICD can result from a number of insults at the molecular level. These insults can be intracellular (cytokine deprivation, genotoxic insult) or extra-cellular (e.g. binding of death receptors such as Fas ligand). Some or all these mechanisms may play an important role in evasion of the immune system by cancer.

How tumours evade the immune system

The treatment of RCC using our knowledge of the immune system

The rationale for using the therapies listed below is based on our understanding of the how the acquired immune system responds to pathogens. As our knowledge base increases, not only of the immune system but also of methods of isolating and/or growing the many different parts of the immune make-up, our repertoire of immune therapeutic agents is also increasing. New agents are then tested in pre-clinical and clinical trials for efficacy and safety. Some of the agents discussed are accepted therapies and others are still undergoing testing.

Interferon

The interferons are natural glycoproteins with antiviral, antiproliferative and immunomodulatory properties. They have a direct effect on the tumour itself as well as important immune modulatory effects, which include the following:

- Antiproliferative effects on renal tumour cells have been shown in vitro.
- Enhanced expression of MHC molecules – thus making the tumour a more 'visible' and better target for the immune system.

- Stimulation of host mononuclear cells including B cells (to enhance the humoral immune system), T cells and natural killer cells (involved in directly killing tumour cells).

Interferon α (IFN-α), which is derived from leukocytes, has an objective response rate of approximately 15% (range 0% to 29%). Preclinical studies have shown synergy between interferons and cytotoxic drugs. In several prospective randomized trials, combinations do not appear to provide major advantages over single-agent therapy. Many different types and preparations of interferons have been used without any difference in efficacy. In a small percentage of patients (about 2% to 5%), the tumour and its metastasis may disappear completely. However, this remission tends to be short-lived (2 to 6 months).

IL-2

A common observation in resected renal cell samples is the presence of large numbers of T cells that have migrated to the tumour. However, under influence of the tumour, the T cells become unresponsive (a state referred to as anergy).

In patients with cancer, the tumour microenvironment and general circulation are hostile to immune cells. This results in immune-mediated cell death and general immuno-compromise.

IL-2 is an activator of and growth factor for T cells. It affects tumour growth by activating lymphoid cells in vivo without affecting tumour proliferation directly. There are a number of ways in which these effects are desirable in the context treating renal cell cancer. That is, IL-2

1. Improves the survival of T cells by promoting the expression of anti-apoptotic proteins.
2. Has been shown to reverse the state of anergy so that the T cells can attack the tumour.
3. Promotes T-cell proliferation. The therapeutic T cells reacting to tumour are also stimulated to proliferate, thus improving their efficacy.

In the initial study by the National Cancer Institute, bolus intravenous infusions of high-dose IL-2 combined with T cells cultured ex vivo in IL-2 (LAK cells) produced objective response rates of 33% (Rosenberg *et al.*, 1985; Rosenberg, 2001). In subsequent multi-centre trials, the response rate was 16%. Subsequent studies also showed that LAK cells add no definite therapeutic benefit and can be eliminated from the treatment. A high-dose regimen (600 000 to 720 000 IU/kg q8h for a maximum of 14 doses) resulted in a 19% response rate, with 5% complete responses. The majority of responses to IL-2 were durable, with a median response duration of 20 months. Eighty percent of patients who responded completely to therapy with IL-2 were alive at 10 years (Rosenberg *et al.*, 1994a; Yang *et al.*, 2003).

Toxic effects associated with high-dose IL-2 are related to increased vascular permeability and secondary cytokine secretion (e.g. IL-1, interferon γ, tumour necrosis factor, nitric oxide). The management of high-dose IL-2 toxicities requires inpatient monitoring, often in an intensive care unit. The major toxic effect of high-dose IL-2 is a sepsis-like syndrome, which includes a progressive decrease in systemic vascular resistance and an associated decrease in intravascular volume due to capillary leak. Other toxic effects are fever, chills, fatigue, infection and hypotension. High-dose IL-2 has been associated with a 1% to 4% incidence of treatment-related death and should be offered only to patients with no cardiac ischaemia or significant impairment of renal or pulmonary function. Management is supportive and includes judicious use of fluids and vasopressor support to maintain blood pressure and intravascular volume as well as avoiding pulmonary toxicity due to non-cardiogenic pulmonary oedema from the capillary leak. This syndrome is normally reversible.

Vaccine therapy

Theoretically, RCC is a good tumour for which to develop vaccine therapy, and there are a number of reasons for this:

1. Renal cancer is immunogenic.
2. Renal cancer responds to immune therapy.

3. Renal cancer is well documented to express many tumour-associated antigens that can be used to target renal cancer.

Vaccine trials are in the early stages of development. One example of vaccine strategy is to utilise the discovery of a tumour antigen found to be expressed at high concentration on the surface of renal cancer; it is referred to as 5T4 (Southall *et al.*, 1990). This antigen was isolated from renal cancer cells and injected in combination with IL-2 into patients with metastatic renal cancer. The vaccine was shown to induce a strong immune response and is currently under further investigation. Other approaches to vaccination include tumour lysates and dendritic cells. Autologous vaccine therapy (inactivated whole tumour cells taken from the patient) is now being tried in combination with cytokine therapy (Pardoll, 1998).

Adopted T cells

T cells are arguably the most important arm of the immune system involved in the eradication of cancer. The advent of techniques to grow large numbers of tumour-infiltrating lymphocytes (TILs) from resected tumours has opened new avenues in the immune treatment of cancers. In early studies, the adoptive transfer of TILs in conjunction with IL-2 in patients who had previously progressed on standard therapies attained response rates of approximately 35%, which was twice the response rate with IL-2 alone (Rosenberg *et al.*, 1988; Rosenberg *et al.*, 1994b). To date, an important limiting factor in the development and wider use of such therapies has been a lack of expertise and resource in being able to isolate adequate numbers of the TILs and, in particular, the tumour-specific T cells that are the likely active part of this therapy. Furthermore, it has been possible to trial this treatment in only a select few tumour groups. A major limitation to the development of such therapy has been the limited number of tumours in which there is T-cell infiltrate in the first place. In fact, with the exception of renal cell cancer and melanoma, very few tumour types have

adequate numbers of T cells infiltrating them to be able to isolate and grow tumour-reactive T cells. Nevertheless, the encouraging experience with TILs and tumour-reactive T cells has led many researchers to develop other techniques to develop such cells. With an increased understanding of how T cells function combined with efficient gene transfer techniques and an ever-increasing list of tumour-associated antigens to act as potential targets, there has been considerable interest in developing 'designer T cells' that are artificially endowed with the ability to react specifically against tumours. These new methods have attempted to negate the need for isolating lymphocytes from tumours. Instead, PBLs can be modified *ex vivo* to make them tumour-specific before being re-infused into their cancer-bearing host. This can be done by either modifying the patient's lymphocytes to express T-cell receptors that are already reactive to the tumour or by generating a receptor with a tumour-recognition domain attached to a signalling domain that can mimic the function of a reactive T-cell receptor. These are referred to as chimeric immune receptors. Both these methodologies have opened up a potential to create a great number of T cells that can potentially react to any targetable tumour. Figures 12.5 and 12.6 demonstrate the chimeric immune receptor. Early trials using these modalities of therapy are currently under way. A summary of the types of adoptive T cells is shown (Fig. 12.7).

Stem-cell transplantation

Nonmyeloablative allogeneic stem-cell transplantation is another research approach. This can induce sustained regression of metastatic RCC in patients who have had no response to conventional immunotherapy. In one recent trial, 19 patients with refractory metastatic RCC who had suitable donors received a preparative regimen of cyclophosphamide and fludarabine, followed by an infusion of peripheral blood stem cells from a human leukocyte antigen (HLA)-identical sibling or a sibling with a mismatch of a single HLA antigen. Patients

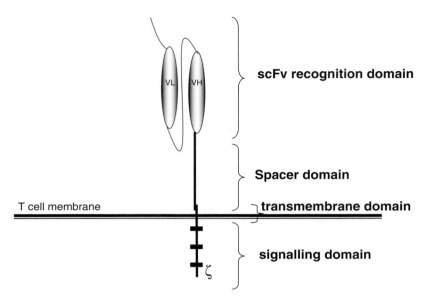

Figure 12.5 The structure of a chimeric immune recceptor (CIR). The CIR comprises a single chain variabie antibody recognition domain (seFv) which recognises cell surface antigen independent of MHC. This is intimately connected to the extra-cellular spacer domain and a transmembrane domain. This communicates distally with the intra-cellular signalling domain which is responsible for activating the T cell expressing the CIR on antigen binding.

with no response received as many as three infusions of donor lymphocytes. Two patients died of transplantation-related causes and 8 died from progressive disease. In 10 patients (53%), metastatic disease regressed; 3 patients had a complete response and 7 had a partial response. The durations of these responses continue to be assessed (Childs *et al.*, 2000). Further trials are needed to confirm these findings and evaluate long-term benefits.

Immune therapy in combination with surgery

Palliative nephrectomy should be considered in patients with metastatic disease for alleviation of symptoms such as pain, haemorrhage, malaise, hypercalcaemia, erythrocytosis or hypertension. Several randomized studies are now showing improved overall survival in patients presenting with metastatic kidney cancer who have nephrectomy followed by either interferon or IL-2 (Flanigan *et al.*, 2001). If the patient has good physiological status, then nephrectomy should be performed prior to immunotherapy. Reports have documented regression of metastatic RCC after removal of the primary tumour. Adjuvant nephrectomy is not recommended for inducing spontaneous regression; rather, it is performed to decrease symptoms or to decrease tumour burden for subsequent therapy in carefully controlled environments.

Multi-kinase inhibitors

The most recent therapeutic agents currently under development and clinical testing have shown considerable promise. These agents specifically target

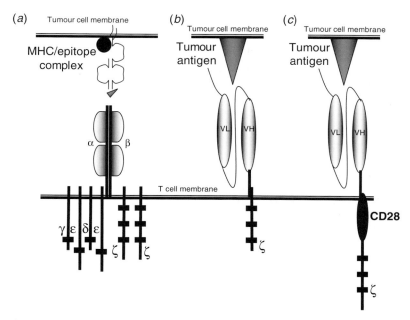

Figure 12.6 Types of chimeric immune receptor. (*a*) The T-cell receptor composed of the α and β chains transmits its signal through the CD3 molecule (γ, ε, δ and ζ moieties) following interaction with MHC/epitope complex. This differs from the chimeric immune receptors; (*b*) the 'classical receptor' is composed of an extracellular single chain antibody recognition domain connected to signalling moiety shown in this example as the CD3 ζ molecule. This is different from the (*c*) fusion receptor which differs from the 'classical receptor' because it expresses part of a co-stimulatory mlolecule (CD28 molecule) proximal to the ζ moiety in the signalling domain. Activation of either chimeric immune receptor can be initiated in the presence of tumour antigen in an MHC independent manner.

multiple pathways that drive the tumour cell growth. Furthermore, a major advantage of these drugs is that they are administrated orally.

Sorafenib targets serine/threonine and receptor tyrosine kinases, including those of receptor activation factor (RAF), vascular endothelial growth factor receptor-2,3 (VEGFR-2,3), platelet-derived growth factor recptor (PDGFR), KIT (receptor tyrosine kinase), FLT-3 and RET. On December 20, 2005, the US Food and Drug Administration (FDA) granted approval for sorafenib (Nexavar) for the treatment of patients with advanced RCC. This is a small molecule that targets two pathways by inhibiting Raf kinase and VEGF multi-receptor kinase. Sorafenib administration in context of metastatic renal cancer has been shown to improve progression-free survival in a large, multinational, randomised double-blind, placebo-controlled phase 3 study and a supportive phase 2 study. The sorafenib phase 3 study was conducted in 769 predominantly male (70%) patients (median age 59) with advanced (unresectable or metastatic) RCC who had received one prior systemic treatment. The median progression-free survival was 167 days in the sorafenib group

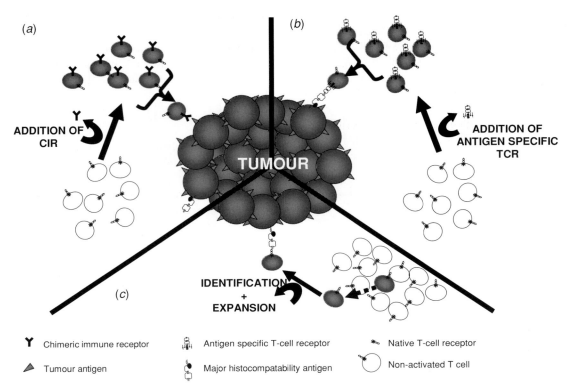

Figure 12.7 Generation of tumour antigen-specific T cells. Different strategies have been employed to endow T cells with the specificity and power to specifically kill tumours. Large numbers of host T cells can be modified to become tumour reactive by transducing them to express. (*a*) chimeric immune receptors or (*b*) tumour specific T-cell receptors using retroviral technology. (*c*) Tumour reactive T cells are identified and grown out of a population of tumour infiltrating lymphocytes. These cells are then expanded for use.

versus 84 days in the placebo control group (HR 0.44; 95% CI for HR: 0.35–0.55, *p* < 0.000001). Tumour response was determined in 672 patients; a partial response was shown in 7 (2%) on sorafenib versus 0 (0%) on placebo. Sorafenib toxicities (based on an updated phase 3 study database of 902 patients) included reversible skin rashes in 40% and hand-foot skin reactions in 30%. Diarrhoea (43%), hypertension (17%) and sensory neuropathy occurred in 13%. Alopecia, oral mucositis and haemorrhage were reported more commonly in the sorafenib arm.

Sunitinib is another multi-kinase inhibitor of VEGFR 1–3 and PDGFR and was approved by the FDA in January 2006 for the treatment of metastatic renal cancer that has become resistant to immunotherapy. This drug has shown high response rates (40% partial responses) and a median time to progression of 8.7 months, with an overall survival of 16.4 months. Major toxicities include fatigue (38%), diarrhoea (24%), nausea (19%), dyspepsia (16%), stomatitis (19%) and decline in cardiac ejection fraction (11%). Dermatitis occurred in 8% and hypertension in 5% of patients. A recent phase 3 study evaluating sunitinib in the first-line setting compared against interferon in patients with metastatic renal cancer demonstrated significant improvement in the response rates compared to the interferon arm.

The future

Future treatment strategies for advanced RCC will likely incorporate a combination of molecular approaches, using multi-drug regimens consisting of small-molecule kinase inhibitors with biological therapies and/or immunomodulatory therapies. A greater understanding and identification of the pathways driving these cancer cells to grow will increase the number of drugs available. The discovery of more tumour-associated antigens that define the tumour cells as different from healthy tissue also makes available more opportunities to target the tumour cells with novel agents such as vaccine and modified immune cells.

For early stage RCC, current and future treatment strategies would utilize these molecular approaches earlier in the adjuvant setting in order to improve overall survival rates.

Clinical scenario

A 55-year-old man with renal carcinoma underwent nephrectomy followed by high-dose (720 000 IU/kg intravenously every 8 h) IL-2 therapy. Within 30 min of commencing therapy, the patient became dyspnoeic, tachycardic (pulse, 130/min) and hypotensive (BP, 90/50).

What is the differential diagnosis?

Differential diagnosis:
- Myocardial infarction
- Pulmonary embolus
- Sepsis
- Cytokine storm

What investigations would you perform?

ECG, FBC, blood culture, U/Es.

ECG demonstrates sinus rhythm; Hb, 14.6; platelets, 360; WBC, 6.7; urea, 12; creatinine, 99.

What supportive measures are undertaken?

Resuscitate: give the patient intravenous crystalloid and dopamine to improve BP and urine output.

A repeat FBC 12 h later shows Hb,14.9; platelets, 34; WBC, 600.

What is the underlying cause of the deterioration?

Cytokine storm induced by interleukin-2 (IL-2). Although systemic IL-2 can induce complete or partial regression of renal cell cancer (RCC) metastases, in 15% to 20% of patients it is associated with a substantial toxicity, which limits its therapeutic usefulness. It appears to be mediated through pathways common to or distinct from those mediating its anticancer effects. The haematological toxicity induced by IL-2 (thrombocytopaenia and lymphopaenia) is paradoxically associated with increased frequency of clinical responses. The reversal of IL-2–induced toxicity by corticosteroid or anti–TNF-a antibodies blunts its therapeutic effects, suggesting a proinflammatory nature for this association.

Multiple-choice questions

1. Renal cancer
   a. presents with Pel-Ebstein fever.
   b. is resistant to standard cytotoxic chemotherapy due to the over-expression of tyrosine kinase.
   c. is most frequently metastatic to the liver.
   d. originating from the collecting duct is usually indolent.
   e. can be associated with haemangioblastoma.
2. Interferon therapy
   a. is the accepted standard treatment for metastatic renal cancer.
   b. may be given intravenously.
   c. up-regulates class I major histocompatibility complex (MHC) antigen.
   d. can rarely cause lethargy.

e. should be used in conjunction with cytotoxic chemotherapy.

3. IL-2 therapy
   a. directly affects the tumour cells.
   b. has a similar mechanism of action as interferon therapy.
   c. if given in high dose may cause remission of metastatic desease for more than 5 years.
   d. mainly results in non-specific T-cell proliferation.
   e. can cause anuria.

4. T cells
   a. extracted from renal cancers are active.
   b. are the major immune agents involved in tumour regression.
   c. in the unmodified form, require the presence of MHC to activate.
   d. proliferate in the presence of interferon.
   e. may cause autoimmunity in the presence of interferon and IL-2.

5. New developments is the treatment of renal cancer:
   a. are mainly oral drugs.
   b. have been shown to improve overall survival.
   c. have very few toxicities.
   d. have not been tested in phase III trials as yet.
   e. may target carcinoembryonic antigen.

Answers

1: a, F; b, F; c, F; d, F; e, T
2: a, T; b, F; c, T; d, F, e, F
3: a, F; b, F; c, T; d, T; e, T
4: a, F; b, T; c, T; d, F; e, T
5: a, F; b, F; c, F; d, F; e, F

REFERENCES AND FURTHER READING

Boise, L. H., Minn, A. J., Noel, P. J. *et al.* (1995). CD28 costimulation can promote T cell survival by enhancing the expression of Bcl-XL. *Immunity* **3**, 87–98.

Boonen, G. J., van Dijk, A. M., Verdonck, L. F. *et al.* (1999). CD28 induces cell cycle progression by IL-2-independent down-regulation of p27kip1 expression in human peripheral T lymphocytes. *European Journal of Immunology* **29**, 789–98.

Childs, R., Chernoff, A., Contentin, N., Bahceci, E. *et al.* (2000). Regression of metastatic renal-cell carcinoma after nonmyeloablative allogeneic peripheral-blood stem-cell transplantation. *New England Journal of Medicine* **343**, 750–8.

Coley, W. B. (1893). The treatment of malignant tumours by repeated inoculation of erysipelas: with a report of 10 original cases. *American Journal of Medical Science* **105**, 487–511.

Cresswell, P., Ackerman, A. L., Giodini, A. *et al.* (2005). Mechanisms of MHC class I–restricted antigen processing and cross-presentation. *Immunology Review* **207**, 145–57.

Dranoff, G., Jaffee, E., Lazenby, A. *et al.* (1993). Vaccination with irradiated tumor cells engineered to secrete murine granulocyte-macrophage colony-stimulating factor stimulates potent, specific, and long-lasting anti-tumor immunity. *Proceedings of the National Academy of Science of the United States of America* **90**, 3539–43.

Flanigan, R. C., Salmon, S. E., Blumenstein, B. A. *et al.* (2001). Nephrectomy followed by interferon alfa-2b compared with interferon alfa-2b alone for metastatic renal-cell cancer. *New England Journal of Medicine* **345**, 1655–9.

Forman, D., Stockton, D., Moller, H. *et al.* (2003). Cancer prevalence in the UK: results from the EUROPREVAL study. *Annals of Oncology* **14**, 648–54.

Golumbek, P. T., Lazenby, A. J., Levitsky, H. I. *et al.* (1991). Treatment of established renal cancer by tumor cells engineered to secrete interleukin-4. *Science* **254**, 713–6.

Harding, F. A., McArthur, J. G., Gross, J. A. *et al.* (1992). CD28-mediated signalling co-stimulates murine T cells and prevents induction of anergy in T-cell clones. *Nature* **356**, 607–9.

Medzhitov, R., Janeway, C., Jr. (2000). Innate immunity. *New England Journal of Medicine* **343**, 338–44.

Pardoll, D. M. (1998). Cancer vaccines. *Nature Medicine* **4**, 525–31.

Reits, E. A., Vos, J. C., Gromme, M., Neefjes, J. (2000). The major substrates for TAP in vivo are derived from newly synthesized proteins. *Nature* **404**, 774–8.

Rosenberg, S. A. (2001). Progress in human tumour immunology and immunotherapy. *Nature* **411**, 380–4.

Rosenberg, S. A., Lotze, M. T., Muul, L. M. *et al.* (1985). Observations on the systemic administration of autologous lymphokine-activated killer cells and recombinant interleukin-2 to patients with metastatic cancer. *New England Journal of Medicine* **313,** 1485–92.

Rosenberg, S. A., Packard, B. S., Aebersold, P. M. *et al.* (1988). Use of tumor-infiltrating lymphocytes and interleukin-2 in the immunotherapy of patients with metastatic melanoma. A preliminary report. *New England Journal of Medicine* **319,** 1676–80.

Rosenberg, S. A., Yang, J. C., Topalian, S. L. *et al.* (1994a). Treatment of 283 consecutive patients with metastatic melanoma or renal cell cancer using high-dose bolus interleukin 2. *Journal of the American Medical Association* **271,** 907–13.

Rosenberg, S. A., Yannelli, J. R., Yang, J. C. *et al.* (1994b). Treatment of patients with metastatic melanoma with autologous tumor-infiltrating lymphocytes and interleukin 2. *Journal of the National Cancer Institute* **86,** 1159–66.

Schultze, J., Nadler, L. M., Gribben, J. G. (1996). B7-mediated costimulation and the immune response. *Blood Review* **10,** 111–27.

Southall, P. J., Boxer, G. M., Bagshawe, K. D. *et al.* (1990). Immunohistological distribution of 5T4 antigen in normal and malignant tissues. *British Journal of Cancer*, **61,** 89–95.

Viola, A., Schroeder, S., Sakakibara, Y., Lanzavecchia, A. (1999). T lymphocyte costimulation mediated by reorganization of membrane microdomains. *Science* **283,** 680–2.

Wulfing, C., Davis, M. M. (1998). A receptor/cytoskeletal movement triggered by costimulation during T cell activation. *Science* **282,** 2266–9.

Yang, J. C., Sherry, R. M., Steinberg, S. M. *et al.* (2003). Randomized study of high-dose and low-dose interleukin-2 in patients with metastatic renal cancer. *Journal of Clinical Oncology* **21,** 3127–32.

13

Alcoholic liver disease

James Neuberger

Introduction

Alcohol has long been associated with the development of liver damage. The spectrum of liver damage induced by alcohol varies considerably, ranging from minimal changes to cirrhosis and alcoholic hepatitis, There exists considerable individual variation in susceptibility to the effects of alcohol in inducing liver damage. Those factors responsible for this variation remain poorly defined. Treatment remains largely supportive; abstinence is the most effective form of therapy.

Epidemiology of alcohol and alcoholic liver disease

Assessment of alcohol consumption is difficult and often unreliable. An approximate estimate of the consumption of alcohol can be obtained by dividing the amount of alcohol consumed by the population by the number of adults legally permitted to drink; this assumes that only legally sold alcohol is consumed and only adults consume alcohol; it ignores individual variations in alcohol consumption. There is great variation in the pattern of consumption; for example, in the United States, 50% of the alcohol consumed is accounted for by 10% of the drinking population. Overall about one-third of the population are light drinkers and one-third moderate to heavy drinkers; the rest are abstainers. Abstinence is more common among women than men and among older people of both sexes than among younger adults.

Younger people are more likely to drink over sensible limits, even though younger people are more familiar with the concepts of units of alcohol and levels of safe drinking,

Alcohol is associated with a variety of diseases and disorders (Table 13.1), but the greatest risk is alcoholic liver disease. Death rates due to cirrhosis are higher for men than women and higher for non-Whites than Whites. Alcohol also contributes to death by accidents, suicides and homicides. This is particularly marked in men below age 35. Indeed, alcohol is associated not only with half of all violent deaths but also with one-third of drownings and one-quarter of homicides, boating and aviation deaths. Alcohol misuse places a significant burden on resources in the UK, where it is estimated that there are around 1.2 million incidents of alcohol-related crime each year, costing the UK about £1.5 billion. Overall, around 11 million working days are lost each year in the UK from the effects of alcohol abuse, with costs of around £1.2 billion.

In 1998 to 1999 in England, there were 19 200 admissions to hospital for conditions associated with alcoholic liver disease and 78 900 admissions for mental and behavioural disorders associated with alcohol. Alcohol excess contributes to 27% of drug overdoses, 20% of head injuries, 17% of road accidents and 10% of gastrointestinal haemorrhages, The annual mortality in the UK attributed to alcohol is about 25 000, but estimates vary between 50 000 and 40 000; the annual incidence of alcoholic cirrhosis in the UK is about 10 per 100 000, and the mortality from alcoholic liver disease is about

Table 13.1 Extrahepatic manifestations of alcohol toxicity

System	Disease
Gastrointestinal tract	
Oesophagus	Reflux
	Oesophageal cancer
Stomach	Gastritis
	Gastric ulcer
Small intestine	Malabsorption
	Altered motor activity
Pancreas	Pancreatitis (acute and chronic)
	Carcinoma
Cardiovascular system	Congestive cardiomyopathy
	Hypertension
Central nervous system	Cerebellar degeneration
	Wernicke–Korsakoff syndrome
	Polyneuropathy
Muscle	Myopathy: acute/chronic
Haematological	Haemolysis
	Impaired cryothropoeisis
	Abnormal morphology: macrocytosis, triangulocytes
	Neutropenia
	Thrombocytopenia
Endocrinological/ metabolic	Hypogonadism
	Hyperoestrogenaemia
	Pseudo-Cushing's syndrome
	Hypoglycaemia
	Ketoacidosis
	Gout
	Osteopenia
Pregnancy	Fetal alcohol syndrome
	Increased risk of abortion and still birth

4 700 deaths per year (this figure is rising – from 2801 in 1988 to 4718 in 1999); about 600 deaths were attributed to alcohol toxicity, cardiomyopathy and dependence syndrome in 1999. Nonetheless, many studies have shown a consistent J-shaped association of alcohol intake with overall mortality. At higher levels of alcohol consumption, the increased mortality is due to increased risk of cancer, liver disease, cardiomyopathy and stroke. The reduced mortality is due to a reduction in deaths from coronary heart disease, possibly due to the beneficial effect of alcohol on HDL cholesterol (see below).

The financial cost in the UK of alcohol excess in 1999 was estimated to be £2 293 million, including £1 881 million to industry costs, £207 million to costs to the NHS and £73 million from criminal activities. This needs to be balanced against the tax revenue from alcoholic drink in 1999 of £11 237 million, representing 3.4% of the total tax revenue and consumer expenditure on alcoholic drinks in that year of £28 091 million.

Alcohol and the liver

It has long been recognised that there is a close relationship between the amount of alcohol consumed and alcoholic liver disease. There is a broad consensus that there is a 'safe-limit'; below 14 units per week for women and below 21 units per week for men, the risk of developing alcoholic liver disease is small. Above these limits, the risks rise proportionally. A study from Italy shows that alcoholic liver disease does not occur when the lifetime ingestion of alcohol is below 100 kg (equivalent to an average daily alcohol consumption of two glasses of wine (30 g alcohol). This Dionysos study also showed that above this limit, there is a linear increase in the risk of alcoholic liver disease with the amount of alcohol consumed, irrespective of the type of alcohol. However, the pattern of drinking was important, with those who drank alcohol outside mealtimes having a three- to fivefold increased risk of developing cirrhosis. Alcohol has many effects, and some, such as the effect on cardiovascular disease, may be beneficial.

Alcohol metabolism

Absorption

Ethanol is absorbed from the gastrointestinal tract by simple diffusion primarily from the duodenum and upper jejunum. The rate of absorption of ethanol is affected by the gastric emptying time and by the presence of the intestinal contents. Thus, in patients with gastroenterostomies, the rate of absorption is increased, whereas in the presence of food, absorption is reduced. Animal studies have suggested that carbohydrates, amino acids and peptides will enhance ethanol absorption. Alcohol given in a more concentrated form (as in whisky) has a greater rate of absorption than in a dilute form (as in beer or wine).

Distribution

Alcohol is relatively lipid-insoluble and is therefore distributed throughout the body, but relatively little is distributed in fat.

Excretion

The average man is able to excrete about 1g of alcohol per hour per 10 kg body weight. The rate of excretion varies considerably. Over 90% of alcohol is oxidised and secreted as carbon dioxide and water (see below). Smaller amounts of alcohol are eliminated via urine (less than 1%) and breath (1 to 3%). The distribution of alcohol between blood and expired air is 2 100: l.

Site of alcohol metabolism

Although alcohol is metabolised in the kidney, stomach, intestine and bone marrow cells, the main site of alcohol metabolism is the liver. There are three main pathways for alcohol metabolism (Fig. 13.2):

Alcohol dehydrogenase
The mitochondrial ethanol oxidising system (MEOS)
Catalase

The main pathway for ethanol metabolism is via the enzyme alcohol dehydrogenase, which metabolises ethanol to acetaldehyde with the production of reduced NAD (NADH) (Fig. 13.1). This takes place in the cytosol: acetaldehyde diffuses into the mitochondria, where it is converted by acetaldehyde dehydrogenase to acetate. The acetate is released into the blood and oxidised by the peripheral tissues with the production of carbon dioxide, water and fatty acids.

Alcohol dehydrogenase

Alcohol dehydrogenase (ADH) plays a central role in the metabolism of alcohol. There exists considerable polymorphism in ADH, which has been related to alcohol metabolism, alcohol dependence and alcoholic liver disease. The three classes of alcohol dehydrogenase isoenzymes are shown in Table 13.2. Hepatic alcohol dehydrogenase activity is low in foetal life, but adult levels are reached by the age of 5 years. The pH optimum for ADH oxidation of ethanol is near 11, so that, physiologically, the rate of reaction is less than half that of maximum with a K_m for ethanol less than 1 mmol. Thus, ethanol is metabolised from the blood at a constant rate until very low blood levels are achieved.

Oxidation of alcohol to acetaldehyde by alcohol dehydrogenase requires NAD as a co-factor, which

Alcohol dehydrogenase

$$C_2H_5OH + NAD^+ \longrightarrow CH_3CHO + NADH + H^+$$

MEOS

$$C_2H_5OH + NADPH + H^+ + O_2 \longrightarrow CH_3CHO + NADP^+ + 2H_2O$$

Catalase

$$C_2H_5OH + H_2O \longrightarrow CH_3CHO + 2H_2O$$

Figure 13.1 Major routes of ethanol metabolism.

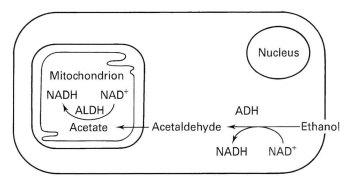

Figure 13.2 Ethanol metabolism by alcohol dehydrogenase (ADH). ALDH, acetaldehyde dehydrogenase.

is reduced to NADH. Since NADH reduction exceeds its rate of re-oxidation under normal conditions, the increased ratio of NADH to NAD is associated with a significant reduction in the redox state of the liver, This is thought to account for the major metabolic effects of ethanol metabolism, which includes inhibition of hepatic gluconeogenesis, decrease of fatty oxidation and decrease in activity of the citric acid cycle. This results in, among other consequences, raised blood lactate, hyperuricaemia and ketosis, or hepatic trapping of triglycerides.

In addition to polymorphism of ADH (discussed below), several factors may affect the activity of ADH. These include intracellular acetaldehyde concentration, shuttle mechanisms transporting reduced equivalents into the mitochondria and the rate of mitochondrial respiratory chain. That the rate of alcohol elimination *in vivo* correlates with the basal metabolic rate suggests that the rate of mitochondrial NADH oxidation is the major limiting factor in the ADH pathway. However, the situation is less clear-cut, since in renal failure, where hepatic ADH activity is increased, blood ethanol clearance remains normal.

Other factors that inhibit the rate of alcohol elimination include prolonged fasting, which reduces alcohol clearance, whereas fructose (sometimes used for hangovers) and corticosteroids enhance alcohol elimination. This may be related to the increased conversion of NADH to NAD. Alcohol metabolism can be inhibited by a number of factors, of which the best known are the ADH inhibitors, so that pyrazole and its derivatives may lead to high blood pressure.

MEOS system

The MEOS system is located in the endoplasmic reticulum and requires NADPH and oxygen. The importance of the MEOS system in alcohol metabolism overall remains uncertain. The cytochrome responsible for the MEOS system is designated P4502EI. This has been characterised and localised to chromosome 7. The MEOS system has also been demonstrated in mucosal cells of the upper gastrointestinal tract and the colon.

Table 13.2 Isozymes of ADH

Class	Locus	Peptide
I	ADH1	
	ADH2	$\beta_1, \beta_2, \beta_3$
	ADH3	γ_1, γ_2
II	ADH4	
III	ADH5	
IV	ADH7	
V	ADH6	

Catalase

Catalase is a haemoprotein located in the periox-omes and is capable of oxidising ethanol *in vitro* in the presence of hydrogen peroxide, but its physiological role remains uncertain.

Acetaldehyde metabolism

Acetaldehyde is oxidised rapidly under normal circumstances, Over 90% is metabolised to acetate in the liver by the enzyme aldehyde dehydrogenase; this enzyme is NAD-dependent and has a very low Km value and a high reaction rate so that, under normal circumstances, very little acetaldehyde is found outside the liver. Acetaldehyde dehydrogenase activity is found in the microsomes, mitochondria and cytoplasm, but the functional activity is probably entirely a mitochondrial process. There are two varieties of aldehyde dehydrogenase (Table 13.3).

Oxidation of acetaldehyde to acetate results in reduction of the cytosolic and mitochondrial redox state. This low redox state is associated with increases in liver and blood lactate-to-pyruvate and β hydroxybutarate–to-acetoacetate ratios.

Aldehyde dehydrogenase (ALDH) may be inhibited by a number of compounds including disulphiram (Antabuse); this is a tetramethylthiouram sulphide and is used because the unpleasant side effects of acetaldehyde are marked when the two agents are taken together. Similar reactions may occur when sulphonurylureas are administered. Metronidazole

Table 13.3 Isozymes of aldehyde dehydrogenase

Class	Isozyme	Distribution
E1	ALDH1	Cytosolic
E2	ALDH2	Mitochondrial periportal > perivenous
E3		Not involved in acetaldehyde oxidation
E4		Not involved in acetaldehyde oxidation

and cefamandole may also inhibit ALDH, resulting in increased production of acetaldehyde and leading to the so-called sensitising reactions. Patients on these agents are at increased risk of developing alcohol flush syndrome. The reaction is characterised by pulsating headaches, tachycardia and erythema of the face and upper chest. In severe cases, asthma, hypotension, angioedema and vascular collapse can occur. These reactions are probably a direct consequence of acetaldehyde toxicity.

Alcohol and liver damage

In general, animal models of alcoholic liver injury have not been helpful in defining the mechanisms of human disease: studies have usually been relatively short term. Although many animal models do show the features of fatty liver, few have shown the longer-term effects of fibrosis, alcoholic hepatitis or cirrhosis. As indicated above, alcohol toxicity is in general compatible with features of a direct or predictable toxin. However, there remains a large variation in sensitivity to alcohol toxicity: only 8% to 30% of people who abuse alcohol in the long term develop cirrhosis; in some patients, liver damage will not progress beyond the stage of fatty liver even in the face of continued alcohol excess. Of those who drink about one bottle of spirits a day, only half will develop a cirrhosis over two decades.

To explain the direct relationship between the linear effect of alcohol consumption and the probability of developing severe liver damage, which has been reliably demonstrated in many populations) and the apparently contradictory data derived from individual studies, it is important to understand not only the direct metabolic mechanisms of ethanol toxicity but also the idiosyncratic mechanisms that account for host variation: these factors are either genetic or immunological.

Factors determining susceptibility to alcoholic liver damage

Although within the population there is a clear dose–response relationship, there is considerable variation in the hepatic susceptibility to damage from alcohol consumption. How alcohol is consumed affects the risk of liver damage: taking alcohol other than at mealtimes, using several types of alcoholic beverage and daily drinking are all associated with an increased risk of liver disease. It remains controversial whether wine, especially red wine, is more beneficial than other drinks.

The diet may play an important role in susceptibility to liver damage: animal models where animals are given diets high in polyunsaturated fat and iron and low in carbohydrate are at greater risk of liver damage. This may explain why those with poorly controlled diabetes mellitus or obesity are at greater risk, since the cytochrome CYP2E1 is induced and the high fat content will be a substrate for lipid peroxidation.

Metabolism of alcohol is dependent on many factors, including whether alcohol is consumed fasted or with food, rates of gastric emptying (which may be affected by fats or hypertonic solutions), the extent of metabolism by the gastric or intestinal mucosa, presence of drugs, the extent of chronic alcohol ingestion, age, body habitus and even time of day. That immune reactions may be implicated in determining the rate of progression or development of alcoholic liver disease is suggested by a number of factors, including evidence of disturbance of the immune system and the clinical observation that liver damage may progress even when alcohol consumption is stopped. Nevertheless, when these factors are considered, variation within an individual shows that rates of metabolism of alcohol vary by less than 10%. In contrast, when individuals are compared, there may be up to a three-fold difference in rates of alcohol metabolism that cannot be explained by the above factors.

Genetic factors in alcohol metabolism

The importance of genetic factors in alcohol metabolism has been shown by studies in mono- and dizygotic twins. Nearly two-thirds of the variability in peak blood alcohol concentration and nearly half of the variability in elimination rates may be due to genetic factors. In contrast, about 10% of the variation in peak blood alcohol concentration could be attributed to differences in alcohol intake and the effects of age, weight and degree of fat. The difference in alcohol susceptibility between males and females is largely related to the different volumes of distribution. Thus, research has concentrated on the importance of the alcohol-metabolising enzymes. There is increasing evidence, however, that other genetic factors are also important in determining susceptibility to alcoholic liver damage (Table 13.4). The dopamine D2 receptor has been linked to alcohol addiction, and some of the genes associated with fibrosis, namely for collagen type I (COLIAI and COL IA2), are important.

HLA antigens

The importance of HLA antigens has remained confusing; part of the problem arises from the fact that the distribution of HLA antigen varies among different populations. Most studies have relied on serotyping, which is unreliable for HLA assignment, and many were done before the recognition of other factors, such as co-infection with hepatitis C virus, which increases liver damage. It is difficult to control for many of the other factors, already described, that might reflect susceptibility. An association between HLA B8 and the development of alcoholic cirrhosis has been described, but data are conflicting. Other

Table 13.4 Genes that may influence susceptibility to alcohol

	Genes
Alcohol metabolism	For ADH
	For aldehyde dehydrogenase
	For cytochrome P450IIE2
Fibrosis	Type I collagen genes
	(COL1A1, COL1A2)
Immune system	HLA alleles
Addiction	Dopamine receptor gene
Other	Gene for α_1-antitrypsin,
	TNF polymorphism

studies have implicated HLA B5, BI5 and B40. One meta-analysis concluded that there was no major association between any one HLA genotype and alcoholic liver disease.

Alcohol dehydrogenase isoenzymes

Alcohol dehydrogenase (ADH) consists of dimeric molecules with sub-units of 40 000 Da. Currently seven different ADH genes have been identified, with five classes of enzymes. These have been sequenced, and analysis of data suggests that there are two functional classes, one with α, β and γ subunits and second with pi, psi and sigma. Furthermore, polymorphisms occur at ADH and ALDH. The differences are due to two amino acid substitutions, which results in different co-enzyme binding sites and affect the kinetic constants. ADH II and III appear with different frequencies in different racial groups. Thus, within ADH II, polymorphism β l is predominant in Black and White populations, whereas β II is predominant in the Chinese and Japanese. β III appears in 25% of the Black population. With respect to ADH III polymorphism, the two γ alleles appear with equal frequencies among Whites, but γ I dominates in the Japanese, Chinese and Black populations.

Acetaldehyde dehydrogenase isoenzymes

As with alcohol dehydrogenase, there are multiple molecular forms of aldehyde dehydrogenase. Of these, only El and E2 are important in acetaldehyde metabolism. Both ALDHI and ALDH2 are tetrameric molecules with sub-units of about 500 amino acids. Polymorphism has been identified for both isoenzymes.

Isoenzymes in relation to alcoholic liver disease

A number of studies have shown that the rates of alcohol excess and of alcoholic liver disease vary between populations, and some of this has been attributed to genetic patterns of alcohol metabolism. Many of the early studies were hampered by the fact that subjects were not specifically genotyped and other factors, such as viral infections, were not considered.

Facial flushing after alcohol consumption is well recognised in the Chinese and Japanese; this has been attributed to elevated acetaldehyde levels and is highly correlated with ALDH2 deficiency. Those who are homozygous for ALDH2*2 have the most severe alcohol flush reaction and higher acid acetaldehyde levels than those with other genotypes of the enzyme. These reactions occur when acetaldehyde concentrations reach between 40 and 60 mmol/L. Among the Japanese, nearly three-quarters report flushing after alcohol; the vast majority of these are ALDH2-deficient. In contrast, nearly all those who do not flush are ALDH2-active. However, this situation is not clear-cut, since around 10% of Whites also report facial flushing following alcohol ingestion, but the ALDH2 *2 isoenzyme has not been found in Whites. A number of studies have shown that those who flush and are ALDH2-deficient are less likely to be heavy alcohol drinkers. However, among alcoholics who are ALDH2-deficient, drinking problems occur later in life.

Mechanisms of alcoholic liver damage

The mechanisms of alcohol toxicity remain poorly understood. A number of mechanisms have been identified but the role of alcohol and its metabolites in direct toxicity compared with the immune involvement and production of cytokines has not been fully explained. The chronic nature of the disease and the great variability in patterns of response have not fully been elucidated.

Factors that may lead to hepatocellular damage and hepatic fibrosis include the following, which probably all contribute to the liver damage:

Increased gut permeability to endotoxins: this may directly stimulate the release of reactive oxygen species (ROS) and cytokines from Kupffer cells.
Toxicity of alcohol metabolites.
Immune activation.

Metabolic toxicity

Ethanol toxicity

Ethanol (Table 13.5) will alter membrane fluidity, but the consequences of this in the pathogenesis of the disease remain uncertain.

Toxicity of acetaldehyde

The effect of alteration in hepatocyte redox levels from ethanol metabolism, as indicated above, results in increased amounts of reduced NAD. This has a number of effects on the liver and general metabolism.

Hyperlactatemia

The enhanced NADH/NAD ratio results in an increased ratio of lactate to pyruvate as a consequence of decreased utilisation and enhanced production of lactate within the liver. The highly increased level of lactate contributes to the generalised acidosis and reduces renal uric acid excretion, resulting in hyperuricaemia. This may lead to gout. The effect of alcohol in causing ketosis will also promote raised uric acid levels.

Depressed lipid oxidation and enhanced lipogenesis

The increased NADH/NAD ratio increases the concentration of alphaglycerophosphate, leading to

Table 13.5 Possible mechanisms of alcohol toxicity

Membrane Alterations
Membrane Lipid Peroxidation
Enzyme Dysfunction
Abnormal Redox State
Decreased cytoprotection
Increased cellular oxygen requirement
Inflammation
Fibrogenesis

retention of triglycerides within the hepatocyte as a consequence of the trapping of fatty acids. Excess NADH also enhances fatty acid synthesis. Because mitochrondia preferentially use hydrogen equivalents from ethanol rather than those from the oxidation of fatty acids, there is decreased fatty acid oxidation, resulting in the accumulation of fat within the liver and the development of megamitochondria. Clinically, serum triglycerides may be grossly elevated: this requires a reduction in alcohol consumption rather than additional medication.

Protein metabolism

Whereas *in vitro* ethanol will inhibit protein synthesis, the effect in humans is less clear-cut. The malnutrition seen in patients with alcoholic liver disease is largely related to poor dietary intake and liver cell failure.

Glucose metabolism

The effect of alcohol and glucose metabolism is complex, since ethanol may either inhibit hepatic gluconeogenesis as a consequence of an increased NADH/INAD ratio when glycogen stores are released. Under other circumstances, gluconeogenesis is actually accelerated, but the mechanisms remain complex.

Hepatic hypoxia

Histologically the main lesions of alcohol in the liver are detected by the centrilobular or perivenular zone, where the PO_2 is least. Ethanol induces an increase in hepatic portal blood flow (as indeed will any meal), but in the situation of chronic alcohol consumption there appears to be defective oxygen utilisation. Again, tissue hypoxia will enhance the amount of NADH and increase the lactate: pyruvate ratio. Furthermore, since there is more ADH in those hepatocytes in the perivenular zone, it is likely that more toxic metabolites of ethanol are generated by metabolism.

Consequences of alcoholic enzyme induction

Alcohol is a potent enzyme inducer; in particular, cytochrome P4502EI is enhanced (Fig. 13.3). Thus, compounds metabolised by this enzyme to potentially toxic intermediates are produced in greater quantity. For example, paracetamol is metabolised to a toxic intermediate (NAPQI), which, if not removed by glutathione, accumulates in the liver, resulting in increased toxicity. In patients with chronic alcohol consumption, cytochrome P450 activity is enhanced, leading to a greater generation of metabolites, which results in increased toxicity of paracetamol. Other clinically important interactions include those with oral contraceptives (potentially leading to reduced contraceptive effect) and warfarin (leading to reduced anticoagulation). In contrast, acute ingestion of alcohol may inhibit enzyme activity and so reduce paracetamol toxicity as less toxic metabolites are generated.

Toxic effects of acetaldehyde adducts

Acetaldehyde may form reactive metabolites that can result in

Increased complement activation
Generation of neoantigens
Toxic effects, including alterations in microtubules and lipid peroxidation (Table 13.6)

Acetaldehyde binds to cysteine and glutathione, resulting in reduced levels of glutathione in the hepatocyte. Since glutathione is a free radical scavenger, the radicals produced by, among other compounds,

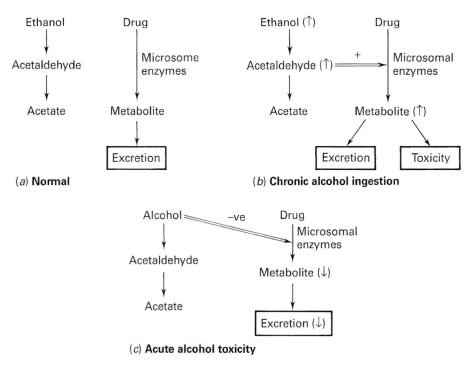

Figure 13.3 Effect of ethanol on drug metabolism. (*a*) Normal. (*b*) Chronic alcohol ingestion. (*c*) Acute alcohol toxicity.

Table 13.6 Possible consequences of acetaldehyde-protein adducts

Neoantigen formation
Complement activation
Disruption of microtubule formation
Inhibition of Enzyme activity

ethanol metabolism by the MEOS system may make the cell more susceptible to lipid peroxidation damage. Acetaldehyde also interferes directly or indirectly with other enzyme activities.

As indicated above, patients with alcoholic liver disease have evidence of disturbance of the immune system, with abnormal immunoglobulin levels and organ specific and non-specific auto-antibodies. The extent to which these are secondary to liver and other target-cell damage more involved in the pathogenesis remains unclear. Nonetheless, there is increasing evidence that some immune mechanisms may be involved with mechanisms of liver damage.

Complement activation

As indicated above, acetaldehyde has been shown to form adducts with plasma membranes, which activate complement *in vitro*. This may result in organ damage.

Damage mediated by white cells

In patients with alcoholic liver damage there is increased appearance of the three main endothelial adhesion molecules (such as ICAM-I, VCAM-I and E selectin). In alcoholic hepatitis, E-selectin is found on inflamed endothelium at the site of neutrophil infiltration and increased ICAM and VCAM on sinusoidal endothelium. In contrast, in cirrhosis, ICAM-l and VCAM-l are strongly expressed on sinusoidal endothelium. Thus, in alcoholic hepatitis and cirrhosis, the distribution would allow the T cells and monocytes to transmigrate.

It is possible that these adhesion molecules are induced by TNF-α, which is secreted in increased amounts in alcoholic hepatitis and cirrhosis. It has been suggested that the increased TNF is produced by predominantly by macrophages and Kupffer cells, stimulated by endotoxin reaching the systemic circulation from alcohol-induced gut damage. Kupffer cells also release other cytokines, ROS and prostaglandin E2, which will stimulate oxygen consumption by the hepatocytes.

Alcohol and fibrosis

One of the key features of alcoholic-induced liver injury is the proliferation of perisinusoidal cells, including myofibroblasts, fibroblasts and transitional cells. The most important of these are the stellate cells (lipocytes, Ito cells or vitamin A–containing cells). These cells contain alcohol dehydrogenase and therefore are able to metabolise ethanol; lipid peroxidation, lactate and acetaldehyde may stimulate the stellate cells directly. Stimulation of the stellate cells may also occur from hepatocyte-derived factors such as transforming growth factor α or insulin-like growth factor or following activation of Kupffer cells. The Kupffer cells may be stimulated by the lipopolysaccharide absorbed from the bowel, where permeability is increased by the toxic effects of alcohol. Stellate cells transform to a myofibroblastic phenotype when they secrete matrix proteins such as collagens types I, II and IV laminin into the space of Disse, with resulting pericellular fibrosis. Because these cells are located in greatest concentration in the perivenular region, damage from alcohol to these cells may explain the distribution of fibrosis.

The mechanisms by which alcohol induces collagen formation is unclear. These may relate to inflammation from alcohol or acetaldehyde or the associated hyperlactataemia. Liver cell necrosis and activation by ROS, cytokines and other mediators of hepatic stellate cells and myofibroblasts will contribute. The increased deposition of collagen in the space of Disse results in reduced blood flow and features of portal hypertension. Thus portal hypertension may be present before the onset of frank cirrhosis. *In vitro*, acetaldehyde and other aldehydes will stimulate these cells.

Finally, alcohol may lead to hepatocellular death by stimulating apoptosis, probably through stimulation of Fas/Fas ligand system–mediated caspase-3 activation and the stress- and mitogen-activated protein kinase (MAPK) cascades.

Clinical aspects

History

The history in patients with possible alcohol liver-related damage is divided into two aspects: (1) obtaining an alcohol history and looking for evidence and (2) determining the extent of target-organ damage. Alcohol dependence and alcoholic liver damage do not necessarily occur together.

It is often very difficult to take an accurate drinking history, since patterns of drinking will vary throughout the life of the individual and it may be difficult accurately to recall patterns of drinking 10 to 15 years earlier. Furthermore, alcohol intake is rarely regular, and the extent and frequency of binges may be difficult to determine. Traditionally the amount of alcohol consumed is measured by units, with one unit of alcohol being approximately half of pint of beer, one pub measure of spirits or one wine glass of wine. This corresponds to about 10 g of alcohol. The use of units is now moderately well understood by the general public, but care must be taken to avoid over-reliance on this, since pub measures of spirits may vary and the strength of spirits and beers may vary considerably. The amount of alcohol in one unit varies from country to country and ranges from 8–16 g alcohol. Evidence of alcohol dependency should be sought and the simple CAGE questionnaire administered as a useful guide to the possibility of alcohol dependence (Table 13.7). Other instruments that have been developed include the Michigan Alcohol Screening Test (MAST), the Paddington Alcohol Test (PAT) and the Alcohol Use Disorders Identification Test (AUDIT). Symptoms of organ failure should be sought.

Table 13.7 Cage questionnaire: two or more positive answers imply a possibility of alcohol dependence

C	Have you ever felt you should cut down on your drinking?
A	Have you felt annoyed when others have criticised your drinking?
G	Do you feel guilty about your drinking?
E	Do you ever have an eye opener (an early morning drink to steady your nerves)?

Clinically the patient may show evidence of alcohol consumption with alcohol on the breath or features of intoxication. Nutritional deficiencies are common. The features of chronic liver disease are well described; they include jaundice, spider naevi, hepatosplenomegaly, ascites, leuconychia and, rarely, encephalopathy. Differentiation between alcohol intoxication, withdrawal and hepatic encephalopathy may be difficult, but withdrawal tends to be associated with stimulation and excitement. None of these clinical features is specific to alcoholic liver disease. Dupuytren's contractures (palmar fasciitis) are not associated with alcoholic liver disease.

Alcoholic and other conditions

It is now clear that patients with chronic viral hepatitis (due to either viral hepatitis B or C) are at greater risk of alcohol-induced liver damage; fibrosis develops more rapidly in such individuals, suggesting clear synergy. Furthermore, alcohol consumption is associated with increased replication of hepatitis B virus. Those patients who are heterozygous or homozygous for haemochromatosis and those with α_1 antitrypsin deficiency are also at greater risk of alcohol-induced liver damage. Whether this represents a combination of two different toxins to the liver or whether there is a more involved interaction remains to be determined.

Obesity itself may mimic alcoholic liver disease; indeed, it is not possible to distinguish between alcohol and non-alcoholic liver disease biochemically

Table 13.8 Blood markers associated with alcoholic liver disease

	Specificity	Usefulness
Raised mean cell volume	+	+++
γ-glutamyl transpeptidase	+	+++
γ-aminobutyric acid	++	+
Carbohydrate-deficient transferrin (CDT)	++	+
Mitochondrial aspartate aminotransferase	++	+
Acetate	++	+
Aspartate, aminotransferase/alanine aminotransferase ratio	++	++

or histologically; the term NAFLD (non-alcoholic fatty liver disease) has been used and may be associated with obesity, diabetes and some drugs. The mechanism of liver damage is probably similar. Obesity may exacerbate alcoholic liver disease.

Blood tests

There are no specific tests to show alcoholic liver damage, but simple screening tests may point to the possibility (Table 13.8).

Haematology

Alcohol is toxic to the bone marrow, and this may result in a pancytopenia and macrocytosis. It must be remembered that there are many other causes of macrocytosis, including folate and vitamin B12 deficiency, hyperlipidaemia and hypothyroidism. Morphologically abnormal red cells may be seen, and a finding of triangulocytes is said to be characteristic of alcoholic liver disease. Both the mean cell volume and the morphological changes slowly resolve after alcohol withdrawal.

Liver tests

GGT

The γ glutamyl transferase (GGT) is the most commonly used biochemical marker of alcohol con-

sumption. This is an inducible enzyme of hepatic origin and may be increased due to any enzyme-inducing agent, including some drugs, such as anticonvulsants. Increases may also be due to biliary or hepatocellular damage, hyperlipidaemia typeIV, diabetes, trauma, obesity and pregnancy. Although the GGT is a marker of enzyme induction, it poorly reflects the degree of liver cell damage. This enzyme plays an important physiological role in counteracting oxidative stress by breaking down extracellular glutathione and making its components available to the cell. There is a close association between GGT and the risk of coronary heart disease, stroke and type II diabetes.

Transaminases

Serum aspartate aminotransferase (AST) and alanine transferase (ALT) are elevated in up to three-quarters of alcohol abusers but rarely exceeds five times the upper limit of normal. In alcoholic liver damage (ALD) , the AST is generally higher than the ALT, in contrast to other types of hepatitis, where serum AST is lower than ALT, but this difference is not diagnostic. There is a selective increase in the mitochondrial isoenzyme of AST, a marker of the mitochondrial damage discussed earlier.

The plasma proteins may be reduced (albumin, haptoglobins and transferrin), whereas acute-phase proteins such as α_2 macroglobulin and caeruloplasmin may be increased. Plasma lipids may be increased; in particular, hypertriglyceridaemia may be a feature of acute alcoholic liver disease, with the values reaching 20 mmol/L or more. High-density-lipoprotein cholesterol (HDL-C), phospholipids and apolipoproteins AI and A2 are increased by ethanol.

Alcohol is also associated with increased iron stores and increased serum ferritin: the extent to which this iron overload is harmful is uncertain. In some instances, it may be clinically very difficult to distinguish iron overload associated with alcohol from the iron overload associated with genetic haemochromatosis.

Other tests of alcoholic liver damage

Alcohol is an enzyme inducer, as outlined above; therefore enhanced glucaric excretion may be found in those who are induced. Similarly, aminopyrine clearance may be increased.

The serum transferrin may be increased in those drinking excessively and a carbohydrate deficient form (CDT) has been reported to be a useful marker. Current techniques of determining this are unreliable, although this diagnostic test has not achieved widespread use.

Overall, there are no specific features of alcoholic liver damage, although a combination of biochemical and haematological tests may point to the diagnosis.

Immunological abnormalities in alcoholic liver disease

Of the auto-antibodies in patients with liver disease, elevation of serum IgA has been recognised for many years. IgA (mainly the IgA 1 subclass) may be deposited in the kidneys, giving rise to IgA nephropathy and leading to glomerulonephritis and renal failure. Monomeric IgA is also present in the hepatic sinusoids of patients with alcoholic liver disease but does not correlate with serum levels of IgA. Other reports have emphasised the importance of elevated serum levels of IgG. The hyper-gammaglobulinaemia associated with liver disease may be due to the increased availability of gut-derived antigens as consequence of reduced Kupffer cell function and porto-systemic shunting. This is confirmed by the presence of increased titres to gut-derived antigens. An alternative explanation is that the hypergammaglobulinaemia is consequent on impaired suppressor cell function.

Non-organ-specific auto-antibodies are also present in increased concentrations in patients with alcoholic liver disease. These include the smooth muscle antibodies and anti-nuclear antibodies. These are found usually in low titres, more commonly in women than in men, of the organ-specific antibodies. Liver-specific antibodies (both IgG and IgA) include those that read with liver membrane antigens, the liver-specific Iipoprotein and the asialoglycoprotein receptor. Of greater interest has been the presence of antibodies to alcohol-altered liver cell determinants. These antibodies, which can induce antibody-dependent cell-mediated toxicity, appear to be related to neo-antigens associated with acetaldehyde rather than with ethanol. Thus acetaldehyde may act as a hapten or induce structural alteration to other proteins, leading to the development of neo-antigens.

Cell-mediated immunity

Delayed hypersensitivity is reduced in patients with alcoholic liver disease, and reactivity is reduced to all recall antigens. Patients with alcoholic hepatitis and cirrhosis have a reduced number of circulating lymphocytes, primarily due to a reduction in T cells while the B-cell numbers are relatively well preserved. This may be due to sequestration of T cells within the liver. Functional studies have shown that in patients with liver disease, lymphocyte transformation is increased when ethanol or acetaldehyde is reduced only in those patients with alcoholic liver disease, and leucocyle migration to acetaldehyde is reduced only in those patients with alcoholic hepatitis. Thus, lymphocytes from patients with alcoholic liver disease can be shown to be sensitised to antigens in normal liver, alcohol hyaline and alcohol-treated liver. It is difficult to determine whether these immune reactions are primary or secondary to alcohol-mediated liver damage.

The reticuloendothelial system

A decreased phagocytic capacity is found in patients with alcoholic liver disease. This may be a direct consequence of alcohol on the cells of the reticuloendothelial system (RES) or blockade by circulating immune complexes. Decreased RES activity is associated with an increased susceptibility to infections, particularly bacterial.

Cytokines and inflammatory markers

Alcoholic liver disease shows features of an inflammatory response with increased circulatory levels of inflammatory cytokines and increased tissue expression of inflammatory and adhesion molecules. Thus, in patients with alcoholic hepatitis, levels of tumour necrosis factor α (TNF-α) and interleukins-1, 6, 8 and 18 are increased. The former two cytokines remain elevated for several months, whereas IL-6 falls with recovery. In general, the degree of elevation of these cytokines correlates with the severity of the liver damage. Whether these (and other) cytokines are implicated in the generation or perpetuation of liver or extra-hepatic organ damage or these changes represent a healing response to alcohol-induced liver damage remains uncertain. However, many of the clinical features of alcoholic hepatitis can be attributed to the effect of these cytokines, including anorexia (TNF also induces leptin gene expression), catabolism, cholestasis, pyrexia and neutrophilia.

Other investigations

The technetium liver scan is now performed rarely and findings are non-specific, although in the presence of alcoholic hepatitis there may be a complete 'white out', where there is no uptake of radioisotope by the liver. This is found only in alcoholic hepatitis and in acute Wilson's disease. The ultrasound may show an enlarged liver with a bright echo due to fat infiltration. The most useful investigation is liver biopsy, which not only helps make the diagnosis and establish the severity of alcoholic liver damage but also excludes other causes of abnormal liver tests.

Liver histology

There are three main liver lesions in alcoholic liver disease:

Fatty liver
Alcoholic hepatitis
Fibrosis and cirrhosis

The lesions tend to be most marked in the perivenular region. This may be a consequence of the possible hypermetabolic state of the hepatocytes in people consuming excess ethanol, because of the effect of ethanol on hepatic oxygenation or may reflect the tissue distribution of the oxygen metabolising enzymes.

Fatty liver

Fatty liver (Fig. 13.4) is characterised by accumulation of fatty droplets within the hepatocytes; commonly this is in a macrovesicular pattern, but when

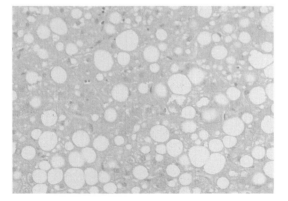

Figure 13.4 Alcohol liver disease, fatty liver. (See colour plate section.)

there is a microvesicular pattern, it is associated with a poor prognosis. Fatty accumulation normally starts in the perivenular area around the central vein. The hepatocytes enlarge and may compress the sinusoids. This may contribute to the portal hypertension seen in patients with fatty liver in the absence of fibrosis.

There are many other causes of fatty liver, including obesity, diabetes, malnutrition, inflammatory disease and toxic reactions, so the lesion is not specific for alcohol.

Clinically, the patients are well and usually asymptomatic; the condition is often detected on routine examination. In the great majority, the lesion resolves on alcohol withdrawal.

However, a proportion will show features of additional steatohepatitis, which is associated with a more aggressive course of disease (see the discussion of hepatitis, below).

Alcoholic hepatitis

Alcoholic hepatitis (Fig. 13.5), also called sclerosing hyaline necrosis, may lead to cirrhosis. Fatty infiltration is usually present, as are ballooned hepatocytes, often containing Mallory bodies. The three features of alcoholic hepatitis are fibrosis, inflammation and parenchymal cell damage. The inflammatory

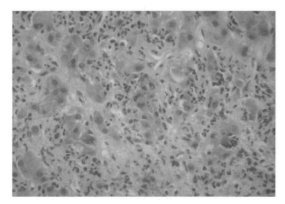

Figure 13.5 Alcohol hepatitis (severe). (See colour plate section.)

response consists predominantly of polymorphonuclear leucocytes. These inflammatory cells are found around the damaged hepatocytes. Fibrosis is always present and is usually pericellular in distribution. Other types of fibrosis include perivenular fibrosis or sclerosis with lesions of the terminal hepatic vein (the central vein). This may lead to veno-occlusive–type lesions but is not specific for alcoholic hepatitis and may be found in cirrhosis.

Parenchymal damage is characterised by swelling of hepatocyte cytoplasm, resulting in balloon degeneration and necrosis. The ballooned hepatocytes are believed to result from a decreased endocytosis and decreased microtubular assembly as a consequence of alcohol metabolites. This leads to a switch in the production of the normal hepatocyte cytokeratin to bile duct–type cytokeratin and is associated with cell swelling and Mallory body formation. The cell swelling compresses sinusoids. Megamitochondria may be seen, and this may be a reflection of recent heavy alcohol consumption. Of interest are that the megamitochondria in peri-portal hepatocytes are differ in shape from those in the centrilobular hepatocytes. The peri-portal megamitochondria are not specific to alcohol and may be found in steatohepatitis from any cause, whereas the focal centrilobular megamitochondria are more specific for alcoholic liver disease. Megamitochondria are associated with a poor outcome.

Mallory bodies or alcohol hyaline may be associated with cholestasis of any cause, but Mallory bodies are frequently found in patients with alcoholic hepatitis and end-stage cirrhosis. These bodies appear to be aggregates of altered intermediate cytoskeleton filaments. Again, these features of alcoholic hepatitis are not specific to alcohol and may be found in chronic cholestasis and Wilson's disease. Pericellular fibrosis and fatty liver with polymorphonuclear infiltration may be also be seen in obesity, diabetes, gastrointestinal bypass and following the effect of drugs such as amiodarone or perhexaline. Pericellular fibrosis may also be found following chemotherapy or with vitamin A toxicosis.

Clinically, the patient may be well but is usually ill with jaundice, fever and right-upper-quadrant abdominal pain. Encephalopathy carries a poor prognosis. The blood tests show a characteristic pattern with a high polymorphonuclear leucocytosis (up to 50×10^9/l), with a high serum bilirubin (which may exceed 900 μmol/L) but a near normal alkaline phosphatase and transaminases. These patients may present after many years of heavy alcohol consumption (mean alcohol consumption of 250 g/day over 25 years!). There is evidence of cytokine activation, especially of IL-8 and IL-B, but the mechanism of the condition is uncertain at present. The severity of the illness is measured by the Glasgow score or the Maddrey score (based on the serum bilirubin and prolongation of the prothrombin time).

Cirrhosis

Cirrhosis (see Fig. 13.6) is characteristically micronodular in nature and is defined as transformation of the normal architecture with hepatocyte necrosis and regeneration nodules surrounded by fibrous septa. There are often features of fatty liver or alcoholic hepatitis. The cirrhosis is usually micronodular. There may be overload of iron, so that differentiation from haemochromatosis may be difficult. Clinically, the patient may present with any of the complications of cirrhosis, such as bleeding oesophageal varices, ascites or jaundice.

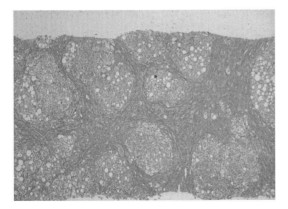

Figure 13.6 Alcoholic liver disease, micronodular cirrhoris. (See colour plate section.)

Treatment

It is important that all health care professionals put in place a screening strategy for identification of harmful drinkers and have protocols in place for intervention. Brief interventions have been shown to be cost-effective. The mainstay of treatment of alcoholic liver disease is abstinence. This is associated with a marked improvement in prognosis and often resolution of the abnormal liver function tests. In the early stages of withdrawal, patients may have severe adverse reactions, including delirium tremens and seizures. Withdrawal should be covered with benzodiazepines. There are many agencies that can offer support for the patient and family; the patient should be formally assessed and referral offered. There is preliminary evidence that naltrexone, a narcotic analogue, may reduce cravings; other studies suggest that, in selected patients, acamprosate may be effective; this is a synthetic GABA analogue that helps maintain abstinence by reducing the properties of alcohol leading to dependence. The rationale for disulphiram is discussed above.

Nutritional support is important: most patients with alcoholic liver disease are malnourished even though alcohol is rich in calories (7.1 kcal/g). Malnutrition arises either from poor intake or secondary to maladsorption or maldigestion (alcohol-induced small bowel damage or pancreatitis). Enteral or rarely parenteral nutritional supplementation may be required, which may be enhanced by anabolic steroids such as oxandrolone.

The increased understanding of the mechanisms of alcoholic liver disease has stimulated many studies of therapeutic agents: at the present time, few of these have been shown to have significant efficacy, which is in part a reflection of the difficulties of running such studies. A number of agents – including propylthiouracil (to counteract the enhanced metabolism and hypoxia of cells), chlorpromazine and S-adenosyl methionine (to stabilise cell membranes), corticosteroids, anabolic steroids and anticytokine treatment (to reduce the immune effects) – have been tried. The role of corticosteroids (such as prednisolone 40 to 60 mg/day for 6 weeks) remains controversial: some analyses suggest a benefit in those with severe alcoholic hepatitis but without sepsis or gastrointestinal bleeding; an early fall in serum bilirubin may be a good predictor of a therapeutic response.

Several strategies to reduce TNF production have been adopted: prednisolone, colchicine, prostaglandin analogues, pentoxifyline, ursodeoxycholic acid and N-acetyl-cysteine. There have been several studies using anti-TNF, but these have usually been relatively small and the findings inconclusive, but the use of the chimeric antibody preparation may be contra-indicated by the associated increased susceptibility to infection. Gut sterilisation and selective bowel decontamination have been tried to reduce the absorption of endotoxin. Propylthiouracil may be helpful in chronic liver disease, and high-dose corticosteroids may reduce the 30-day mortality among those with severe alcoholic hepatitis. In these cases, N-acetyl cysteine has also been advocated, with some benefit.

Membrane-stabilising drugs and anti-oxidants such as cyanidanol-3, polyunsaturated phosphatidylcholine, silymarin, vitamin E and selenium may also have some therapeutic benefit.

Summary

Alcohol can affect every organ and system within the body; hepatotoxicity of alcohol results primarily from metabolism within the liver and to a lesser extent within other organs. The main metabolic pathway is via alcohol dehydrogenase, with generation of acetaldehyde and reduced hepatic NADH; within the liver, there is stimulation of hepatic stellate cells, which results in collagen formation and deposition, leading to cirrhosis. Acetaldehyde may also be generated by the microsomal ethanol oxidizing system (MEOS) leading to the formation of free oxygen radicals, which may lead to further liver damage. Although there is a good correlation between the amount of alcohol drunk and the probability of developing liver disease, there are significant individual variations. Susceptibility to alcoholic liver disease is affected by other hepatotoxins, such as hepatitis B or C, viral disease and host factors, some of which are genetic. Patients with alcoholic liver damage have a variety of both cellular and humoral abnormalities of the immune system, but the extent to which these are involved in the pathogenesis of liver disease rather than the consequence of liver disease remains uncertain.

Treatment of alcoholic liver disease remains primarily that of abstinence: drug therapy has been tried, including corticosteroids, anti-TNF agents (such as antibodies and oxypentiphyline) and N-acetyl cysteine for alcoholic hepatitis, colchicine and propylthiouracil, but none yet has been shown to reverse the liver damage.

Clinical scenario

A 40-year-old woman was referred to the medical assessment unit by her GP with swollen ankles, abdominal distension and jaundice. Although previously well with a young family, on questioning she admitted to drinking between $1^{1}/_{2}$ and 2 bottles of wine each night for at least 15 years. On examination she was thin and jaundiced. There was palmar erythema and a number of spider naevi on her chest and back. There was shifting dullness in her abdomen suggestive of ascites.

Investigations

Sodium 129 mmol/L	Potassium 3.7 mmol/L
Urea 2.8 mmol/L	Creatinine 78 μmol/L
Albumin 31 g/L	Total protein 58 g/L
Bilirubin 33 μmol/L	Alanine aminotransferase 165 IU/L
Alkaline phosphatase 250iu/L	Haemoglobin 10g/dL
Mean cell Volume 101fL	Platelets 120×10^9/L
Prothrombin time 14 seconds	White cell count 16×10^9/L

Questions

1. What is the diagnosis?
2. What initial investigations are indicated?
3. What treatment would you instigate?

Answers

1. The diagnosis in this case is likely to be decompensating alcoholic liver disease.
2. The shifting dullness on examination probably represents ascites. As such, an ascitic tap is indicated. The ascitic fluid needs to be examined for protein and glucose levels and also evidence of infection. The patient's white cell count is elevated, and this may represent spontaneous bacterial peritonitis.
3. Early treatment is aimed at stabilisation of the patient. Due to her dependence on alcohol, she will need replacement with the benzodiazepine chlordiazepoxide. She needs nutritional supplementation, which may be intravenous or oral. If spontaneous bacterial peritonitis is suspected, cefuroxime and metronidazole are indicated. Spironolactone may also be used as a diuretic.

Multiple-choice questions

1. Alcohol is implicated in:
   a. Half of all violent deaths.
   b. A quarter of drug overdoses.
   c. Half of gastrointestinal haemorrhages.
   d. Up to 40 000 deaths a year in the UK.
   e. The loss of 11 million working days per year in the UK.
2. Regarding histological changes in the liver caused by alcohol:
   a. Portal hypertension is caused by enlargement of the sinusoids.
   b. A microvesicular pattern of lipid droplets in hepatocytes is associated with a good prognosis.
   c. Megamitochondria are associated with a good prognosis.
   d. Fibrosis is always present in alcoholic hepatitis.
   e. Cirrhosis is usually macronodular.
3. Successful treatment of the patient with alcoholic hepatitis may include:
   a. High-dose corticosteroids.

b. Abstinence from alcohol.
c. Anti–IL-1.
d. N-acetylcysteine.
e. Nutritional support.
4. During the metabolism of alcohol:
   a. The majority of alcohol absorption is from the stomach.
   b. The end products of alcohol metabolism are excreted via the urine.
   c. Acetaldehyde dehydrogenase is localised to the endoplasmic reticulum. Disulphiram inhibits alcohol dehydrogenase.
   d. Facial flushing after alcohol consumption is associated with acetaldehyde dehydrogenase 2 deficiency.

Answers

1: a, T; b, T; c, F; d, T; e, T
2: a, F; b, F; c, F; d, T, e, F
3: a, T; b, T; c, F; d, T; e, T
4: a, F; b, F; c, F; d, F; e, T

FURTHER READING

Agarwal, K., Kontorinis, N., Dieterich, D. T. (2004). Hepatitis. *Current Treatment Options in Gastroenterology* **7,** 451–8.

Bellantani, S., Tiribelli, C. (2001). The spectrum of liver disease in the general population: lesson from the Dionysos study. *Journal of Hepatology* **35,** 531–7.

Bautista, A. P. Impact of alcohol on the ability of Kupffer cells to produce chemokines and its role in alcoholic liver disease. *Journal of Gastroenterology and Hepatology* **15,** 349–56.

Casey, C. A., Nanji, A., Cederbaum, A. L. *et al.* (2001). Alcoholic liver disease and apoptosis. *Alcoholism, Clinical and Experimental Research* **25 (5 Suppl ISBRA),** 49S–53S.

Day, C. P. (2000). Who gets alcoholic liver disease: nature or nurture? *Journal of the Royal College of Physicians, London* **34,** 557–62.

Department of Health. (2001). Statistics on alcohol: England, 1978 onward. London: Office of National Statistics.

Diehl, A. M. (2004). Obesity and alcohol. *Alcohol* **34,** 81–87.

Eriksson, C. J. (2001).The role of acetaldehyde in the actions of alcohol (update 2000). *Alcoholism, Clinical and Experimental Research* **25 (5 Suppl ISBRA)**, 15S-32S.

Grove J., Daly, A. K., Bassendine, M. F. *et al.* (2000). Interleukin 10 promoter region polymorphisms and susceptibility to advanced alcoholic liver disease. *Gut* **46,** 540–5.

Levistky, J., Mailliard, M. E. (2004). Diagnosis and therapy of alcoholic liver disease. *Seminars in Liver Disease* **24,** 233–47.

Mathurin, P, Mendenhall, C. L., Carithers, R. L. *et al.* (2002). Corticosteroids improve short-term survival in patients with severe alcoholic hepatitis (AH): individual data analysis of the three randomised placebo controlled double blind trials of corticosteroids in severe AH. *Journal of Hepatology* **36,** 480–7.

McClain, C. J., Song, Z., Barve, S. S. *et al.* (2004). Recent advances in alcoholic liver disease: IV. Dysregulated cytokine metabolism in alcoholic liver disease. *American Journal of Physiology, Gastrointestinal and Liver Physiology* **287,** G497–502.

Monzoni, A. Masutti, F., Saccoccio, G. *et al.* (2001). Genetic determinants of ethanol-induced liver damage. *Molecular Medicine* **7,** 255–62.

Royal College of Physicians (2001). Alcohol – Can the NHS Afford It? Report of a working party. London: Royal College of Physicians.

Room, R., Babor, T., Rehm, J. (2005). Alcohol and public health. *Lancet* **365,** 519–30.

Stewart, S., Jones, D., Day, C. P. (2001). Alcoholic liver disease: new insights into mechanisms and preventative strategies. *Trends in Molecular Medicine* **7,** 408–13.

Tome, S., Lucey, M. R. (2004). Review article: current management of alcoholic liver disease. *Alimentary Pharmacology and Therapeutics* **19,** 707–714.

14

Diet, health and disease

Michael E. J. Lean

Introduction

It is beyond the scope of this chapter to reproduce a textbook of human nutrition. Instead, basic principles are discussed, with illustrative examples. (See also Further Reading.)

Throughout most of the history of humankind, the assumption has been that the whole process of disease is beyond our control. Our dominant management strategy has been attempts to appease or reward the gods. Elements of this behaviour can be traced up to the present day at a personal or family level for individual afflictions, at a group or community level for epidemics or for the illnesses of our leaders. The concepts of science and of internal medicine emerged from the universities in the fourth century BC in Athens to challenge the gods and provide prognoses and diagnoses based on an empirical evidence base coupled with a theoretical framework. Treatment was a later development, initially based on concepts of allopathic or homeopathic magic, and only quite lately based empirically on observations. The concept of a disease mechanism is very recent indeed. In the twentieth century, the discovery of microbial pathogens and of antibiotics led to a pharmaceutically driven concept of pathogenesis. A disease was not worth considering if there was no treatment. The treatment did not need to be complete, but it had to be marketable.

The role of diet in disease long antedates drugs in medical practice. Many drugs were derived from herbal approaches involving sympathetic magic, homeopathy and allopathy – the only remedies available before drugs. A few remedies proved, when tested scientifically, to promote recovery or reduce symptoms – they actually worked – which raised the question 'how?' Some herbal or dietary remedies had bioactive properties, which might now be considered pharmaceutical. Others contained nutrients that, in retrospect, could plausibly be mechanistically important. Dietary and nutritional factors in aetiology and treatment were eclipsed by drugs in the second half of the twentieth century because of their major and highly marketable short-term effects. That was totally understandable: for the first time medical treatment could offer a cure for some acute illness and a complete reversal of symptoms in some conditions. However, there has been a constant backdrop of concern that modern medicine has been failing to address the entire disease process or seeking to explain why some people, and not others, develop diseases at particular times. This concern, which led to a pursuit of 'holistic' treatments from alternative practitioners, is becoming the dominant issue for conventional medicine in the twenty-first century.

The twentieth-century model for the diagnosis and conceptualisation of disease mechanisms was a horizontal grid of categories (e.g. inherited/acquired; acute/chronic; inflammatory/infectious; neoplastic/degenerative). This grid helped to explore alternative diagnoses but failed to contextualise the individual with time, place or society and, as a consequence, provided only limited insight into the processes of disease development.

In the twenty-first century, medicine still uses diagnostic grids, since the need to offer *diagnosis, prognosis* and *treatment* is still paramount. However, there is a new need to offer *prevention*, and for that an understanding is required of disease mechanism. Interventions to change things are needed at a pre-clinical stage. Moreover, an understanding is required of the patterns of diseases likely to be faced by an individual or population such that preventive interventions directed at a particular disease can confidently be expected to reduce the entire profile of illness throughout life.

These are testing demands. It is easier to settle back into the twentieth-century interventional or prescriptive model of medical practice. An example can be drawn from diabetes. At one level (indeed as diagnostically defined) diabetes is a disease related to elevated blood glucose affecting eyes, kidneys and nerves through microangiopathy. However, type 2 diabetes also encompasses the (possibly separate) disease process of impaired glucose tolerance, whose clinical importance is a massive increase in ischaemic heart disease, stroke and peripheral vascular disease. A broader understanding of the disease is that of a global disorder of nutrient storage. It is necessary to become overweight to reveal impaired glucose tolerance (IGT) and also the hypertension and dyslipidaemia characteristic of the so-called metabolic syndrome. An even more fundamental understanding of diabetes is required to accommodate observations of increased cancer rates in people with diabetes in large surveys and of elevated inflammatory markers with reduced antioxidant status, reduced vitamin C levels and markers of free radical–mediated molecular damage.

Diabetes is now better conceptualised as a part of a disease process with multiple pathological consequences at different stages. The clinical course of an individual depends on his or her genetic endowment to provide a catalogue of predispositions (including a more or less complete expression of the metabolic syndrome). The timing and grouping of clinical manifestations of diabetes then depend on the influence of diet and lifestyle factors – potentially psychological and cultural as well as physical – that present stresses. People with diabetes can thus now be categorised (in retrospect) as those with exaggerated

or more pathogenic responses to stressful life exposures. Specifically, these include (1) excess net calorie consumption leading to overweight (IGT/type 2 diabetes is extremely rare at BMI 21 to 22 kg/m^2); (2) physical inactivity, and (3) a dietary mix that is low in fruit and vegetables, low in fish and high in foods high in saturated fat and sugars. The age of onset and rate of progression through IGT to type 2 diabetes and the development of vascular complications depend on the resolution of equations including extent of genetic predisposition, age and the duration and severity of all these diet and lifestyle factors (Fig. 14.1). Given a strong genetic predisposition, type 2 diabetes can now be recognised in obese, inactive children.

Since we cannot change genes, medical efforts to prevent, delay or reduce the impact of diabetes should primarily be addressing the diet and lifestyle component of its aetiology. As evidenced by the United Kingdom Prospective Diabetes Study (UKPDS) results, the benefits of drug therapy at a late clinical stage of disease are certainly of value, but they are quite limited. Most drug therapies do not address the underlying predisposition to diabetes or the pathways involved in progression. These fall within the realm of human nutrition (Table 14.1). If researched with similar levels of funding to pharmaceutical trials, it would be expected that nutritional intervention would lead to major clinical benefit. Extreme nutritional interventions have dramatic results. For example, major weight loss in obese patients who need insulin to control type 2 diabetes can restore entirely normal glucose tolerance as well as reducing elevated blood pressure and lipids.

Dietary requirements

All living organisms have needs that must be satisfied from external supply.

Energy and macronutrients

For any living thing there is a need to import energy. Plants can do this from the sun by photosynthesis,

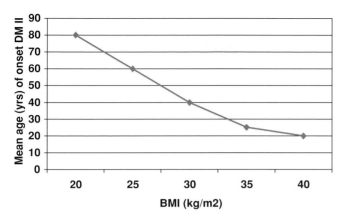

Figure 14.1 Relation of BMI and age at diagnosis among people with newly diagnosed type 2 diabetes.

Table 14.1 The three pillars of human nutrition (What we are; What we eat; What we (can) do in the example of type 2 diabetes

---

1. **'What we are' – Body composition**
Exaggerated intra-abdominal fat deposition
Intra-muscular and hepatic lipid deposition
Muscle atrophy
Increased percentage of body fat
Reduced body magnesium

2. **'What we eat' – Diet composition**
Positive energy balance (20–50 kcal/day) causing weight gain and fat accumulation
Excess saturated fat, impairing insulin sensivity
Low dietary antioxidants, allowing chronic inflammation
High proportion of glycolytic type 2 fast-twitch muscle fibre
Low proportion of type 1 slow-twitch oxidation

3. **'What we (can) do' – functional capacity**
Reduced capacity for fat oxidation
Low adiponectin and excess fatty acids impair insulin sensitivity and glucose storage and oxidation
Low capacity for endurance activity
Tendency to inactivity
Chronic minor appetite excess above the need for energy balance

---

but all other species, humans included, need to access calories from foods. Specifically, energy must be obtained from the 'macronutrients' (fat, carbohydrates and proteins), which are ultimately oxidised to generate adenosine triphosphate (ATP). These components are found in varying proportions, in all natural foods. For energy provision alone, there is no fixed requirement for specific macronutrients, so a wide range of proportions of the macronutrients can provide energy. The optimal balance of macronutrients for health is determined by other biological proportions of the macronutrients (e.g. an upper limit for fat, and specifically saturated fatty acids, is recommended principally because of the impact of fats on coronary heart disease (CHD)/IGT, that is, diabetes and obesity.

There probably is a small demand for dietary carbohydrates to provide glucose for the brain, about 50 g/day. There is a biological need for exogenous 'essential' fatty acids of the n-6 series at about 3% of total calorie consumption. Dietary protein need is again relatively small (about 10% of dietary energy) to provide for the small losses in the normal continuous turnover of proteins. However, most protein is broken down to amino acids, which are then metabolised in the same way as carbohydrates, the

Table 14.2 Requirements of macronutrients as a percentage of energy

	Minimal needs (%E)	Optimal	Usual human diets
Fat (essential fatty acids)	3%	20%–35%	20% – 40% (total fat, 5%– 10% essential fatty acids)
Carbohydrates	5%–10%	45%–55%	40% – 60%
Proteins	5% – 8%	10% –15%	10% – 20%

nitrogen-containing amino group being excreted as urea. The body's requirements is determined by the much smaller requirement for 'essential' amino acids (the ones that are not synthesised adequately within the body) and thus also on the composition of the dietary proteins that provide them. The absolute requirement is thus lower for proteins whose proportions of component amino acids best match the needs of the body.

For each of the macronutrients, the absolute dietary requirement is much less than the amounts provided by almost all normal human diets (Table 14.2).

In relation to long-term health, there are other considerations for macronutrient balance related to minimising the risk or delaying the onset of a range of diet-related (preventable) diseases. There is no single, closely defined ideal diet composition, but upper limits can be set, mainly on epidemiological evidence with a certain amount of interventional corroboration, to give the ranges for a 'prudent' or 'healthful' diet composition shown in Table 14.2. These ranges of macronutrient needs are agreed by a range of scientific bodies worldwide as representing the optimal pattern in relation to a range of diseases. Although originally determined for dietary advice to reduce CHD and stroke, the same advice is optimal to reduce obesity, diabetes and a variety of cancers.

The absolute energy needs of the body vary with growth, activity and disease. As people get bigger (taller and heavier), the metabolic rate increases and the requirement for energy rises. Obese individuals require more calories than thinner people to avoid weight loss. Basal metabolic rate is usually 50% to 75% of the 24-h metabolic rate. Physical activity usually comprises 25% to 50% of total metabolic rate (energy need). It can increase. Illness can have a variety of effects. Classically, acute stress and shock suppress metabolism for up to a day or so; thereafter metabolic rate and energy requirements tend to rise as long as inflammation and repair processes are active. This has been described as the 'ebb and flow' pattern of metabolism. The elevation of metabolic rate by inflammation can be up to 100% in conditions such as severe burns, but more usually acute infections increase metabolism by only about 10% to 20%, which is compensated by reduced physical activity. The weight loss that accompanies acute and repeated infections or chronic inflammation is more related to loss of appetite.

The mechanism for illness increasing energy expenditure/metabolism or metabolism include the catecholamines, (balanced against corticosteroids, which tend to suppress metabolic rate) and the pro-inflammatory cytokines [e.g. tumor necrosis factor (TNF) and the interleukins IL-1, IL-2 and IL-8], which form part of the acute-phase response to illness. Their effect on metabolism and simultaneous suppression of appetite can to some extent be modified by specific antisera or by treatment with non-steroidal anti-inflammatory drugs. It is difficult to overcome these mechanisms by trying to coax patients to eat more.

Dietary provision

The influence of diet on health is complicated both as an area of research to unravel disease mechanisms and also as in the context of interventions for disease management.

Although biological and biochemical processes need nutrients, people consume foods or diets, not isolated nutrients. Foods are rarely eaten in isolation or as a single source of nutrition for any length of time. They are eaten in combination with other foods and in patterns influenced by cultural factors, habit and fashion or marketing. Food supply is thus variable and thereby nutrient supply can vary widely, although it is possible to derive the same provision of nutrients from a huge range of foods combined in different ways.

Given the long time course of influences from diet on health and the variability of provision and choice, a useful biological concept to link food and health is 'dietary exposure' (e.g. 5 apples per week for 25 years or 240 g pizza per week for 10 years). However, what the body sees is not foods but nutrients, having reached the point of absorption (e.g. exposure to a high-saturated-fat diet greater than 10% of total energy (E) intake for so many years). The absorbed nutrients are usually very similar to those consumed (i.e. provision minus wastage), but some losses in the processes of digestion. Many food components are digested to smaller units (e.g. triglycerides to fatty acids and monoglycerides protein to amino acids). For some nutrients (e.g. plant phenolics), there is extensive metabolism within the gut lumen. The 'available' nutrients in foods are usually a little less than the total in the food. Absorption is usually nearly 100%, but malabsorption is a failure of a number of diseases. Malabsorption may be clinically apparent with identifiable food passing through the gut, or it may be subclinical. Malabsorption may also be specific to certain nutrients (e.g. loss of pancreatic lipase results in fat malabsorption), which is clinically obvious as steatorrhea when above about 7 g per meal, or it may be subclinical, with a lower but metabolically important loss of ingested fats (and calories) at lower levels. Malabsorption may be a non-specific feature of gastrointestinal or other diseases. For example, reduced food intake for any reason leads to gastrointestinal mucosal atrophy and a reduction in lactase-producing capacity, such that milk consumption may result in incomplete absorption of lactose from milk. Diarrhoea is a consequence of lactate fermentation in the colon.

Whereas research has provided detailed information about the absorption, digestion and overall availability of nutrients from foods, our methods for establishing what foods people eat in free-living situations are much weaker. They have to depend mainly on self-reported food consumption, and this introduces a consistent cross-cultural bias towards overweight people claiming to eat less than is physiologically possible. A second difficulty is the long pre-clinical period of most diet-related diseases. For these reasons much of our understanding of the relationship between food exposure and consumption must depend on observational data and ecological analyses of 'food disappearance' and disease patterns. Randomised clinical trials are possible in some areas but not widely applicable. Furthermore, most diet-related diseases are multi-factorial. They depend on severity and duration of dietary exposure to accelerate or delay onset and progression.

A consequence of these limitations to research is that gene–diet or gene–nutrient interactions are hard to identify.

Diseases of nutritional deficiency

The classical nutritional disorders were those of nutrient deficiency, usually in extreme and obviously deprived circumstances.

There is biological need for a surprisingly small number of *essential* elements (Fig. 14.2). All life on earth arises from only about 20 of the elements, but different species have slightly different biochemical capacities, demanding external provision of species-specific complex molecules. These form their nutrient requirements.

Plants can harness energy (from the sun) by photosynthesis and store that energy in chemical bonds, in carbohydrate, fat and protein. Animals require supplies of these 'macronutrients' to provide energy, but these molecules also provide most chemical units needed for the synthetic processes of growth, repair and reproduction. A number of fatty acids and amino acids are termed 'essential', meaning that they are required for health but that we do not have the capacity for their synthesis. When they are not provided in adequate amounts, the processes for

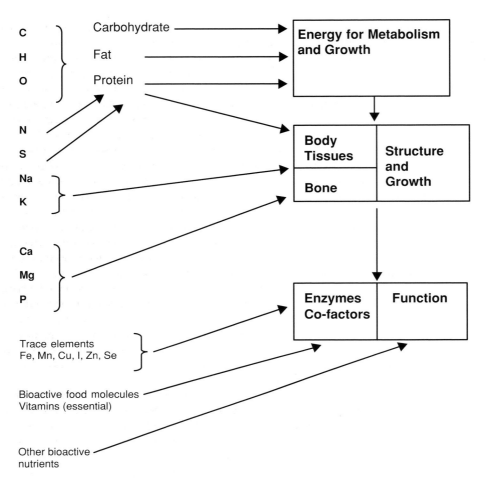

Figure 14.2 Elemental contributions to human nutrition and health.

which they are needed slow down or stop. In the case of essential fatty acids, other non-essential fatty acids may be incorporated into processes, conferring different properties on the end product. The amino acids are much more specific, but within the body there are potential supplies of amino acids from proteins that are consistently undergoing re-modelling. The distribution of amino acids within the body varies during times of essential amino acid deficiency. The quantitative requirements for amino acids and essential amino acids are generally low, but they may vary during illness because of losses or through increased metabolic and synthetic require-ments. The capacity of the body to synthesise amino acids that are normally 'non-essential' may be compromised during illness, making them temporarily 'essential'. An example of this is glycine, which is normally synthesised within the body from pre-cursors obtained from foods or from protein re-modelling. In infancy the demand for glycine is greater and the capacity to synthesise it may be reduced by illness. A normally adequate glycine supply can become a limiting factor in the processes of recovery and growth. It is therefore preferable to consider the term 'essential', when applied to nutrients, as describing a process rather as defining specific compounds.

Aside from the macronutrients, there are a small number of other food compounds that are essential, grouped as vitamins and essential trace elements (Fig. 14.2). Most of the vitamins were discovered to be essential dietary compounds in the investigation of clinical manifestations of malnutrition. The history of their discoveries is interesting because this work formed a large part of what has developed into biochemistry and molecular biology. The discovery of vitamins also fuelled the imagination of people who like to believe in magic and particularly in the magical properties of specific foods in relation to health, reproductive capacity and longevity. The classical vitamin deficiency diseases certainly exist and in some cases have formed endemic disease patterns, but usually dietary deficiency states are characterised by multiple deficiencies; therefore the clinical manifestations are often complicated. Both vitamins and essential trace elements are mainly required as co-factors for enzymes. Their deficiencies place a brake or even a halt on specific biochemical pathways, and in some cases this results in limited and easily recognisable clinical manifestations (e.g. vitamin B1 deficiency leading to beri-beri and Wernicke's encephalopathy or iron deficiency leading to microcytic anaemia).

For other vitamin and trace element deficiencies, the clinical manifestations are more general or widespread. For example, zinc is required in over 100 enzyme systems. Its deficiency leads to multiple effects. In extreme situations, there is the characteristic clinical presentation with de-pigmentation and wiry consistency of the hair and skin ulcers around the mouth and anus. However, lesser degrees of zinc deficiency place limitations on tissue growth and repair, which may become manifest only as delayed healing from wounds such as burns and increased susceptibility to infection, which are difficult to attribute in an individual case.

There are a number of conservation mechanisms available to minimise the impact of reduced nutrient supply. Essential processes like respiration are protected, but others such as growth, reproductive function, gastrointestinal mucosal cell turnover, and immune function are nutrient-costly and can be slowed down in a hierarchical manner. As dietary provision is reduced or distorted away from the optimal provision for health and 'goodness of fit' is compromised, function is impaired and ultimately health suffers unless there are in-built mechanisms to buffer the system by storage and regulated absorption.

Dietary deficiency of a nutrient is thus not necessarily the same as a nutritional deficiency state. Like many animals, humans eat in meals, usually two or three main meals a day with variable periods in between. There is obviously a need for nutrients to be stored in between meals and for that storage to cope with expected periods of food deprivation. Humans have also adapted to cope with nutritional fluctuations resulting from seasonal variations in supply. The two potential strategies for doing this are to vary synthetic and other metabolic activities in the body according to supply or to develop storage capacity for nutrients whose supply may be variable. These two strategies do not always seem well harmonised to the human food supply. Thus, for example, we have very large stores of iron in the liver, bone marrow in particular, which can provide adequate supplies of iron for four weeks. For zinc, however, a nutrient required in very similar absolute amounts to iron, there are no stores at all; therefore the only possible response to dietary deficiency is to limit the synthetic processes that require zinc. Nutrients can be broadly divided into those whose storage capacity allows for function over minutes, hours, days, weeks and months (Table 14.3).

A final strategy available for some nutrients is to recover or re-synthesise those nutrients from waste

Table 14.3 Storage capacity for essential nutrients

Minutes	Oxygen
Hours	Water, carbohydrate
Days	Zinc, magnesium
	Vitamin C, selenium and most water-soluble vitamins, amino acids
Weeks and months	Fat-soluble vitamins, iron, iodine, vitamin B12

products. This happens to a small degree, which may occasionally be important for survival with respect to the amino acids. The pathways of protein turnover result in net losses from the body of nitrogen in the form of ammonia in the bowel. Bowel bacteria have some capacity to re-synthesise amino acids from excreted ammonia, and this can be reabsorbed from the large bowel. One of the mysteries regarding the survival of vegetarians is where they obtain vitamin B12, given that vitamin B12 is an essential nutrient and the only essential nutrient found exclusively in animal food products. Vitamin B12 is the only functional form of the essential trace element cobalt. Cobalt is found in a variety of other forms in foods and passes through the bowel into the colon, where bacteria are able to synthesise vitamin B12 in sufficient amounts for its adequate absorption from the colon.

Deficiency diseases always reflect the balance between nutrient supply (in available form) and its losses from the body, either through metabolism or through pathological losses from wounds (particularly inflamed or infected wounds with high rates of exudation) by malabsorptive diarrhoea. At a clinical diagnostic level it is often difficult to quantify losses, and intake can only be estimated from a patient's memory. Usually disease sufficient to generate important nutrient losses from the body will also reduce appetite and food consumption. In western medical practice, therefore, nutrient deficiency is commonly multi-factorial. A state of nutrient deficiency commonly indicates serious pathology. For example, iron deficiency, manifest as microcystic anaemia, is more frequent in individuals with low iron consumption (classically the 'bread, jam and tea' diet of the urban deprived). However, as iron status falls, capacity to absorb iron increases through gut adaptation. Therefore, clinically evident iron-deficiency anaemia often points to occult blood loss from a bowel tumour.

This capacity to increase absorption during times of limited supply is not seen with all nutrients. It applies only when the usual absorption is low (10% to 40% of dietary supply in the case of iron) and where uncontrolled absorption could be hazardous.

Iron is a potent oxidant and potentially toxic: a modest over-dose of ferrous sulphate tablets can be fatal. Thus gastrointestinal absorption is regulated by active transport mechanisms (involving transferrin and the copper containing enzyme caeruloplasmin). The expression and function of iron transport mechanisms are regulated by iron status. Similar regulations exists for copper and for calcium. During pregnancy, when demand for these trace elements is increased, their absorption also increases. Similar bio-modulation occurs in the placenta to ensure adequate supply, even up a gradient, to the fetus.

Management of deficiency diseases

Logical and effective management of deficiency disease has a number of key components that reflect or augment other medical considerations.

In an individual case, the diagnosis is usually made on clinical suspicion, from history and examination, with little help from diagnostic tests unless the disease is very advanced. As deficiencies develop, functional capacity is lost at an early stage and overt pathology often occurs before there are major changes in blood biochemistry. In some cases, biochemistry can be extremely misleading. For example, as zinc deficiency advances, there is tissue catabolism with release of hitherto functional zinc into the plasma, so plasma levels can be high.

The circulating levels of many vitamins and minerals are influenced by acute-phase changes. Thus plasma levels of many nutrients fall during any inflammatory state even if the whole-body or tissue status is good. In the past it was observed that serum albumin commonly changes in parallel with plasma nutrients, and this was interpreted as meaning that albumin was a nutritional marker. It is not; indeed, serum albumin remains at normal levels even in advanced starvation. Instead, both albumin and nutrient levels vary with inflammation and illness non-specifically. Once a diagnosis of a nutrient deficiency is made, it is necessary to consider the inter-relationships of nutrients in foods and in the body and to assess whether it is a single, isolated deficiency (unusual) or part of a more general state of under nutrition. Recorded patterns of weight change are thus important.

Treatment can take the form of physiological, dietary, dose replacement or pharmacological therapy. These may be provided in isolation or as part of a composite nutritional supplement. It is important to recognise the upper safe limits for nutrient consumption as well as the scale of body stores available to take up excess supply. Thus, for example, it makes sense to provide supra-dietary doses of iron, folic acid and vitamins A or B12 to a deficient individual because they are large stores that could valuably be filled. On the other hand, it makes little sense to supply very high doses of zinc or vitamin C to correct deficiency, since there are no stores.

Moreover, clinical recovery from nutrient deficiency is usually relatively slow and not influenced by dosage. The striking exception to this is thiamine (vitamin B1) deficiency, most frequently met in alcoholics who eat insufficient wholemeal bread and cereal-based foods. Deficiency can progress over hours to cause permanent brain damage in Korsakoff's psychosis. Immediate, high-dose parenteral replacement is necessary to circumvent the normally slower biological mechanisms.

When the gastrointestinal tract is not available, it is of course possible to provide partial or complete nutrition intravenously. There are practical problems over formulation that can prevent difficulties such as precipitation or flocculation of feeds and of hyper-osmolarity if full energy requirements are provided (because large complex molecules cannot be given). However parenteral feeding can now be maintained for years by committed and well-supported individuals. Without the normal transport regulation provided by a healthy gut, patients dependent on parenteral nutrition are vulnerable to small variations in nutrient supply or availability. Unusual problems have been reported, such as serious manganese toxicity in children, because standard parenteral micronutrient formulations were excessive for some individuals. Monitoring of plasma concentrations is recommended for that purpose. The main clinical problems faced in patients receiving par-

enteral nutrition, however, are the avoidable ones of sepsis (given that the feed is a perfect bacterial culture medium) and of over-feeding. Our ability to cope with excess nutrient loads is limited by storage capacity and by the speed of processing into stores. Excess energy is converted in the liver into lipid, which is normally transported to adipose tissue stores. If the supply exceeds the limits of this process, fat accumulates in the liver, which can seriously misfunction. The limit is somewhere around 25% to 50% of excess energy (caloric) supply, and transport processes may be impaired by illness. In the past, over-energetic efforts to re-feed undernourished patients have led to serious liver disease and even death. This can be avoided by better understanding of nutritional requirements. Energy requirements can be measured using bedside indirect calorimetry, but for practical purposes, standard equations predict it adequately (Department of Health, 1991).

The process of re-feeding after nutritional depletion needs to avoid another clinical pitfall, the 're-feeding syndrome'. Under-feeding and illness result in a loss of adipose tissue and muscle mass as well as atrophy of most tissues other than brain. During recovery and re-feeding, disproportionately large supplies of intracellular nutrients are needed. The re-feeding syndrome is a characteristic arrest of recovery accompanied by extreme weakness, which results from inadequate supply of potassium, phosphate, zinc and so on. Patients often die. Its manifestations can resemble those of protein or essential amino acid deficiency (seen mainly in experimental animals), but giving more protein makes matters worse.

Classically, dietary nutrient deficiencies were considered in relation to the emergence of the classical deficiency diseases (Table 14.4). However there are other functions of many nutrients that can have more subtle, long-term effects on health. Thus the antioxidant actions of vitamins C and E can be related to protection against CHD and stroke, perhaps by reducing the oxidation of low-density-lipoprotein cholesterol (LDL-C). At a population level, declining fruit and vegetable consumption, hence vitamin C supplies, has been a plausible component of increased CHD in

Table 14.4 Assessment of nutritional deficiencies: vitamins

Vitamin	Method	Comment
A	Clinical	Infections common
		Night blindness is a good indicator
		Corneal lesions are very late-stage findings
	Plasma carotenoids	
	Plasma retinol	Sensitive indicator of liver stores but reduced in infection
Thiamine	Clinical	Neuropathy and optic atrophy are late-stage findings
	HPLC	Specific
	Erythrocyte transketolase	Sensitive but rapidly altered by amount of dietary thiamine
Riboflavin	Clinical	Mouth lesions are non-specific
	Erythrocyte gluthatione reductase	Assay related poorly to clinical state
Niacin	Clinical	Glossitis, stomatitis, dermatitis
	Urinary n-methyl-nicotinamine/creatine excretion	Sensitive. Difficult assay
Folate	Serum folate	Marked changes after dietary intake
	Erythrocyte folate	Sensitive assay of body stores
B12	Plasma vitamin level	Sensitive assay of body stores. Elevated by liver disease
C	Clinical	Specific but occur at late stages only
	Plasma or leucocyte ascorbate (HPLC)	Sensitive. Rapid response to diet. Falls non-specifically in illness
D	Clinical	Rickets, osteomalacia
	Plasma alkaline phosphatase	Non-specific. Sensitivity may be improved by isoenzyme analysis
	Plasma 25-hydroxycholecalciferol	Very specific
	Bone marrow histology	Specific
E	Plasma or eythrocyte tocopherol (HPLC)	Sensitive and specific. Must be corrected for plasma LDL on total cholesterol
K	Prothrombin time	Non-specific, as it is influenced by hepatocellular dysfunction

the twentieth century. Whether treating individuals with vitamin C confers benefit is less clear. Perhaps paradoxically, vitamin E intakes have generally risen, reflecting higher intakes of fats and oils, to which it is added as an industrial antioxidant. Folate, also found in fruits and vegetables, is needed at a certain level to permit normal bone marrow function – its deficiency leads to anaemia and pancytopaenia. However folate is also necessary for normal fetal develop-

ment and methionine metabolism. With insufficient folate, neural tube defects and elevated homocysteine (contributing to CHD) are found. These clinical problems do not occur in every case, however, and it is becoming clear that some common polymorphisms that alter the form of folate-dependent enzymes have the effect of increasing the biological requirement for folic acid. Early in our evolutionary history, consumption of fruits and vegetables was probably sufficient to provide for most individuals, even with polymorphisms that increase demand. Current levels of fruit and vegetable consumption, and supply in many post-industrial countries are so low that whole populations are compromised. A difficulty for medical science and practice lies in determining the extent to which this single factor contributes to a multi-factorial condition like CHD and negative impact and the effort that should be put into increasing such consumption as well as fruits and vegetables in the food supply. Folate supplementation of bread and cereals has been adopted in North America, with early evidence suggesting reductions in neural tube defects and CHD.

Diseases of nutritional excess

Optimal growth, function and reproduction, the basis on which human evolution operated, was driven by a plane of nutrition that undoubtedly included periodic under-feeding and thus a need for nutrient storage. Our evolution was probably not affected by sustained over-nutrition to an important degree. Moreover, much human life is now beyond the reproductive age range over which evolutionary forces would have operated. Over-nutrition places new and potentially unresolvable stress on the species.

Conceptually, overfeeding may be 'balanced' – with an excess of all nutrients in approximately the same proportions as required for health, or unbalanced, with an excess of only some nutrients. The most recognisable consequence, obesity, arises when our weakly regulated upper limit of appetite control allows excess energy intake relative to needs, with excess body fat accumulation. Initially, fat accumulates in adipose tissue, but in many people, particularly those genetically predisposed to the metabolic syndrome, lipid transport mechanisms are overcome and lipid accumulates in the liver. Non-alcoholic hepatic steatosis (NASH) with abnormal liver function tests is just one manifestation of the metabolic syndrome – dyslipidaemia, insulin resistance and hypertension, all conspiring to increase CHD risks.

Obesity has multiple pathological consequences, affecting virtually every organ system in the body (Table 14.5). Many of these effects develop as excessive body-mass index (BMI), or an increase in waist circumference across the normal range, and manifest with minor degrees of overweight before reaching 'obesity'. Some are mainly mediated by physical effects (e.g. arthritis, back pain, leg oedema). Others are metabolic or appear in combination with physical effects. An example is the hypertension associated with obesity, which represents a high proportion of what used to be termed 'essential hypertension'. Permanent alterations in blood pressure regulation seem to occur after a period of obesity, such that the fall in blood pressure with weight loss may be only temporary. One additional contribution may be over-nutrition with sodium as an almost unavoidable accompaniment to food calories. Obese people need to consume more calories than thinner people to avoid weight loss. In doing so, they have increased intakes of sodium, mainly as an additive in processed food, bread and cereals. Evidence is now strong that excess sodium intake resets blood pressure control to higher levels (He et al., 2002).

Obesity and metabolic syndrome (ATP III) are also characterised by low-grade but sustained overproduction of inflammatory markers – many produced in adipose tissue itself – which compound the features of the syndrome. The concept and diagnostic criteria of metabolic syndrome are still evolving. It is believed that a group of genetic variants operate in a common way to cause accelerated CHD by effects on insulin resistance, blood glucose, dyslipidaemia and blood pressure. All these are well-known risk factors for CHD and disease treatment when each individual reaches a threshold level. All are aggravated by weight gain – specifically by increased waist and intra-abdominal fat. Treatment for metabolic syndrome initially calls for weight loss and weight maintenance, for equivalent health benefit need to be started at a lower BMI or waist circumference than for people without metabolic syndrome (Table 14.6).

Other forms of over-nutrition that contribute to disease include the excess provision of saturated fatty acids – either within a normal, acceptable total

Table 14.5 Medical consequences of overweight and obesity

Physical symptoms	Metabolic	Social
Tiredness	Hypertension	Isolation
Breathlessness	NIDDM	Agoraphobia
Varicose veins	Hepatic steatosis	Unemployment
Back pain	Hyperlipidaemia	Family/marital stress
Arthritis	Hypercoagulation	Discrimination
Oedema/cellulitis	Ischemic heart disease and stroke	Financial
Sweating / intertrigo		
Stress incontinence		
Anaesthetic/surgical	**Endocrine**	**Psychological**
Sleep apnoea	Hirsutism	Low self-esteem
Chest infections	Oligomenorrhea /infertility	Self-deception
Wound dehiscence	Metromenorrhea	Cognitive disturbance
Hernia	Oestrogen-dependent	Distorted body image
Venous thrombosis	Cancers: breast, colon, uterus, prostate	Depression

fat intake or, worse, as part of an undesirably elevated fat intake. There is no dietary requirement for saturated fat. Its consumption alters hepatic and whole-body lipoprotein metabolism such that LDL-C forms a greater part of total serum cholesterol. With obesity and inactivity, high-density-lipoprotein cholesterol (HDL-C) is reduced and triglyceride increased; this profile promotes atheroma formation and CHD. A further type of problem associated with over-nutrition is that proportionally greater provision of protective antioxidant dietary compounds appear to be needed.

The balance between pro-oxidant and antioxidant (reducing) compounds within tissues is closely regulated and most functional antioxidants are synthesised endogenously, but vitamin E undoubtedly has an important function in the CNS and probably elsewhere. Serious and permanent damage occurs if it is absent – classically in patients with abetalipoproteinaemia. There is at least a strong likelihood, on current evidence, that the cardio-protective and anti-cancer actions of fruits and vegetables are mediated by antioxidants (vitamin E, vitamin C and phenolics such as flavonoids). Their roles may be especially important in the context of overweight or obesity and when inflammatory stress is intro-

duced chronically. It is worth noting that the classically studied nutrients were the *essential* nutrients but that plant foods contain many other bioactive compounds (e.g. phenolics) that may influence long-term health in susceptible individuals.

Conclusion and implications

Recent re-examination of links between diet and disease have been stimulated by a recognition that drug treatment cannot cure or reverse the major diseases of the industrial world. These diseases are *all* multifactorial and their management should rely on long-term prevention rather than treatment. Diet and nutrition offer benefit for many sick patients, although seldom as dramatically or completely as the pharmaceutical interventions for infection. The future seems set to place a major emphasis on characterising the interactions between genetic predispositions to diseases, within individuals and within populations, and the specific interactions with dietary and nutritional factors. At one level, in the post-genomic age, this understanding could in theory guide specific treatments or preventive dietary strategies for individuals. However, this would be likely

Table 14.6 Clinical identification of metabolic syndrome

Risk factor	ATP III criteria	IDF criteria
	Any three of these:	Large waist plus any two:
Abdominal obesity	Waist circumference	Waist circumference
- Men	102 cm (> 40 in.)	94 cm (> 37 in.)
- Women	88 cm (> 35 in.)	80 cm (> 32 in.)
Fasting triglycerides	150 mg/dl (1.7 mmol/l)	150 mg/dl (1.7 mmol/l)
High-density-lipoprotein (HDL) cholesterol		
- Men	< 40 mg/dl (1.0 mmol/l)	< 40 mg/dl (1.0 mmol/l)
- Women	< 50 mg/dl (1.3 mmol/l)	< 50 mg/dl (1.3 mmol/l)
Blood pressure	130 / 85 mm Hg	130 / 85 mm Hg
Fasting glucose	110 mg/dl (6.1 mmol/l)	100 mg/dl (5.6 mmol/l)

to result in misleading guidance if the full profile of potential disease faced by an individual were not considered or in bewildering confusion if it were.

The most valuable consequence of current research on gene–nutrient interaction is likely instead to be a better informed and more committed approach towards population-directed measures that will reduce total disease burdens on society and ultimate health service costs. The major barriers at present are confusion or ignorance among both the public and health care professionals, and by health policies that in reality are only health care policies. If it is agreed that a change in what people eat would improve health, then education can play a part; but for any improvement, the total food supply must change. At a national level food consumption equals food supply (with minor adjustments for food, wastage and home-grown foods. People can only eat what is put before them, and that is what they do eat: the Industry does not provide foods which are not purchased). This becomes a political task that extends well beyond the brief of conventional health (or health-care) ministers.

Summary

Historically, diet was always considered the mainstay of health, and dietary origins were commonly attributed to diseases. This chapter explores the extent to which diet can still be considered a critical factor in many diseases. Indeed, viewing disease through the eyes of human nutrition (what we are, what we eat and what we do) can clarify some confusing issues – for example, the concept of metabolic syndrome and its treatment. This chapter addresses diseases of over-feeding, under-feeding and of imbalanced feeding – that is, the span from clinical to public health medicine.

Clinical scenario

Following an operation to correct a fractured neck of femur, a diabetic patient was seen on the ward by an endocrinologist. The patient complained of frequent spasms in her leg muscles, which she was convinced were responsible for her recent injury. Her investigations were as follows:

Calcium	1.8 mmol/l
Alkaline phosphatase	650 IU/l
25(OH) cholecalciferol	10.9 ng/ml
1,25(OH)$_2$ cholecalciferol	< 10 ng/ml
Pelvic X-ray	Looser's zones on superior and inferior pubic rami

Questions

1. What is the diagnosis?
2. What investigations are indicated?

Answers

1. The patient has vitamin D deficiency. This has resulted in hypocalcaemia, and the spasms described by are tetany. In vitamin D deficiency, there is insufficient calcium absorption for the body's requirements. As a result, parathyroid hormone levels are increased and calcium is mobilised from the bones. In adults, this leads to osteomalacia. The Looser's zones seen on the pelvic X-ray are characteristic.

2. Investigations should be directed at establishing a cause for the impaired synthesis and absorption of vitamin D. These include inadequate sunlight exposure coeliac disease, inflammatory bowel disease, cystic fibrosis and cholestatic liver disease, renal failure. It should also be noted that, once synthesised, vitamin D is stored in body fat. In obesity, the increase in body fat may reduce the bio-availability of the vitamin despite large stores within adipose tissue.

Multiple-choice questions

1. The defined components of the metabolic syndrome include:
   a. Elevated low-density-lipoprotein (LDL) cholesterol levels
   b. Impaired glucose tolerance
   c. Hypertension
   d. Enlarged waist circumference
   e. Elevated triglyceride levels
2. Conditions occurring as a consequence of obesity include:
   a. Urinary incontinence
   b. Obstructive sleep apnoea
   c. Asthma
   d. Breast cancer
   e. Obsessive compulsive disorder
3. Zinc deficiency can cause:
   a. Delayed wound healing
   b. Mouth ulcers
   c. Skin depigmentation

d. Neuropathy
e. Cardiac conduction defects

4. The following is true of re-feeding syndrome:
   a. It can follow a prolonged period of dietary excess
   b. Nutrients may not properly be absorbed
   c. Weakness results from deficiencies of phosphate and potassium
   d. There may be enhanced deposition of adipose tissue
   e. Treatment is by high protein supplementation

Answers

1: a, F; b, T; c, F; d, T; e, T (fasting glucose > 6.0 mmol/L, BP > 130/85)
2: a, T; b, T; c, F; d, T, e, F
3: a, T; b, T; c, T; d, F; e, T
4: a, F; b, T; c, T; d, F; e, F

FURTHER READING

Department of Health (1991). Dietary Reference Values for Food Energy and Nutrients for the United Kingdom. Report of the panel on Dietary References Values of the Committee on Medical Aspects of Food Policy. London: Department of Health.

Gibney, M.J., Elia, M., Ljungquist, O., Dowsett, J. (2005). *Clinical Nutrition*. Oxford: Blackwell Publishing.

He, F. J., MacGregor, G. A. (2002). Effect of modest salt reduction on blood pressure: a meta-analysis of randomised trials. Implications for public health. *Journal of Human Hypertension* **16,** 761–70.

Hillier, T. A., Pedula, K. L. (2001). Characteristics of an adult population with newly diagnosed type 2 diabetes: the relation of obesity and age of onset. *Diabetes Care* **24,** 1522–27.

International Diabetes Federation. www.idf.org

Mann, J., Truswell, A. S. (eds.) (2007). *Essentials of Human Nutrition*, 3rd edn. Oxford: Oxford University Press.

National Cholesterol Education Program (2001). Third report of the expert panel on detection, evaluation and treatment of high blood cholesterol in adults (adult treatment panel III). *JAMA* 285, 2486–97.

15

Trauma

Nick Payne and David W. Yates

Introduction and epidemiology

Trauma has always been a major source of morbidity and mortality for man, and as other disease such as infection is either conquered or controlled, the relative importance of trauma grows.

Some 10% of global mortality is due to injury. In 1990, road accidents ranked as the ninth most important cause of death worldwide, but even this dire figure is expected to rise, to sixth place (at 8.4 million people per year) by 2020. In 2020, road accidents are expected to be the third most common cause of disability (Murray and Lopez, 1997). The main cause of trauma today are:

Accidents, especially road accidents

Homicide, suicide and assault

War

Burns

In 2003 the number of deaths in England and Wales from road accidents alone was 2 274 males and 751 females. In the under-45 age group, over 1 500 males and over 330 females were killed on the road (Office of National Statistics, 2003). This is a huge loss of fit, healthy life, and *all* preventable and unnecessary. Between 1996 and 2002, the deaths rates per 100 000 for road accidents have remained reasonably constant, between 8.8 and 9.4 for males of all ages, and 2.8 and 3.5 for females of all ages (Office of National Statistics, 2003).

These figures relate just to deaths, which, although tragic, do not result in ongoing problems. The number of injured and disabled who live with constant pain, difficulty and expense for many years is thought to be as much as 10 times these figures, although these numbers are more difficult to quantify with confidence. There is thus a major impact on public health, with huge resource implications. There is a societal cost as well as an individual cost.

Many people will be familiar with the trimodal distribution, or three-peak model, proposed by Trunkey (1983). This divides deaths into:

Immediate, about which the doctor can do little (but the legislator a lot)

Early, which with good resuscitation can be reduced

Late, due to sepsis and organ failure

This model has been challenged (Lecky *et al.*, 2000), and a new model has been derived from the Trauma Audit and Research Network (TARN) database, which shows an exponential decline in deaths with time, and no late peaks. Some 25% of deaths occur within the first $2\frac{1}{2}$ hours and 50% within the first day.

Reducing the burden

There are ways in which to improve the shocking and unacceptable amount of death and disability. The approaches can be divided into the following:

- *Primary prevention*, not letting an incident occur. Enforcing speed limits, public education, the increasing unacceptability of drink driving and social improvement to reduce the violence in society. This should reduce the 'immediate' group of deaths.

- *Secondary prevention*, minimising injury when incident does occur. The compulsory wearing of seatbelts and motorbike helmets, the self-help of wearing pedal-bike helmets (which should also be compulsory), driving cars with supplementary restraint systems and corporate help such as giving adequate protective clothing to those in the firing line, such as police officers. This should also reduce the 'immediate' group of deaths.

- *Tertiary prevention*, optimising outcome through improved treatment when incident and trauma does occur. Increased availability and improved standards of pre-hospital care (such as British Association Immediate Care, or BASICS), better and more widespread training of emergency staff (such as Advanced Trauma Life Support, or ATLS), and the setting up of dedicated trauma centres. Although the efficacy of trauma centres is unproven, it is known that there is a variation in outcome at different centres, and work needs to be done to elicit the reasons and then correct this discrepancy. Improvements in tertiary prevention should help in the 'early' group, probably the 'late' group, and possibly a very few of the 'immediate' group if help is very prompt.

Box 15.1

NAME	Kevin Neil Platt

AGE	19 years
VEHICLE	12-year-old saloon car

No head restraint, no airbag and seatbelt not worn.

INCIDENT	Lost control at roundabout, 40 mph, into lamppost

Fortunately no other vehicle or pedestrian involved.

Blood alcohol found to be 180 mg/dl

INJURIES	Blunt head injury on windscreen, GCS E1, M4, V2: Glasgow Coma Score Eye response 1, Motor response 4, Verbal response 2.

Hyperextension injury to the cervical spine

Chest into the steering wheel with multiple rib fractures and a left-sided flail segment (an area of paradoxical movement, reducing tidal volume), haemopneumothorax, lung and cardiac contusions

Right-upper-quadrant abdominal crush injury

Compound fracture/dislocation right ankle

The accident

To put trauma in perspective, let us imagine a typical road crash.

This previously healthy young man has sustained monstrous polytrauma. His chances of survival are slim, and if he does survive, he will have the effects of this evening's error with him for the rest of his life.

Immediate effects of injuries

Box 15.2

AIRWAY	At risk due to his reduced GCS and neck trauma
BREATHING	Decreased gas exchange and lung volume

Decreased air entry due to flail segment

CIRCULATION	Decreased cardiac contractility and blood volume

(Blood volume loss both apparent and occult, in his chest and abdomen)

Mechanical inhibition of heart filling due to pneumothorax

Before we discuss how to help Kevin, we must start to understand what is happening at a cellular level.

Macro-physiology

The cardiovascular response to blood loss

There is obviously great difficulty in doing human research in this area. Most of the work has been done on laboratory animals, (with extrapolated conclusions), simulated by lower body suction (where negative pressure is applied to pool blood in the legs) or in observational studies. As the vast majority of trauma that we see in the UK is blunt, (only 3.9% of trauma deaths are due to penetrating injury, (Lecky *et al.*, 2000) research should reflect this, and on the whole it tries to. In applying the research that has been done to real life, it must be remembered that simple haemorrhage (the usual research model) is not directly comparable to tissue injury, which – as explained below – is much more complex.

Currently in the UK we are seeing an increase in penetrating trauma (more the North American picture). We are at the low-velocity, knives and hand-guns stage. The injuries resulting from high-velocity weapons are seen only rarely in this country. High-velocity injuries result in

- Greater tissue destruction (energy is dissipated from the projectile and this energy is proportional to the square of the velocity).
- Greater tissue contamination (as debris is sucked into the wound).
- Damage away from the tract of the projectile (due to pressure waves).
- An unpredictable wound tract (as the projectile spirals).

The teaching used to be that volume of blood loss had a simple relationship with increasing pulse and decreasing blood pressure. It is not this straight-forward. Research by Little and colleagues (Little *et al.*, 2005) has shown that we need to look at the whole picture: the injury itself, blood pressure, pulse rate, respiratory rate, level of consciousness, capillary refill, urine output. Laboratory measurements such as lactate, blood gases and oxygen debt also need to be considered in this complicated equation.

The three basic reflexes that apply to simple haemorrhage are as follows.

The arterial baroreceptor reflex

The Basics

This is operational during the initial blood loss, up to 15% total blood volume. Its aim is to maintain arterial blood pressure. In the aortic arch and the carotid sinus there are stretch receptors, which are *less* stimulated as the pulse pressure drops. This information reaches the brain via the vagus and glossopharyngeal nerves, which responds by reducing vagal inhibitory efferents to the heart and increasing sympathetic efferents to vessels. There is thus a tachycardia and vasoconstriction. Total peripheral resistance and blood pressure rise.

Also

The vasoconstriction is more marked in some systems than others. The gut is an important example,

and decreased flow results in increased gut wall permeability as local relative ischaemia causes mucosal damage. This is an important consideration in the origins of sepsis and the consequent development of multiple organ failure. The body will try to maintain blood flow to the brain and heart.

There is a shift of fluid from the extra-vascular to the intra-vascular space, which also improves the blood pressure. This is due to a change in the pressure gradient between these compartments. Remember that this fluid from the extra-vascular space will need to be replaced at some point.

As blood loss continues, there is suddenly a precipitous drop in blood pressure. This is due to the depressor reflex.

The depressor reflex

The basics

This occurs after about 20% of blood volume is lost. Mechano-chemo receptors in the left ventricle are stimulated as the filling pressure drops. This information reaches the brain via the vagal C-fibres, and the brain responds by increasing vagal activity to the heart and decreasing sympathetic vasoconstrictor tone. There is thus a bradycardia and vasodilatation. Total peripheral resistance drops, and blood pressure falls dramatically. This is decompensation.

Also

This is a very complex and poorly understood reflex. It may be viewed as a last-ditch attempt by the body to preserve the heart, and if cardiac arrest is not to occur very soon, there must be a rapid replacement of circulating volume.

The baroreceptor and depressor reflexes together constitute the *biphasic response*.

The chemoreceptor reflex

The basics

Chemoreceptors in the aortic and carotid bodies are stimulated by a fall in oxygen tension and they inform the brain. This results in an increased respiratory rate as well as a decreased heart rate via the vagus nerve and sympathetically induced vasoconstriction.

Also

As CO_2 tension rises and pH falls, the body becomes more sensitive to falls in O_2 tension.

The increased respiratory activity blunts the vagal bradycardia and the sympathetic vasoconstriction.

As the blood pressure drops due to the depressor reflex, this chemoreceptor reflex is stimulated, maintains blood pressure and blunts the vagal bradycardia.

Tissue damage

Thus it can be seen that there are some complicated reflexes that interact during *blood loss*. There is also *tissue damage*, and this has a further effect. There is an alpha adrenoceptor sympathetic vasoconstrictor response to direct tissue damage. This results in an increase in blood pressure, total peripheral resistance and heart rate. This is the familiar "fight or flight" response. Glomerular filtration rate (and thus the more measurable urine output) drops, gut blood flow drops (resulting in local hypoxia and decreased barrier function) and the sensitivity of baroreceptors drops, resulting in a persistent tachycardia. When decompensation (i.e. bradycardia) does occur, it is pre-terminal. The overall outcome of haemorrhage with tissue damage is worse than that due to haemorrhage alone.

Tissue damage also results in noradrenaline release in the thermoregulatory centres in the hypothalamus, resulting in desensitisation of control and inhibition of both heat loss and production. Severely injured patients are thus prone to hypothermia.

Alcohol

In common with many people involved in road crashes, Kevin has been drinking. This has the following effects:

Inhibits baroreceptor reflex
Potentiates depressor reflex

This combined effect thus will accentuate the bradycardia and hypotension, which in turn will make a cardiac arrest more likely, and the prognosis in a traumatic cardiac arrest is very poor indeed.

The cytokine response

This is an inadequately understood area, with some of the evidence being of poor quality, variable and contradictory. There is also little research on this type of trauma, so that much of what we know has been applied from other areas, such as burns or elective surgery. What is known, however, is that the immune system is critically involved in the response to trauma. When we know more, we may be able to manipulate this response to improve survival.

Cytokines

Cytokines are small (15 to 30 kDa) glycoprotein messengers, which are released from a huge variety of cells in response to an equally wide variety of stimuli (Rixen *et al.*, 2000; Fosse *et al.*, 1998). The stimuli in this case are direct trauma and the consequences of that trauma (such as hypoxia and acidosis), but it may also be infective or toxic (released from damaged gut), hormonal, developmental, inflammatory, etc.

Cytokines bind to cell wall receptors, and their action may be defined as:

Autocrine (i.e. acting on the cell that produces them)
Paracrine (i.e. acting on cells near to the production site)
Endocrine (i.e. acting on distant cells)

Cytokines such as interleukin-6 (IL-6), IL-8 and IL-1 are inflammatory, and indeed IL-6 is responsible for the rise in acute-phase proteins such as C-reactive protein and fibrinogen. This rise is of course seen later, after at least 6 h, as protein takes time to make. The acute-phase proteins are then concerned with wound repair. The degree of IL-6 production is related to the degree of tissue damage.

IL-8 is a chemo-attractant agent and helps to get macrophages and neutrophils to the site of the damage.

IL-1 affects the anterior hypothalamus and produces a fever. Thermoregulation is damaged in trauma, and more of this is discussed later.

Some cytokines are, however, anti-inflammatory, such as IL-10, but its role is even less clear than that of the other cytokines. There is some laboratory evidence that release of this cytokine is influenced by sex steroids (Angele *et al.*, 2001).

Complement activation

This follows immediately after trauma, and with sepsis, hypoxia and endothelial damage. The amount of activation is proportional to the degree of trauma and a worsening base excess but is not related to the location of the injury. Increasing complement is associated with an increasing risk of multi-organ failure (MOF) and acute respiratory distress syndrome (ARDS). Increasing levels of IL-6 and IL-8 are also related to increasing risk of ARDS.

The endocrine response

Although the endocrine response involves nearly all hormone levels changing and interacting, here is a summary of the most important effects of trauma on the neuroendocrine system. It will be seen that the overall shift is towards glucose usage, which for the brain is obligatory.

Cortisol

Released from the adrenal cortex in response to increased adrenocorticotrophic hormone (ACTH) release from the anterior pituitary, cortisol rises in proportion to the degree of trauma sustained until, in very severe trauma, the levels drop again, possibly due to decreased adrenal blood flow. Cortisol promotes gluconeogenesis; it stimulates fatty acid and glycerol release from adipose and amino acids from protein. All this causes a rise in blood glucose. Cortisol also antagonises insulin effects at a cellular level, reducing glucose uptake. The body is in a state of catabolic hyperglycaemia.

Cortisol also increases the vascular sensitivity to vasoconstrictive stimuli and thus helps avoid hypotension.

Adrenaline and noradrenaline

Release of both is increased due to sympathetic stimulation and direct tissue damage. The rise is proportional to the degree of tissue damage.

Insulin and glucagon

Release of insulin from the pancreas is reduced acutely, mediated by adrenaline acting at alpha receptors and worsening the hyperglycaemia. The degree of the resulting hyperglycaemia increases with the degree of trauma. After a few days, insulin levels are supranormal, but there is still a hyperglycaemia due to insulin resistance. Glucagon levels rise acutely (mediated by beta adrenoceptors) but return to normal within a few days.

Immediate management

The evidence base on which trauma management is founded is an area of huge growth, ongoing in the form of TARN (Trauma Audit Research Network). This collates details of patients who suffer trauma and provides analysis of outcome, based on the patients' injuries and physiological status, using scoring systems such as the Injury Severity Score, (ISS) and Revised Trauma Score (RTS). This information is disseminated back to the hospitals, enabling them to audit and improve care.

There are many excellent texts and courses that cover the emergency management of trauma; the most prominent of these is the North American system of Advanced Trauma Life Support (ATLS) (American College of Surgeons, 2004). This is a regularly updated system that has become standard in the UK and is considered core for those working in Accident and Emergency. It was developed in Nebraska in the 1970s, after an orthopaedic surgeon had crashed his private plane and found that the care of his surviving family members was inadequate. The whole system of history, examination and investigation was turned on its head, and now in trauma the doctor acts directly on what is found, without a firm diagnosis. The immediately correctable is corrected in a firmly established order of priorities, beginning with the 'ABCs': airway, breathing and circulation.

For details of how to manage trauma, the student should refer to the ATLS course manual (7th edition). There are a few points that need be emphasized.

A team approach

This has to occur
- In the resuscitation room (with a small co-ordinated team)
- Within the hospital (early referral to relevant specialties for definitive treatment)
- Between hospitals (in the case of safe transfer to tertiary referral centres)

The normalization of physiology

The principle is to get oxygen to the tissues for their normal metabolism and the removal of cellular waste to avoid cell death. This is why the airway (with protection of the cervical spine) and breathing are prioritised, with haemorrhage control and fluid replacement soon after. There is controversy regarding how to normalise the circulation.
- *Which fluid?* (Yates *et al.*, 1999) There is ongoing debate as to the relative merits of crystalloids and colloids. Proponents of each side have ample ammunition to throw at the other. Crystalloids do not cause anaphylaxis, and the extra-vascular fluid volume (into which a large part of the saline goes) needs to be replaced anyway. Colloids leak through altered capillary membranes and may make pulmonary oedema worse, and clot quality may be worse after colloid (Vincent, 2000). On the other hand, less colloid is required than crystalloid, and

there are some studies showing *less* pulmonary oedema with colloid. The typically British compromise is for clinicians to use a bit of both, which fails to advance the argument. Blood would seem the logical ideal, but apart from questions of availability, compatibility and sterility, a lower haematocrit (0.3 to 0.35) is associated with improved tissue oxygenation, either due to better flow or increased oxygen uptake. Normovolaemia is more important to attain than the correction of anaemia. Synthetic oxygen carriers are not available yet. They may provide another option, but not as yet.
- *Hypo- or normo-tensive resuscitation?* (Bickell *et al.*, 1994; Girolami *et al.*, 2002). There may be a place for maintaining an artificially low blood pressure, as at a higher blood pressure any clots that may have formed are more likely to dislodge and vasoconstriction will be reversed. Work has been done in penetrating trauma to support this, but in blunt trauma it appears that aggressive fluid resuscitation in line with ATLS guidelines leads to a better outcome. Hypotension leads to poorer tissue perfusion, local acidosis, cell membrane leakage and gut bacteria invasion of the portal veins. What is clear is the importance of *surgical haemorrhage control* in association with fluid replacement. This haemorrhage may be obvious (onto the floor) or occult (into the chest, abdomen, pelvis and long bones), and this ongoing occult haemorrhage must be recognized and treated promptly by definitive surgery. In the case of isolated head injury, hypotension is proven to be detrimental and therefore must be corrected (Chestnut *et al.*, 1990).

Monitoring trauma patients

As mentioned above, there is no simple relationship between volume of blood loss and the usual physiological parameters measured in the resuscitation room. The work by Little and colleagues (1995) drew attention to the shock index (SI). This is

Shock index = heart rate (beats per minute)/
systolic blood pressure (mm Hg)
Systolic blood pressure (BP)

There is a more direct correlation between volume of blood lost and the SI than with BP and pulse. The other physiological parameters should all be measured, as should the pulse oximetry (but this may be inaccurate if the patient is cold or grossly anaemic) and the whole picture assessed.

Blood tests

The normal range of blood tests would include full blood count (FBC), urea and electrolytes (U & E's), glucose, and a cross-match. What is often forgotten is an arterial blood gas (ABG), which will give a measure of the base excess (BE). This is a measure of oxygen debt. It has been shown that the worse a BE becomes (i.e. the more negative it becomes), the more likely are increases in IL-6, IL-8 and IL-1, with earlier ARDS and a higher mortality. The critical threshold appears to be a BE of 6.6 mmol/l. The ABG will also tell you PaO_2, $PaCO_2$ (which helps on decisions to ventilate), Ph and bicarbonate.

The FBC will give a lot of haematological information, but of most use are the haemoglobin, platelets and haematocrit. It used to be said that the haemoglobin would drop only after a matter of hours and was thus of little value. This is not so. Haemoglobin may drop quickly, and an idea of blood volume lost may be gained from initial haemoglobin (Bruns *et al.*, 2007). Platelets must be monitored, as they are utilised rapidly and there may be later clotting problems (especially with large transfusions). The value of haematocrit with respect to tissue oxygenation has been mentioned.

Glasgow Coma Scale (GCS)

This is a measurement of level of consciousness as judged by the following three criteria.

1. Eye opening
   Spontaneous = 4
   To voice = 3
   To pain = 2
   None = 1
2. Motor response
   Obeys commands = 6
   Localizes pain = 5
   Withdraws to pain = 4
   Decorticate = 3
   Decerebrate = 2
   None = 1
3. Verbal response
   Orientated = 5
   Confused = 4
   Inappropriate = 3
   Incomprehensible = 2
   None = 1

This is a reproducible clinical tool that is best used not as a single reading but for observing a change over time. Thus the lowest GCS score possible, even if dead, is 3, and any patient whose score is 8 or less is said to be in coma. The GCS score is also used as an audit tool; for example, in the Revised Trauma Score, with systolic blood pressure and respiratory rate.

Most cases (80%) of brain injury are mild, with a GCS score of 13 to 15 at the time of assessment, but some of these patients may still have sustained significant trauma; they may have had altered consciousness or be suffering amnesia. They are candidates to suffer concussion syndrome, which may result in great disability or loss of earnings. Using an extended GCS, (GCS-E) (Nell *et al.*, 2000). with scoring for the degree of amnesia, it may be possible to identify more sensitively this sub-group and direct them to appropriate rehabilitation services. There is also work by Townend and Ingebrigtsen (2006) studying S100B, a 21-kDa protein released from glial cells in brain injury, which may act as a marker to identify those patients who appear to have mild injury but are at risk of long-term disability. This measure is used as a negative predictor to exclude severe brain injury.

What do we do with Kevin?

This unfortunate young man will require the following:

1. A rapid-sequence induction of anaesthesia and endotracheal intubation (to secure his airway)

with subsequent ventilation. This must be done with care so as not to worsen his neck injury.

2. A left-sided chest drain to drain the blood and air already there and ensure that he does not develop a tension pneumothorax.
3. Fluid and blood replacement via at least two wide-bore intravenous cannulae. Volumes must be guided by his injuries and physiological measurements initially and then the results of blood tests.
4. Reduction and covering of his compound fracture/dislocation.
5. Analgesia.
6. X-rays of his cervical spine, chest, pelvis and right lower leg and a computed tomography (CT) scan of his brain once he is stable.
7. Referral (and safe transfer) to definitive care.

Multi-organ failure and acute respiratory distress syndrome

This is a complicated and controversial area yet crucial to understand if trauma deaths are to be reduced. There is much research ongoing.

The origins are multifactorial – it occurs after trauma and surgery, sepsis, hypoxia and acidosis.

The pathways are poorly understood – cytokines, super-oxides from activated neutrophils and bacteria may all play a role.

Typically the strategies to deal with MOF and ARDS are thus also multiple and controversial. Steroids, antibiotics, inotropic support, prone ventilation, inhaled nitric oxide, permissive hypercapnia, nebulised prostacyclin and various different ventilatory methods all have been tried (including extracorporeal gas exchange) and all in conjunction with support of other systems. Attempts to produce a system of integrated emergency and intensive care seem to produce the best outcome, but the mortality remains high.

The student would be well advised to read a review of published papers (Ware and Matthay, 2000) and discuss any patient experience with a practicing intensivist.

Clinical scenarios

Scenario 1

An otherwise fit young man sustains a crossbow bolt injury to his epigastrium. He had the following parameters on arrival in the emergency department:

Airway – patent and self-supported

Breathing – chest clear with good and equal air entry and a respiratory rate of 28 breaths per minute

Circulation – blood pressure 95 systolic, pulse rate 120 bpm and capillary refill 5 s

GCS score – 15

Questions

What are your initial six actions as an emergency department junior doctor?

What do you NOT do, and why?

Why is the patient's respiratory rate abnormal?

From where may he be losing blood?

Scenario 2

You admit to your department an otherwise healthy 21-year-old woman who has been involved in a traffic accident. She was the only survivor of a head-on crash. She has seat-belt marks to her chest and abdomen (left shoulder to RUQ) and a frontal/facial haematoma. She arrives in the emergency department with the following parameters:

Airway – snoring

Breathing – decreased air entry on the left, respiratory rate 25 per min

Circulation – blood pressure 110 systolic, pulse rate 130 bpm and capillary refill 4 s

GCS score – E1, M4, V2 (E = eye opening, M = motor response, V = verbal response)

Questions

What are your initial three actions as an emergency department junior doctor?

Give four reasons for her decreased air entry.

State eight places from which she may be losing blood.

What may happen to her circulation soon?

Give three reasons why her GCS is decreased.

Scenario 3

A 35-year-old builder has been struck on the right-hand side of his head by a piece of scaffolding that was swinging from a crane. He had no helmet on. There are no other injuries, and he is otherwise fit and well. He arrives in the emergency department with the following parameters:

Airway – snoring

Breathing – chest clear with good and equal air entry, respiratory rate 14 per min

Circulation – blood pressure 190 systolic, pulse rate 39 bpm and capillary refill <2 s

GCS score – E1, M2, V1

Questions

What are your initial 3 actions as an emergency department junior doctor?

In what way and why are this man's cardiovascular parameters abnormal?

What imaging needs to be done?

What is decerebrate posturing, and what other physical signs may you find?

Scenario 4

A 30-year-old intravenous drug user has been stabbed in the right side of the chest during an argument and arrives in the emergency department screaming abuse. He has the following parameters:

Airway – obviously patent and self-supporting

Breathing – initially unable to assess further than the noise

Circulation – blood pressure 110 systolic, pulse rate 140 bpm and capillary refill 3 s

GCS score – 15

Before having his chest X-ray the patient becomes quiet. You notice that he has decreased air entry on the right side of his chest, which is hyper-resonant. His blood pressure is 90 systolic with a pulse of 180 bpm, and his GCS score has dropped to E3, M6, V4.

Questions

What are your initial three actions as an emergency department junior doctor?

Why do you think he is rapidly becoming very ill?

Why has his GCS score dropped?

Your registrar arrives and performs what procedure?

Answers

Scenario 1

Your initial six actions are:

1. Call for help.
2. Give supplemental oxygen.
3. Gain wide-bore intravenous access.
4. Take blood for FBC, U&E'S, glucose and cross-match, and ABGs.
5. Give fluid replacement, either crystalloid or colloid.
6. Give analgesia.

You do NOT try to remove the bolt. This may result in massive, uncontrollable haemorrhage. The bolt should be removed only in the operating theatre.

His respiratory rate is abnormal because he is hypovolaemic and acidotic, anxious and in pain.

Think of the anatomy along that path. Any organ or combination of organs can be damaged. Most of his loss will be occult, into his abdominal cavity; thus he may lose his entire circulating volume with little to see.

Scenario 2

Your initial three actions are:

1. Call for help.
2. Maintain the airway, which is partially obstructed (remembering cervical spine control) and give supplemental oxygen.
3. Gain wide bore intravenous access.

Reasons for decreased air entry are:
1. Haemopneumothorax
2. Tension pneumothorax
3. Lung contusion
4. Flail segment resulting in paradoxical movement
She may be losing blood from:
1. Disrupted major vessels
2. Lung parenchyma
3. Intercostal vessels
4. Liver
5. Spleen
6. Splanchnic bed
7. Any external wounds
8. Any so far unnoticed long bone fractures

At the moment her systolic blood pressure is satisfactory, and she is compensating for her blood loss. However, at any moment she may have a hypovolaemic cardiac arrest, as her baroreceptor reflex fails, her depressor reflex occurs and she decompensates.

Her GCS score is decreased because:
1. She is hypoxic secondary to her A and B problems.
2. She is hypovolaemic due to her bleeding.
3. She has a head injury.

It is relevant that she was the only survivor, as it gives an idea of the forces involved. Death of another occupant, ejection from the vehicle and rollovers are indicators of severity, and a review of other factors indicates cabin intrusion, extrication time, internal structure deformation, speed and restraint use as important in serious versus non-serious injury (Verteegh *et al.*, 2005).

Scenario 3

Your initial three actions are:
1. Call for help.
2. Maintain the airway, which is partially obstructed (remembering cervical spine control) and give supplemental oxygen.
3. Gain wide-bore intravenous access.

This man has hypertension and bradycardia. He is well perfused peripherally, but the rising intracranial pressure causes reduced perfusion of his

brainstem. The brainstem reacts in terms of a hypovolaemia problem and tries to compensate.

Any head injury requires additional CT of the cervical spine to rule out fracture or dislocation. This may or may not be normal in this case. He does NOT require an X-ray of his skull because he will be having an urgent CT scan of his brain. This must be done only when he has been stabilised, as interventions cannot be performed in the CT scanner.

Decerebrate posturing is extension of both arms and both legs in response to painful stimuli. The classical eye sign to expect with intracranial haematoma is initially an ipsilateral mildly dilated pupil with sluggish reactivity, progressing to a fixed dilated pupil. This is due to third cranial nerve compression as the uncus herniates through the tentorium due to rises in intracerebral pressure. There may also be contra-lateral hemiplegia as the pyramidal tracts are compressed. These are late signs. The most common sign of raised intracranial pressure is a decreased level of consciousness.

Scenario 4

Your initial three actions are:
1. Call for help.
2. Check the airway and give supplemental oxygen.
3. Try to gain any intravenous access. In an IVDU (intravenous drug user), this can be almost impossible.

This man has developed a tension pneumothorax. There is a dual problem in that both his breathing and circulation are compromised. The right lung has collapsed, so he will be hypoxic from reduced gas transfer, and there is a mechanical obstruction to heart filling despite adequate venous pressure, causing a cardiogenic shock. This will cause hypotension, tachycardia and a tissue acidosis. It must be corrected quickly if cardiac arrest is to be avoided.

His GCS score has lowered because he is hypoxic.

The immediate life-saving procedure is a needle thoracocentesis, which will decompress the tension pneumothorax temporarily. This is performed by inserting a cannula into the second intercostals space in the mid-clavicular line on the affected side. The definitive procedure, which should be done when there is intravenous access (in case of haemothorax), is insertion of a chest drain.

REFERENCES

American College of Surgeons (2004). *Advanced Trauma Life Support Course Manual*, 7th ed.

Angele, M. K. *et al*. (2001). Testosterone and oestrogen differently affect Th1 and T2 cytokine release following trauma-haemorrhage. *Cytokine* 16, 22–30.

Bickell *et al*. (1994). Immediate versus delayed fluid resuscitation for hypotensive patients with penetrating torso injuries. *New England Journal of Medicine* **221,** 1105–9.

Bruns, B. *et al*. (2007). Hemoglobin drops within minutes of injuries and predicts need for an intervention to stop hemorrhage. *Journal of Trauma* **63,** 312–5.

Chestnut *et al*. (1990). The role of secondary brain injury in determining outcome from severe head injury. *Journal of Trauma* **34,** 216–20.

Fosse, E. *et al*. (1998). Complement activation in injured patients occurs immediately and is dependent on the severity of the trauma. *Injury* **29,** 509–14.

Girolami *et al*. (2002). Haemodynamic responses to fluid resuscitation after blunt trauma. *Critical Care Medicine* **30,** 385–92.

Lecky, F. *et al*. (2000). Trends in trauma care in England and Wales 1989–97. UK Trauma Audit and Research Network. *Lancet* **355**:1771–5.

Little, R.A. *et al*. (1995). Preventable deaths after injury: why are the traditional "vital" signs poor indicators of blood loss? *Journal of Accident & Emergency Medicine* **12,** 1–14.

Murray, C. J., Lopez, A. D. (1997). Alternative projections of mortality and disability by cause, 1990–2020: Global Burden of Disease Study. *Lancet* **24,** 349:1498–504.

Nell, V., Yates, D.W., Kruger J. (2000). An extended Glasgow Coma Scale (GCS-E) with enhanced sensitivity to mild brain injury. *Archives of Physical Medicine and Rehabilitation* **81,** 614–7.

Rixen, D. *et al*. (2000). Metabolic correlates of oxygen debt predict post trauma early acute respiratory distress syndrome and the related cytokine response. *Journal of Trauma*, **49,** 392–403.

Savola, O. *et al*. (2004). Effects of head and extra cranial injuries on serum protein S100B levels in trauma patients. *Journal of Trauma* **56,** 1229–34.

Townend, W., Ingebrigtsen, T. (2006). Head injury outcome prediction: a role for protein S-100B? *Injury* **37,** 1098–108.

Trunkey, D.D. (1983). Trauma. *Scientific American Lancet* **249,** 25–35.

Versteegh, S. L. *et al*. (2005). Using crash information to improve the treatment of crash injuries. CASR Report Series, CASR014. Adelaide, Australia: University of Adelaide.

Vincent, J. L. (2000). Issues in contemporary fluid management. *Critical Care* **4,** S1–2.

Ware, L. B., Matthay, M. A. (2000). The acute respiratory distress syndrome. *New England Journal of Medicine* **342,** 1334–49.

16

The interaction between organic and psychiatric disease

Else Guthrie

Introduction

Psychiatric illness is approximately twice as prevalent in patients with organic disease than in the general population. The relationship between psychiatric disorder and organic disease is complex. It is important not to conceptualise organic illness as being 'physical' and psychiatric illness as 'all in the mind'. Changes in psychological states are determined by underlying physiological processes, the mechanisms of which are being slowly revealed as new and more powerful brain imaging techniques are developed. This chapter describes the main ways in which psychiatric illness and medical disorders interact. Because depressive disorders are the most common psychiatric conditions that occur in the medically ill, greater emphasis is placed upon the discussion of these disorders. The chapter begins with a description of the normal range of psychological responses to medical illness because it is difficult to identify abnormality without an understanding of normal processes.

Normal response to organic illness

Physical illness is stressful and worrying. There is no single 'normal' response, each individual is likely to react differently. Coping with illness is a dynamic process that changes over time. People need to manage the initial emotional shock of diagnosis, assimilate information and construct an understanding of the illness and the limitations or the demands it imposes upon them; then they can begin to formulate ways to cope. Common emotional responses and coping strategies are listed in Box 16.1.

Box 16.1 Common responses to illness

Emotional responses
Worry
Fear of death
Anger
Despair
Sense of loss
Guilt
Depression
Wish to die

Coping strategies
Seeking information
Seeking support
Helping others
Developing new interests or skills if former ones are
    compromised by illness
Making plans for the future
Sharing anxieties and worries about the illness with friends
    and family
Expressing anger
Managing loss

The degree of stress associated with organic illness is more dependent upon the patient's perception of the illness than upon the illness itself (Leventhal *et al.*, 1992; Scharloo *et al.*, 1998). Individuals with similar organic conditions can develop very different psychological responses depending upon their perception of the condition. This can then affect their care, as patients who are very anxious or worried may not be able to take in appropriate information and advice about treatment.

Worry and emotional distress should be regarded as *normal* responses to illness. Most individuals, however, manage to adjust to physical disease, given time and support. As a rule of thumb, it takes approximately 6 months to adjust psychologically to a major life change.

Effective communication should help doctors to elicit patient's concerns and identify particular coping strategies in each individual. Those who cope by gaining a sense of control over their condition will require detailed information about their illness and treatment possibilities. However, people who cope by distancing themselves from problems may find too much information intrusive and distressing. Any single coping strategy carried to an extreme is probably unhelpful, and most people have a repertoire of responses.

Other factors that affect peoples' response to illness include the following:

- Personality – e.g. pre-morbid history of anxiety traits or hypochondriacal concerns.
- Prior experience of serious illness in family member – e.g. death of a close relative with condition similar to the patient's.
- Psychological status at the onset of illness – e.g. depression or anxiety that precedes the onset of organic illness is predictive of a poorer psychological response (Nickel *et al.*, 2002).
- The type of illness – certain conditions such as cancer or conditions which involve the brain are associated with a greater degree of psychological distress.
- The chronicity of the illness – chronic illness requires the individual to make not just one but a series of psychological adjustments.
- Interpersonal factors and support by family and caregivers.
- High-quality emotional support can help to ameliorate the stress of physical disease.

Psychiatric disorder and organic disease

In the past, the lack of diagnostic tests for psychiatric disorders resulted in much confusion as to what was meant by 'depression' or 'anxiety disorder'. As a way of ensuring consistency in diagnosis, structured diagnostic systems have been developed over the last 20 to 30 years. The American classification system is termed the 'DSM' system, which stands for 'Diagnostic and Statistical Manual', of which currently there is a fourth edition (the *Diagnostic and Statistical Manual of Mental Disorders*, fourth edition, 1994), but work has already begun on the fifth edition, which is scheduled to be published in 2011. The World Health Organisation has also published a diagnostic manual for mental disorders; it is included in the *International Classification of Diseases* (10th edition). In each manual, the categorical criteria for a particular psychiatric disorder are specified. The manuals are of most used for research purposes, where diagnostic consistency is a pre-requisite for the internal validity of any study of mental disorder. In clinical practice, they provide a useful framework for diagnosis, but rigid adherence can be unhelpful, particularly in relation to psychiatric conditions occurring in the context of physical disorder. For example, a diabetic patient with a relatively mild eating disorder that does not fulfill criteria for bulimia nervosa may have severe problems with glycaemic control, with potentially serious long-term consequences.

There are four ways in which psychiatric disorder can be associated with organic disease:

1. Psychiatric disorder that develops as a direct consequence of organic disease
2. Psychiatric symptoms that are a manifestation of underlying organic disease
3. Psychiatric disorders that cause organic illness or increase the risk of developing organic disorder
4. Independent concurrence of physical illness and psychiatric disorder

In reality, the relationship between a psychiatric disorder and physical disease is more complex than that of a simple causal relationship, whatever the direction of causality. For example, a patient who abuses alcohol for many years may develop early signs of brain damage with memory loss. The patient may also develop alcoholic liver disease with subsequent delirium. On recovery, he may become depressed in response to his poor health status, and he may be more vulnerable to depression because of the organic brain impairment. In this example, at least three of the above four types of interaction between psychiatric disorder and organic disease, are relevant.

The association of psychiatric disorder and physical disorder is probably mediated by a variety of genetic, physiological and social factors. In the above example, the patient may be more vulnerable than others to developing alcoholism because of a combination of genetic and environmental factors; equally, he may be more vulnerable to developing alcoholic liver disease because of the particular genetic and environmental factors affecting him.

For the sake of clarity, each of the four ways in which psychiatric disorder and organic disease can interact are discussed below as if they were separate and discrete mechanisms. It is important to remember, however, more than one mechanism may be relevant that in most patients and that a circular, fluid pattern of interaction between psychiatric and organic states is most likely.

Psychiatric disorder that develops as a direct consequence of organic disease

There are two major ways in which psychiatric disorder can develop as a direct consequence of organic disease. The first involves a psychological reaction to organic illness that becomes more severe or prolonged than normal. The second involves the development of psychiatric illness as a consequence of underlying organic brain disorder.

Reaction to illness

The most common psychiatric disorder that develops as a consequence of organic disease is major depression, although anxiety states, post-traumatic stress disorder, conditioned responses, body image problems, hazardous drinking and sexual problems can also occur. Patients can become depressed as a reaction to the disease itself or as a result of the treatment of the disease (e.g. radical surgery, drugs that depress mood). Major depression is associated

with significant morbidity and mortality. Depressive disorders are inadequately detected and treated by hospital doctors and often continue following discharge without receiving treatment from the general practitioner. Apart from alleviating the severe distress experienced by the patient with depression, there are several other important reasons for treating depression in the medical setting.

Depressed patients are more likely than non-depressed patients to
- commit suicide (Hoyer *et al.*, 2000).
- spend more time in hospital and have more outpatient visits, even adjusting for the confounding severity of physical illness (Koenig and Kuchibhatla, 1998).
- have greater disability (Pohjasvaara *et al.*, 2001).
- have a poorer quality of life (Robinson-Smith *et al.*, 2000).
- have an increased risk of early mortality (Pennix *et al.*, 2001; Abas *et al.*, 2002).

Characteristics of depression

Depressive disorders are all characterized by a severe and persistent lowering of mood. Symptoms can be divided into three main areas: mood and motivation, cognitive changes, and biological features (Box 16.2).

Box 16.2 Depressive symptoms

Mood and motivation symptoms
Persistently lowered mood (may be worse in the morning)
Diminished interest or pleasure in almost all activities (anhedonia)
Social withdrawal
Loss of energy
Poor concentration
Cognitive changes
Depressive ideation: feelings of guilt, worthlessness, self-blame
Suicidal thoughts
Hopelessness
Biological symptoms
Poor appetite, loss of enjoyment of food

Significant weight loss when not dieting

Sleep disturbance most days (either initial insomnia or early morning waking)

Retardation or agitation

Decreased sex drive

Symptoms must be persistent and present for at least 2 weeks.

The following points should raise awareness of the possibility of depression:

- Does the person's distress appear to be very severe?
- Is there evidence of a failure to adjust to the illness? (e.g. Does the person feel just as bad as he or she did when the illness was first diagnosed?)
- Is the person expressing suicidal ideas?
- Is the person's physical function poorer than expected?
- Is the person's recovery from illness slower than expected or is rehabilitation difficult?
- Is there poor social interaction? (e.g. Does the person fail to respond to relatives visiting, staff or other patients on the ward?)

In the setting of physical disease, particular attention should be given to the non-biological symptoms of depression (affective and cognitive symptoms, Box 16.2). It is important to note that suicidal feelings should always be taken very seriously and are very rarely a normal reaction to physical illness. Some patients with terminal illness may decide that they wish to die, but there is usually evidence of careful and thoughtful deliberation over a period of months. This is very different from the attitude of a patient on a medical ward who suddenly tells staff that he or she wants to end his or her life.

Three symptoms of depression provide particularly good discrimination between depressed and non-depressed medical patients (Hawton *et al.*, 1990) (Box 16.3).

Box 16.3 Symptoms of depression that provide good discrimination between depressed and non-depressed medical patients

Depressed mood

Morning depression

Hopelessness

A variety of screening measures are available to detect depression in the medically ill; however, simple, direct enquiries can result in the detection of most cases of depression in the general medical setting (Chochinov *et al.*, 1997) (Box 16.4).

Box 16.4 Simple questions to elicit depression

'How are you feeling in yourself?'

'Are you feeling down or depressed?'

The view that depression is at least in part a biological phenomenon is based upon the monoamine theory of depression, which proposes that reduced availability of the monoamine serotonin (5HT) and to a lesser extent noradrenaline (and dopamine) is important in the pathogenesis of depression. Evidence for this includes the finding of reduced metabolites of these neurotransmitters in the cerebrospinal fluid and urine of depressed patients and reduced serotonin in the post-mortem brains of suicide victims. The mechanism of action of antidepressant drugs is based on their ability to increase synaptic serotonin and noradrenaline.

The main class of antidepressants are the monoamine reuptake inhibitors, which increase 5HT levels in the synapse by blocking the normal reuptake of 5HT into the presynaptic nerve ending. A second class, monoamine oxidase inhibitors, increase 5HT by blocking its normal enzymatic breakdown. A third approach, with only weak clinical effects, is to increase 5HT production in the presynaptic neuron by giving L-tryptophan, a precursor amino acid.

The regions in the brain most commonly found to be abnormal in functional brain imaging studies of major depression are the prefrontal cortex, anterior cingulate gyrus and temporal lobe. It has been hypothesized that dorsal brain structures have decreased activity in depression while ventral structures show increased activity in the symptomatic depressed state. Studies examining activity change from before and after short-term medication treatment of major depression have generally found normalization of brain activity in the regions cited.

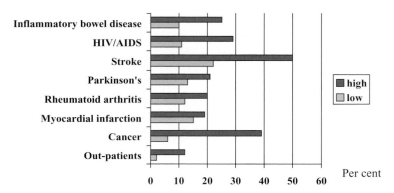

Figure 16.1 Prevalence of psychiatric disorder in different organic conditions. (Bars show the highest and lowest recorded rates.)

The prevalence of depression is particularly high in certain physical conditions or groups of patients. These include the following:

- Illnesses that affect the brain, such as stroke, Parkinson's disease, HIV/AIDs (Fig. 16.1)
- Life-threatening disorders such as cancer
- Chronic, painful, disabling illnesses that impede self-care (e.g. rheumatoid arthritis)
- Patients undergoing unpleasant treatments (e.g. chemotherapy)
- Old age

A wide range of drug treatments for physical illness can produce a lowering in mood and cause depression in the medically ill, including cardiac drugs, antihypertensives, endocrine agents, anticonvulsants and drugs used in the treatment of cancer (Fasullo *et al.*, 2004).

A clear association between implementation of the drug regime and the development of depression should be demonstrable before consideration is given to altering the patient's treatment or the addition of antidepressant medication.

Anxiety states as a response to organic illness

Normal worry plays an important role in motivating people to solve dilemmas or problems. Excessive worry or problematic worrying, however, becomes disabling and counter-productive. Problematic worries, in comparison with normal worries, are more intense and uncontrollable. Anxiety disorders are states of mind characterized by excessive or problematic worrying, as a consequence of which individuals become distressed or dysfunctional. The main disorders include panic disorder, agoraphobia, generalized anxiety disorder, simple phobias, social phobia, obsessive compulsive disorder and post-traumatic stress disorder. The main features of each disorder are summarized in Table 16.1. There is much overlap between these conditions, and co-morbidity for depression is high.

Pure anxiety states are much less common than depression in the medically ill but are more likely to be recognized by hospital staff. Patients with ischaemic heart disease may present with episodes of panic and chest pain, which are difficult to distinguish clinically from angina. Individuals with type I diabetes may develop a phobic reaction to injecting themselves with insulin (needle phobia). Symptoms of post-traumatic stress disorder are frequent in patients with non-severe stroke and may be accompanied by a depressive and anxious state (Bruggimann *et al.*, 2006).

Acute injury as a consequence of a traffic accident or some other trauma is associated with high levels of anxiety. Flashbacks or vivid dreams are common and should not be regarded as pathological in the

Table 16.1 The main features of the different anxiety disorders

Type of disorder	Main features
Panic disorder	Recurrent and unexpected panic attacks with or without anxiety in between attacks.
Agoraphobia	Fear or anxiety about being in public places or enclosed situations from which escape may be difficult.
Generalized anxiety disorder	Excessive anxiety and worry.
Specific phobia	Marked and persistent fear of specific objects or situations.
Social phobia	Marked and persistent fear of social situations in which embarrassment may occur.
Obsessive compulsive disorder	Persistent, intrusive, unwanted thoughts or images that are difficult to ignore and are recognized by the person as their own. Associated ritualistic behaviour may develop.
Post-traumatic stress disorder	Intrusive, recurrent thoughts or images of a traumatic experience associated with avoidance of stimuli associated with the trauma as well as generalized background anxiety.

immediate aftermath of severe trauma. These feelings and experiences, however, usually subside within 6 to 8 weeks. Post-traumatic stress disorder and other anxiety states such as phobic anxiety disorder are well recognised psychiatric complications of such experiences and occur in up to one-third of cases (Mayou and Bryant, 2001).

The development of psychiatric illness as a consequence of underlying organic brain disorder

Medical conditions such as stroke or head injury are associated with high rates of psychiatric disorder, particularly depression. Although depression can develop in these conditions as a psychological response to illness (see above), structural brain lesions appear to be associated with a very long term risk of depressive disorder.

Head injury in early adulthood is associated with an increased lifetime risk of depression, and this risk of depression remains elevated for decades following the initial trauma. After accounting for potential confounders such as alcohol abuse, cardiac disease, stroke, age and education, the risk of depression is highest among those who have sustained a severe head injury (Holsinger et al., 2002).

Psychiatric symptoms as a manifestation of underlying organic disease

Certain medical conditions, usually those involving the neuroendocrine system, can cause severe changes in mood, which are probably caused by alterations in the balance of the hypothalamic–pituitary axis.

For example, depression is a prominent feature of hypothyroidism and may be the presenting complaint. Depressive symptoms are usually present in severe cases of hypothyroidism. Furthermore, patients with subclinical hypothyroidism have been noted to have a higher-than-normal lifetime prevalence of depression. In depressed populations, the rates of subclinical hypothyroidsim (8% to 17%) are two to three times higher than in the normal population (5%); in refractory depression, the presence of thyroid abnormalities is even greater (30%) (Howland, 1993). A recent study suggests that patients with bipolar affective disorder who have a lower free thyroxine index and higher levels of thyroid-stimulating hormone than other patients with similar psychiatric symptoms have a poorer response to treatment (Cole et al., 2002).

Approximately 50% of patients with Cushing's syndrome have symptoms of atypical depressive disorder prior to diagnosis of the condition and 12% have a major affective disorder. There is an improvement in psychological symptoms following treatment of hypercortisolism. It has been hypothesised that glucocorticoid-induced suppression of hypothalamic secretion of corticotropin-releasing hormone may be the cause of atypical depression before and after correction of hypercortisolism (Dorn *et al.*, 1997).

Delirium

The central feature of an acute brain syndrome is clouding of consciousness. In a mild form the patient can appear virtually normal, but on detailed examination he or she will display an inability to attend to simple tasks and will be disoriented for time, place and person. In a severe form, the patient may be very drowsy or even unconscious. Typically, the level of consciousness varies, with the patient often being more drowsy and disoriented at night. During the day, he or she may have lucid spells and appear relatively normal unless asked to perform detailed cognitive tests. The physical cause will be successfully

found in 90% of cases. Older patients are most at risk. Surveys show rates in general medical wards to be 10% to 20%, rising to 50% in geriatric wards. The sudden development of a functional psychotic disorder in an individual with no previous history is extremely rare, and visual hallucinations are relatively rare in functional psychoses but are strongly suggestive of an underlying brain syndrome. Table 16.2 summarises the main features of delirium and Table 16.3 shows the most common causes.

Elderly patients or those with underlying degenerative brain disease are more prone to developing toxic confusional states than are younger patients. Particular care is required in using sedation, and much smaller dosages should be used than those usually recommended for younger adult patients.

Psychiatric disorders that cause organic illness or increase the risk of developing organic disorder

There are three ways in which psychiatric conditions can be causally related to organic illness. First, many patients with chronic psychiatric

Table 16.2 Mental state abnormalities in delirium

Aspect of mental state	Signs
Appearance and behaviour	Dishevelled, self-neglect
	Behaviour either overactive with restlessness, wandering and disinhibition or underactive with somnolence. Sterotypies and perseverative behaviour (e.g. plucking at bed sheets). Agitation.
Speech	May be reduced or mute; or loud. Usually disjointed.
	Dysarthria.
Mood	Labile: mood swings rapidly over minutes; irritable. Fear and anxiety can occur in response to visual hallucinations.
Abnormal beliefs	Often transient ideas of reference or persecution.
Abnormal perceptions	Visual hallucinations and illusions frequent. Tactile and olfactory hallucinations also occur.
Cognition	The following are usually impaired: immediate memory (digit span); concentration (serial sevens); orientation for time, day and place; recent memory. Remote memory is usually intact.
Insight	Impaired.

Table 16.3 Common causes of delirium

System	Examples
Drug toxicity	Complex treatment regimes involving polypharmacy
	Minor tranquillisers/ benzodiazepines
	Anticholinergic drugs
	Tricyclic antidepressants
	Digoxin
	Lithium
	Anticonvulsants
	SSRIs
	Antiparkinsonian drugs
	Diuretics
	Steroids
	Antihypertensives
Drug withdrawal	Alcohol
	Barbiturates
Deliberate self-harm	Many drugs taken in excessive quantities
Metabolic	Renal failure
	Hepatic encephalopathy
	Hypoglycaemia
Trauma	Head injury
	Sub-dural haematoma
Infection	Encephalitis
	Meningitis
	Septicaemia
	Chest infection
	Urinary tract infection
Vascular	Stroke
Other	Cerebral tumour or cerebral metastases,
	post-ictal state, endocrine disturbance,
	AIDS, dehydration, any major systemic illness

disorders (e.g. chronic depression or schizophrenia) have adverse health behaviours (e.g. smoking, obesity, lack of exercise) that put them at higher risk of organic disorder than the general population. Second, particular psychiatric disorders such as alcohol abuse or eating disorders can cause medical disease. Third, psychiatric disorder may be a risk factor for the development of particular medical conditions.

Health behaviours and psychiatric disorder

There is a high prevalence of cigarette smoking among patients with psychiatric disorders, particularly those with schizophrenia, alcohol disorders and depression. In a recent study of community residents, 65% of women and 80% of men with a history of major depression were regular smokers. Also, among those individuals with a lifetime history of major depression, less than 14% of smokers were able to stop smoking and remain abstinent. Such high rates of smoking clearly place patients with psychiatric disorder at risk of long-term cardio-respiratory disease, including lung cancer and chronic obstructive pulmonary disease. It has been hypothesized that the high rates of addiction to smoking in subjects prone to depression may be a form of self-medication. Cigarette smoke contains a substance that inhibits monoamine oxidase (MAO), and it also contains nicotine, which is an agonist at nicotinic receptors. MAO inhibitors are effective antidepressants and antidepressant-like properties of nicotinic agonists have been demonstrated in a rat model. Cigarette smoking affects noradrenergic proteins in the locus caoeruleus, which are similar to changes in animals produced by long-term antidepressants treatment (Klimek *et al.*, 2001).

Further work is required to tease out the psychological, physiological and environmental factors that result in high rates of smoking among psychiatric patients.

High rates of smoking and obesity are common health behaviour problems in schizophrenia. Both result in increased medical problems in later life for patients with this disorder. Weight gain is a particular problem in schizophrenia; it may result from the effects of the illness, which produces an amotivational state associated with over-eating and a lack of exercise. In addition, many of the drugs used to treat schizophrenia, including the newer atypicals, cause weight gain and an increased incidence of hyperlipidemia and diabetes (Lublin *et al.*, 2005).

Psychiatric disorders associated with physical ill health

Alcohol misuse

Alcohol misuse is the most common psychiatric disorder to cause physical illness, contributing to approximately 20% to 25% of all general hospital admissions (Jarman and Kellett, 1979; Lloyd et al., 1982). Between 37% and 50% of all patients attending emergency departments have consumed alcohol prior to presentation, and, when followed over a 5-year period, those who presented in an intoxicated state had a mortality rate 2.4 times that of the normal population (Davidson et al., 1997). It is estimated that in Great Britain in 1999 there were 16 830 casualties in traffic accidents involving illegal alcohol levels, representing 5% of all traffic accident casualties. There has been a 200% increase in alcohol consumption in the UK since 1950, and in recent years there has been a sharp increase in the number of women who drink excessively (from 9% to 12%). The number of males who drink excessively has remained relatively stable over the last 10 years at approximately 27%.

A unit of alcohol is 8 g of ethanol, which is contained in

- A half pint of normal-strength beer, lager or cider
- A quarter pint of extra-strong beer, lager or cider
- A small (125-ml) glass of wine
- A 50-ml glass of sherry or port
- A single pub measure (25 ml) of spirits

Sensible drinking is up to 21 units for men or 14 units for women weekly, spread over 4 or more days. Drinking above these levels is termed 'alcohol misuse'. Hazardous drinking occurs over 35 units per week for men or 21 units for women. Dependence is more likely over 50 units per week for men or 35 units for women.

In the general hospital setting, alcohol misuse is often undetected. Some 35% of patients with alcoholic liver disease have never received advice about alcohol consumption, and less than half have been advised by their general practitioner to stop drinking. Only 22% have ever been referred for treatment for alcohol abuse. By the time patients develop alcoholic liver disease, effective intervention may be

more difficult. A high index of suspicion is required for patients presenting with a variety of medical disorders, so that alcohol problems can be detected at an early stage of the process, where intervention is more likely to be effective. Table 16.4 shows some of the ways in which patients with alcohol problems can present to physicians. A detailed review of the physical sequelae of alcohol misuse is not provided in this chapter.

Drug abuse

The most common physical sequelae following drug abuse in the general hospital setting are the consequences of intravenous drug use rather than the adverse effects of the drug itself. Sequelae include abscesses, infected needle sites, septicaemia, emboli, HIV and AIDS.

Deliberate self-harm (DSH)

This is one of the most frequent examples of psychiatric disorder resulting in physical illness. An estimated 140 000 cases present to general hospitals in England and Wales each year (Hawton et al., 1997). The majority of episodes involve self-poisoning, commonly with analgesics or psychotropic agents, and these appear to be on the increase (O'Loughlin and Sherwood, 2005) . Suicidal intent (the extent to which a person wished to die) can vary greatly and may not be reflected in the physical danger of the act. Many people are unaware of the relative dangers of different types of medication taken in overdose, and physical danger should therefore not be assumed to indicate intent. The other frequent method of DSH is self-cutting, usually with little threat to life. A minority of episodes, however, involve deep cutting, which endangers major blood vessels and nerves.

Schizophrenia/hypomania

Patients with schizophrenia or hypomania may suffer severe injuries as a result of acting upon their voices or delusions. It is not uncommon for a patient

Table 16.4 Ways in which patients with alcohol problems can present in a general hospital setting

Trauma	Neurological
Accidents (e.g. fracture while intoxicated)	Blackouts
Accidental arson (e.g. falling asleep while smoking)	Seizures
Fights	Tremor
Traffic accidents	Paraesthesia/peripheral neuropathy
	Muscular weakness/ alcoholic myopathy
	Ataxia/cerebellar degeneration
	Alcoholic amblyopia
Gastrointestinal	Unexpected alcohol withdrawal syndrome while an in-patient
Gastritis/pain, nausea	Coarse tremor
Haematemesis	Tachycardia
Hepatitis	Sweating
Pancreatitis	Disorientation and clouding of consciousness
Alcoholic liver disease	Seizures
	Hallucinations, predominantly visual
Organic psychosyndromes	Haematology
Wernicke-Korsakoff syndrome	Unexplained macrocytosis
Alcoholic dementia and cerebral degeneration	Anaemia

with schizophrenia to be admitted to an orthopaedic ward with multiple injuries after jumping off a high building.

Eating disorders

There are two major forms of eating disorder, both of which can result in physical complications. Anorexia nervosa is characterised by the following symptoms: body mass index less than 17.5 (18.5 is suggestive of low weight), a morbid fear of fatness, a distorted body image and amenorrhoea for a period of at least 3 months. Body mass index is calculated by the following formula: weight (kg)/height (in metres)^2. The key symptoms of bulimia nervosa are recurrent episodes of binge eating, a lack of control over eating during binges, recurrent inappropriate compensatory behaviour to prevent weight gain (e.g. self-induced vomiting, laxatives, fasting, excessive exercise), a minimum average of two binges per week for 3 months, persistent over-concern with body shape and weight. Patients with severe anorexia ner-

vosa may need admission to a medical ward for the treatment of severe starvation. This may include the correction of electrolyte imbalance and rehydration as well as feeding with a nasogastric tube. The major physical sequelae of eating disorders are shown in Table 16.5.

Psychiatric disorder as a risk factor for the development of medical disease

Depression can result in a large range of adverse health consequences, including impaired physical function, increased morbidity and an increased risk of death, which cannot be explained by suicide alone (Beekman et al., 1997). Of current major interest is the relationship between depression and cardiac mortality.

Among patients hospitalised with a myocardial infarction, a diagnosis of major depression has been shown to be associated with a two- to four-fold increased risk for cardiac mortality, and the mortality risk increases with the severity of depression

Table 16.5 Physical sequelae associated with eating disorders

Decreased body temperature	Additional consequences of self-induced vomiting:
Compensatory lanugo body hair	Electrolyte imbalance
Decrease heart rate	Cardiac arrythmias
Decreased respiration rate	Dehydration
Decreased metabolic rate	Loss of tooth enamel
Hypocalcaemia/decreased bone density	Callous formation on dorsum of phalanges
Decreased calcium from teeth	Additional consequences of purgative abuse:
Decreased libido or failure to develop	Hypokalaemia
libido if condition begins around puberty	Cardiac arrest
Poor tolerance of the cold	Melanosis coli
Poor peripheral circulation resulting in chilblains	
Sleep disturbance	
Oedema	
Gastrointestinal discomfort	
Coarse and dry skin, hair loss	

(Pennix *et al.*, 2001); that is, individuals with major depression are at greater risk than those with subclinical depressive symptoms (Figure 16.2). In addition, patients with established coronary artery disease appear to be at higher risk than those without such a history (Glassman and Shapiro, 1998), although some of the literature is conflicting in this area due to the different populations and settings in which studies have been carried out.

Two main mechanisms have been proposed for the relationship between depression and cardiac mortality (Table 16.6). The first may be related to lifestyle factors. Depression may be associated with a number of risk factors that increase morbidity and

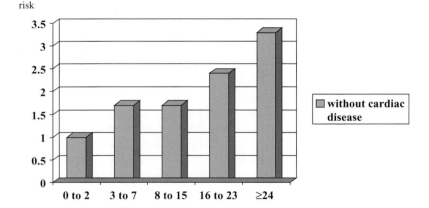

Figure 16.2 Relative risk for cardiac death according to level of depressive symptoms. (Adapted from Pennix *et al.*, 2001.)

Table 16.6 Potential mechanisms that may account for the link between depression and cardiac mortality

Impairment of platelet function.

Decreased heart rate variability.

Immune activation and hypercortisolaemia as stress responses to depression may result in decreased insulin resistance and increased steroid production and blood pressure.

Unhealthy lifestyles (smoking, alcohol consumption, poor diet and lack of exercise) are more common in patients with depression and are increased risk factors for cardiac disease.

Depressed patients may be less compliant with treatment.

Antidepressant treatment may have cardiotoxic effects.

mortality from cardiovascular and other physical disease. This may include smoking, excessive alcohol consumption and a lack of exercise. Although in statistical analyses such factors are treated as confounders, they are in reality intermediary factors on the same common pathway. If depression makes you smoke more, your physical health will be jeopardized. The second mechanism relates to biological change that occurs during depression. Increased cortisol and platelet coagulability and changes in heart rate variability are known to be associated with depression. Such effects may produce a more vulnerable cardiovascular system.

Independent concurrence of physical illness and psychiatric disorder

Because of the relatively high prevalence of psychiatric disorder and medical disease in the general population, it is possible for the two to occur together without any major association. For example, a patient with schizophrenia may develop rheumatoid arthritis or diabetes. Although there may be no causal association between the two conditions, it is likely that the subsequent management and treatment of the patient's medical condition, including compli-

ance with treatment, may be influenced by the status of his or her mental health.

Summary

The relationship between psychiatric illness and organic illness is complex. Psychiatric illness can develop as a consequence of organic illness, but equally psychiatric illness can itself be a risk factor for organic illness. In any patient, several different mechanisms may be relevant. The most common psychiatric illness in the general hospital setting is depression. This is often undetected by medical staff but can be identified by one or two brief questions. Depression in organic illness is associated with increased disability, a poorer quality of life, longer hospital stays and increased mortality. It is important that it be detected and treated appropriately.

Clinical scenarios and multiple-choice questions

Scenario 1

A 39-year-old woman with inflammatory bowel disease is admitted to hospital for investigation of recurrent abdominal pain. While in hospital she appears down and does not interact with other patients on the ward. She confides in one of the nurses that she is 'fed up with being ill' and would rather be dead. She feels tired all the time, cannot sleep because of the pain and has lost over 7 kg in weight. She feels low all of the time, particularly when she first wakes up, and feels she will never get better and has nothing to look forward to. She has even thought of ending her life.

Questions

1. The following symptoms in the above case are the most reliable indicators of a depressive disorder:
   a. Insomnia
   b. Lethargy
   c. Hopelessness

d. Morning depression

e. Weight loss

2. In order to receive a diagnosis of major depressive disorder, the patient must have had symptoms of low mood for at least

a. 2 days

b. 2 weeks

c. 4 weeks

d. 2 months

e. 6 months

3. The suicidal thoughts that the patient is experiencing

a. are a normal reaction to physical illness.

b. are a symptom of a depressive disorder.

c. an indication that she should receive an urgent assessment from a liaison psychiatrist.

d. should be ignored by staff so as not to encourage her to think in such a fashion.

e. are a sign of attention-seeking behaviour.

4. This patient is more likely than other patients with inflammatory bowel disease who are not depressed but have similar symptoms to

a. commit suicide.

b. have less disability.

c. have a poorer quality of life.

d. spend less time in hospital.

e. have more out-patient contacts.

Answers

1. c, d

Three symptoms of depression provide particularly good discrimination between depressed and non-depressed medical patients. They are depressed mood, morning depression and hopelessness. The other symptoms in this case could be caused by depression but also could be attributable to the patient's physical condition.

2. b

To make a diagnosis of major depressive disorder, continuous symptoms have to be present for at least 2 weeks.

3. b, c

Suicidal ideation should always be taken very seriously and should prompt an urgent referral for psychiatric assessment. This is best carried out by a liaison psychiatrist with experience of the treatment and management of depression in medically ill patients. The suicidal thoughts are most likely the result of a depressive illness, and these negative thoughts will disappear if the depression is treated.

4. a, c, e

Depressed medical patients in comparison with non-depressed patients are more likely to commit suicide, have greater disability and poorer quality of life; they are also more likely to spend more time in hospital and require more out-patient treatment.

Scenario 2

A 56-year-old man is admitted to hospital with chest pain. Tests confirm that he has had a myocardial infarction (MI). In the subsequent weeks he develops biological and cognitive symptoms of depression. He worries constantly about his heart and is fearful of taking exercise despite medical advice to the contrary. He is seen by a psychiatrist who asks him to complete the Beck Depression Inventory. His score is 33. He is started on antidepressant treatment and within 3 weeks begins to show evidence of improvement. He becomes less depressed and less worried about his condition. He begins to exercise and consults his GP about help with stopping smoking.

His health, prior to the recent illness was good. He has no prior history of cardiac disease or hypertension. He did, however, smoke 15 to 20 cigarettes per day.

Questions

1. This patient's risk of mortality in comparison with non-depressed patients who suffer a myocardial infarction is

a. 10 times greater.

b. 100 time greater.

c. at least twice as great.

d. up to 4 times greater.

e. half as much.

2. The following factors in this case increase the risk of mortality post-MI:
   a. Symptoms suggestive of a major depressive disorder
   b. A high score on the Beck Depression Inventory
   c. No prior history of cardiac disease
   d. No prior history of hypertension
   e. Previous good health
3. The following changes are associated with depression post MI:
   a. Abnormal brain function in the anterior cingulate gyrus
   b. Increased heart rate variability
   c. Impairment of platelet function
   d. Increased steroid production
   e. Increased brain function in the motor cortex
4. Treatment of the depression is likely to result in
   a. normalization of brain activity.
   b. normalization of mood.
   c. an increased risk of death because of cardiotoxic effects of antidepressants.
   d. improved quality of life.
   e. poor compliance with medical treatment.

Answers

1. c, d
The increased risk is between two and four times.

2. a, b
Patients with a major depressive disorder as opposed to subclinical depression are at greater risk of mortality post-MI. The Beck Depression Inventory is a rating scale used to measure the severity of depression. A score of 33 on the Beck Depression Inventory is very high and suggests that the patient does not have sub-clinical symptoms. A patient with sub-clinical symptoms would be more likely to have a score of around 15.

3. a, c, d
Depression is associated with abnormal brain function in a variety of areas including the anterior cingulate gyrus but not the motor cortex. There is impaired platelet coagulability and decreased heart rate variability. Steroid production is increased.

4. a, b, d
Treatment of depression is associated with a normalization of brain activity and an improvement in mood and quality of life. It is not associated with an increased risk of death. There is preliminary evidence that treatment of depression post-MI results in a reduced risk of mortality, but further studies are required to confirm this.

Scenario 3

A 28-year-old man is admitted to hospital in an unconscious state with a head injury following a fight in a pub. Investigation reveals that he has a depressed, compound skull fracture. Computed tomography reveals an extradural haematoma, which is removed surgically; he makes a good initial recovery. He admits to drinking 5 pints of beer a day and double this amount at weekends. He has a previous history of violence associated with drinking and was admitted to hospital 2 years earlier with a seizure.

Questions

1. This man in comparison with the general population has
   a. an increased risk of depression in the months following this injury.
   b. no greater risk of depression in the years following this injury.
   c. a very long term risk of depressive disorder.
   d. an increased risk of anorexia nervosa.
   e. an increased risk of epilepsy.
2. This man's reported weekly alcohol consumption is
   a. 45 units.
   b. 90 units.
   c. above the recommended safe limit.
   d. likely to be an over-estimate of how much he drinks.
   e. unlikely to result in dependence in the long term.
3. The head injury this man sustained
   a. is severe.

b. is associated with a greater risk of depression than head injuries that do not result in unconsciousness.
c. would be considered one of the ways in which alcohol problems can present in the general hospital.
d. is associated with a good prognosis if surgery is performed quickly.
e. would be considered minor.

4. Alcohol misuse in the general hospital setting
   a. is often undetected.
   b. requires a high index of suspicion.
   c. is more prevalent in males than females.
   d. is more prevalent in medical in-patients than out-patients.
   e. is more prevalent in the elderly.

Answers

1. a, c, e

This man has an increased short- and long-term risk of depression. The previous history of a seizure in addition to this recent head injury conveys a greater risk of epilepsy.

2. b, c, e

The amount he reports drinking is 90 units per week: 10 units per day during the week plus 20 units on Friday and Saturday. This is well above the recommended safe limit for men, which is 35 units per week. The amount he actually drinks is likely to be more. Drinking above 50 units a week is associated with an increased risk of developing alcohol dependence syndrome.

3. a, b, c, d

Severe head injury is associated with a higher risk of depression than mild head injury. Some 90% of patients make a good recovery following surgery for an extradural haematoma. Seizures and head injuries are among the ways alcohol problems can present in the general hospital.

4. a, b, c, d

Alcohol problems are most prevalent among young male in-patients.

Scenario 4

A 50-year-old woman develops type II diabetes. She is overweight and smokes 30 cigarettes per day. She has suffered from depression for the last 2 years and has been treated with antidepressant medication.

She has always worried about her health and particularly feared developing diabetes as her grandmother suffered from diabetes and developed renal and vascular complications.

She thinks of diabetes in terms of a death sentence and believes her life is over. She finds it difficult to accept her illness and her compliance with treatment is poor. She prefers not to think about it, or her diet and hopes it will go away. Six months later, she is feeling even lower and contemplates suicide.

Questions

1. The following factors may affect this patient's psychological response to developing diabetes:
   a. Pre-morbid obsessional traits.
   b. Prior experience in a family member.
   c. The development of a chronic illness.
   d. The presence of depression at the time of onset of the diabetes.
   e. The presence of pre-morbid hypochondria.

2. The patient's perception of diabetes 'as a death sentence'
   a. will have no bearing on her psychological adjustment.
   b. is the most powerful predictor of a poor psychological response to the illness.
   c. is the usual response to developing diabetes.
   d. suggests a positive outcome.
   e. prevents the development of strategies to cope with the condition.

3. The usual time it takes to adjust to the onset of a serious illness is approximately
   a. six days.
   b. six weeks.
   c. six months.
   d. 12 months.
   e. 5 years.

4. The main coping strategies employed by this woman in relation to her illness are
   a. denial.
   b. making plans for the future.
   c. developing new skills.
   d. seeking information.
   e. hope of a magical cure.

Answers

1. b, c, d, e
This patient has premorbid hypochondriacal traits, a previous family history of diabetes and depression at the time of onset of the illness. All three suggest the possibility of a poorer adjustment to the illness.

2. b, e
The degree of stress associated with organic illness is more dependent upon the patient's perception of illness than on the illness itself. Such a negative view of the illness will prevent the patient from adopting any positive strategies to help adjust to the condition.

3. c
It takes approximately 6 months to adjust to the development of a serious medical condition. For any individual, the actual time course will depend upon a variety of factors.

4. a, e
This patient is coping mainly by denying that she has the condition or by hoping it will vanish or miraculously disappear.

Scenario 5

A 35-year-old man with schizophrenia is admitted to hospital with multiple fractures after he jumped off a bridge. He is confined to bed but is being nursed on an orthopaedic ward on the third floor of the hospital. He has a body mass index of 33. He smokes 40 cigarettes per day but has not been allowed cigarettes since his admission to hospital. He is fearful of staff and believes that they may be plotting to kill him. He appears to be distracted and responding to hallucinations.

Question

How might this man's psychiatric status interact with his the treatment of his physical injuries?

Answers

1. His persecutory ideation regarding staff may make him less likely to accept treatment.
2. He may make further attempts to harm himself or try to get out of bed, causing further injury to himself.
3. His anxiety and tension will be increased by his inability to smoke.
4. If he has negative symptoms of schizophrenia (i.e. an amotivational state) this may make physiotherapy and rehabilitation difficult, as he will lack the motivation to improve.
5. Medication for his psychiatric condition may control his psychotic symptoms but cause extrapyramidal side effects, which could cause pain.
6. He may be less able to give informed consent regarding his treatment because of his fears regarding staff. This may be detrimental to his overall care.

Scenario 6

A 34-year-old woman develops symptoms of anxiety 3 months after being discharged from an intensive care unit. She was admitted following a traffic accident but has no memory of it. She was a passenger in a vehicle in which the driver, her boyfriend, was killed. She sustained severe chest and abdominal injuries requiring surgery. She remained on the intensive care unit for 5 days, during which she was confused and experiencing visual hallucinations. Although she eventually made a good recovery from her physical injuries, she complains of restlessness and irritability. She is fearful and easily frightened by sudden noises. She is unable to sleep and is suffering from nightmares. The nightmares are similar each night and involve her being back on the intensive care unit. She believes that she is in a bed surrounded by demons who are breathing fire over her. She has been unable to drive a car since the accident or even to travel as a passenger. She also feels anxious on buses.

Questions

What psychiatric condition is this woman suffering from?

Why has it arisen?

Answers

This woman has classical symptoms of post-traumatic stress disorder. She has no memory of her accident but has developed a traumatic memory linked to her experience on the intensive care unit, when she was delirious and experiencing visual hallucinations. It is not unusual for symptoms of post-traumatic stress disorder to have a delayed onset.

FURTHER READING

Abas, M., Hotopf, M., Prince, M. (2002). Depression and mortality in a high risk population. 11-Year follow-up of the Medical Research Council Elderly Hypertension Trial. *British Journal of Psychiatry* **181,** 123–8.

Beekman, A. T., Deeg, D. J., Braam, A. W. *et al.* (1997). Consequences of major and depressed mood in later life: a study of disability, well-being and service utilization. *Psychological Medicine* **27,** 1397–409.

Bruggimann, L., Annoni, J. M., Staub, F. *et al.* (2006). Chronic posttraumatic stress symptoms after nonsevere stroke. *Neurology* **66,** 513–6.

Chochinov, H. M., Wilson, K. G., Enns, M. (1997). Are you depressed? Screening for depression in the terminally ill. *American Journal of Psychiatry* **154,** 674–6.

Cole, D. P., Thase, M. E., Mallinger, A. G. *et al.* (2002). Slower treatment response in bipolar depression predicted by lower pretreatment thyroid function. *American Journal Psychiatry***159,** 116–21.

Davidson, P., Koziol-McLain, J., Harrison, L. *et al.* (1997). Intoxicated ED patients: a 5-year follow-up of morbidity and mortality. *Annals of Emergency Medicine* **30,** 593–7.

Fasullo, S., Puccio, D., Fasullo, S., Novo, S. (2004). Pharmacological treatment of depression after acute myocardial infarction. *Italian Heart Journal Supplement* **5,** 839–46.

Glassman, A. H., Shapiro, P. A. (1998). Depression and the course of coronary artery disease. *American Journal of Psychiatry* **155,** 4–11.

Hawton, K., Fagg, J., Simkin, S. *et al.* (1997). Trends in deliberate self-harm in Oxford, 1985–1995. Implications for clinical services and the prevention of suicide. *British Journal of Psychiatry* **171,** 556–60.

Holsinger, T., Steffens, D. C., Phillips, C. *et al.* (2002). Head injury in early adulthood and the lifetime risk of depression. *Archives of General Psychiatry* **59,** 17–22.

Howland, R. H. (1993). Thyroid dysfunction in refractory depression: implications for pathophysiology and treatment. *Journal of Clinical Psychiatry* **54,** 47–54.

Hoyer, E. H., Mortensen, P. B., Olesen, A. V. (2000). Mortality and causes of death in a total national sample of patients with affective disorders admitted for the first time between 1973 and 1993. *British Journal of Psychiatry* **176,** 76–82.

Jarman, C. M. B., Ellett, J. M. (1979). Alcoholism in the general hospital. *British Medical Journal* **88,** 469–72.

Klimek, V., Meng-Yang, Z., Dilley, G. *et al.* (2001). Effects of long-term cigarette smoking on the human locus coeruleus. *Archives of General Psychiatry* **58,** 821–7.

Koenig, H. G., Kuchibhatla, M. (1998). Use of health services by hospitalized medically ill depressed elderly patients. *American Journal of Psychiatry* **155,** 871–7.

Leventhal, H., Leventhal, E. A., Schaefer, P. M. (1992). Vigilant coping and health behavior. In Ory, M. G., Abeles, R. P. (eds.). Aging, Health, and Behavior. Thousand Oaks, CA: Sage Publications, pp. 109–40.

Lloyd, G. G., Chick, J., Crombie, E. (1982). Screening for problem drinkers among medical inpatients. *Drug and Alcohol Dependence* **10,** 355–9.

Lublin, H., Eberhard, J., Levander, S. (2005). Current therapy issues and unmet clinical needs in the treatment of schizophrenia: a review of the new generation antipsychotics. *International Clinical Psychopharmacology* **20,** 183–98.

Mayou, R., Bryant, B. (2001). Outcome in consecutive emergency department attenders following a road traffic accident. *British Journal of Psychiatry* **79,** 528–34.

Nickel, R., Wunsch, A., Egle, U. T. *et al.* (2002). The relevance of anxiety, depression, and coping in patients after liver transplantation. *Liver Transplantation* **8,** 63–71.

O'Loughlin, S., Sherwood, J. (2005). A 20-year review of trends in deliberate self-harm in a British town, 1981–2000. *Social Psychiatry and Psychiatric Epidemiology* **40,** 446–53.

Pennix, B. W., Beekman, A. T., Honig, A. *et al.* (2001). Depression and cardiac mortality: results from a community based longitudinal study. *Archives of General Psychiatry* **58,** 221–7.

Pohjasvaara, T., Vataja R., Leppavuori, A. *et al.* (2001). Depression is an independent predictor of poor long-term functional outcome post-stroke. *European Journal of Neurology* **8,** 315–9.

Robinson-Smith, G., Johnston MV. Allen J. (2000). Self-care self-efficacy, quality of life, and depression after stroke.

Archives of Physical Medicine and Rehabilitation **81,** 460–4.

Scharloo, M., Kaptein, A. A., Weinman, J. *et al.* (1998). Illness perceptions, coping and functioning in patients with rheumatoid arthritis, chronic obstructive pulmonary disease and psoriasis. *Journal of Psychosomatic Research* **44,** 573–85.

Schuckit, M. A., Smith, T. L., Anthenelli, R., Irwin, M. (1993). Clinical course of alcoholism in 636 male inpatients. *American Journal of Psychiatry* **150,** 786–92.

Index

Page numbers followed by '*f*' indicate figures; page numbers followed by '*t*' indicate tables.